Biomaterial-Related Infections

Biomaterial-Related Infections

Editors

Natália Martins
Célia F. Rodrigues

MDPI • Basel • Beijing • Wuhan • Barcelona • Belgrade • Manchester • Tokyo • Cluj • Tianjin

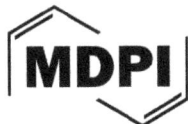

Editors
Natália Martins
Faculty of Medicine,
University of Porto
Portugal
Institute for Research and
Inovation in Health (i3S),
University of Porto
Portugal

Célia F. Rodrigues
LEPABE—Laboratory for
Process Engineering
Environment Biotechnology and Energy,
Department Chemical Engineering,
Faculty of Engineering—University of Porto
Portugal

Editorial Office
MDPI
St. Alban-Anlage 66
4052 Basel, Switzerland

This is a reprint of articles from the Special Issue published online in the open access journal *Journal of Clinical Medicine* (ISSN 2077-0383) (available at: https://www.mdpi.com/journal/jcm/special_issues/biomaterial_related_infections).

For citation purposes, cite each article independently as indicated on the article page online and as indicated below:

LastName, A.A.; LastName, B.B.; LastName, C.C. Article Title. *Journal Name* **Year**, *Article Number*, Page Range.

ISBN 978-3-03943-438-1 (Hbk)
ISBN 978-3-03943-439-8 (PDF)

© 2020 by the authors. Articles in this book are Open Access and distributed under the Creative Commons Attribution (CC BY) license, which allows users to download, copy and build upon published articles, as long as the author and publisher are properly credited, which ensures maximum dissemination and a wider impact of our publications.

The book as a whole is distributed by MDPI under the terms and conditions of the Creative Commons license CC BY-NC-ND.

Contents

About the Editors vii

Natália Martins and Célia F. Rodrigues
Biomaterial-Related Infections
Reprinted from: *J. Clin. Med.* **2020**, *9*, 722, doi:10.3390/jcm9030722 1

Piotr Piszczek, Aleksandra Radtke, Michalina Ehlert, Tomasz Jędrzejewski, Alicja Sznarkowska, Beata Sadowska, Michał Bartmański, Yaşar Kemal Erdoğan, Batur Ercan and Waldemar Jędrzejczyk
Comprehensive Evaluation of the Biological Properties of Surface-Modified Titanium Alloy Implants
Reprinted from: *J. Clin. Med.* **2020**, *9*, 342, doi:10.3390/jcm9020342 5

Bih-Show Lou, Chih-Ho Lai, Teng-Ping Chu, Jang-Hsing Hsieh, Chun-Ming Chen, Yu-Ming Su, Chun-Wei Hou, Pang-Yun Chou and Jyh-Wei Lee
Parameters Affecting the Antimicrobial Properties of Cold Atmospheric Plasma Jet
Reprinted from: *J. Clin. Med.* **2019**, *8*, 1930, doi:10.3390/jcm8111930 35

Alexandru Mihai Grumezescu, Alexandra Elena Stoica, Mihnea-Ștefan Dima-Bălcescu, Cristina Chircov, Sami Gharbia, Cornel Baltă, Marcel Roșu, Hildegard Herman, Alina Maria Holban, Anton Ficai, Bogdan Stefan Vasile, Ecaterina Andronescu, Mariana Carmen Chifiriuc and Anca Hermenean
Electrospun Polyethylene Terephthalate Nanofibers Loaded with Silver Nanoparticles: Novel Approach in Anti-Infective Therapy
Reprinted from: *J. Clin. Med.* **2019**, *8*, 1039, doi:10.3390/jcm8071039 53

Aleksandra Radtke, Marlena Grodzicka, Michalina Ehlert, Tomasz Jędrzejewski, Magdalena Wypij and Patrycja Golińska
"To Be Microbiocidal and Not to Be Cytotoxic at the Same Time . . . "—Silver Nanoparticles and Their Main Role on the Surface of Titanium Alloy Implants
Reprinted from: *J. Clin. Med.* **2019**, *8*, 334, doi:10.3390/jcm8030334 75

Aleksandra Radtke, Michalina Ehlert, Tomasz Jędrzejewski and Michał Bartmański
The Morphology, Structure, Mechanical Properties and Biocompatibility of Nanotubular Titania Coatings before and after Autoclaving Process
Reprinted from: *J. Clin. Med.* **2019**, *8*, 272, doi:10.3390/jcm8020272 99

Célia F. Rodrigues, Alexandra Correia, Manuel Vilanova and Mariana Henriques
Inflammatory Cell Recruitment in *Candida glabrata* Biofilm Cell-Infected Mice Receiving Antifungal Chemotherapy
Reprinted from: *J. Clin. Med.* **2019**, *8*, 142, doi:10.3390/jcm8020142 121

Bahare Salehi, Dorota Kregiel, Gail Mahady, Javad Sharifi-Rad, Natália Martins and Célia F. Rodrigues
Management of *Streptococcus mutans*-*Candida* spp. Oral Biofilms' Infections: Paving the Way for Effective Clinical Interventions
Reprinted from: *J. Clin. Med.* **2020**, *9*, 517, doi:10.3390/jcm9020517 137

Célia F. Rodrigues, Maria Elisa Rodrigues and Mariana Henriques
Candida sp. Infections in Patients with Diabetes Mellitus
Reprinted from: *J. Clin. Med.* **2019**, *8*, 76, doi:10.3390/jcm8010076 153

About the Editors

Natália Martins has an extensive background in dietetics and nutrition, natural product chemistry and biochemistry, drug discovery, phytochemistry, phytopharmacology, functional foods, and nutraceuticals. She has been increasingly focused on the use of naturally occurring bioactives for human health, not only from the point of view of health promotion and disease prevention, but also from the perspective of treatment. Natália holds several specializations in evidence-based medicine, clinical nutrition, and personalized medicine. She has worked as a university professor since 2017. She was an advisor for several MSc and PhD theses, and she is a member of the evaluation panel of the College of Nutritionists (Porto, Portugal). She has participated in various research projects, received several grants and awards, and published more than 120 articles in peer-reviewed, highly reputed, international journals (h-index 22). She has authored 10 book chapters and presented more than 40 communications in national and international conferences. Natália is also a member of the Council for Nutritional and Environmental Medicine (CONEM, Norway), reviewer for more than 50 highly reputed international journals, invited reviewer for several book publishers, and editorial board member of several international journals. She also edited several special issues and research topics in highly reputed journals and is currently editing several books for renowned publishers.

Célia F. Rodrigues is a *Candida* spp. expert, with extensive know-how working with molecular techniques, susceptibility assays, biofilm development, antimicrobial drugs, in vivo assessments, alternative and novel treatments, and biomaterials at LEPABE, Faculty of Engineering, University of Porto. Presently, she is also working on a project related to microorganisms, FISH, and microfluidics. She is an invited assistant professor at CESPU, where she teaches future pharmacists. Célia is a reviewer for more than 40 international journals; she has co-supervised/mentored MSc and PhD Students, organized research conferences/seminars, and served as a juror of Congress. Finally, Célia has won several grants and awards from Portuguese and international entities. (https://www.researchgate.net/profile/Celia_Rodrigues2; Ciência ID: 5F12-D3E1-E028).

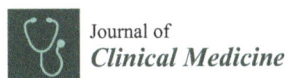

Editorial

Biomaterial-Related Infections

Natália Martins [1,2,*] and Célia F. Rodrigues [3,*]

1. Faculty of Medicine, University of Porto, Alameda Prof. Hernâni Monteiro, 4200-319 Porto, Portugal
2. Institute for Research and Innovation in Health (i3S), University of Porto, 4200-135 Porto, Portugal
3. LEPABE—Laboratory for Process Engineering, Environment, Biotechnology and Energy, Faculty of Engineering, University of Porto, Rua Dr. Roberto Frias, 4200-465 Porto, Portugal
* Correspondence: ncmartins@med.up.pt (N.M.); c.fortunae@gmail.com (C.F.R.)

Received: 4 March 2020; Accepted: 4 March 2020; Published: 7 March 2020

Medical devices are a typical and important part of health care for both diagnostic and therapeutic purposes. Nonetheless, these devices (e.g., catheters, implants, dentures, or prostheses) recurrently lead to the appearance of several types of infections. In fact, there is a high rate of colonization of abiotic surfaces (such as biomaterials from medical devices), due to an induction of biofilm-growing microorganisms, which are progressively resistant to antimicrobial therapies. The biofilm structures are composed of attached and structured microbial communities, surrounded by an exopolymeric matrix. They are the predominant mode of microbial growth, as they offer ecological advantages, such as protection from the environment, nutrient availability, metabolic cooperation, and acquisition of new traits. Furthermore, there are single and multiple-species communities of biofilms, most of them particularly difficult to eradicate and a source of many recalcitrant infections. Undeniably, it is now recognized that most infections are connected to a biofilm etiology.

Numerous methods have been established to fight device-related infections. Among them, there are natural products (e.g., phenolic compounds), surface coating/functionalization of biomaterials (e.g., peptides, β-lactams), or inorganic elements (e.g., copper and silver nanoparticles). These options are recognized mainly as having a broad-spectrum bacterial/fungal activity, being decisive to understand how these infections develop and to progress/find new biomaterials. Antifouling coatings (e.g., repellents or low adhesion to microorganisms, or antimicrobial coatings), improvement of biomaterials' functionalization strategies, and support tissues' bio-integration are some of them.

Eight papers were published in this issue, six of them being research papers with promising new developments. The reports describe the bioactivity of amorphous titania nanoporous and nanotubular coatings [1], the use of a method to increase the antimicrobial efficiency of a cold atmospheric plasma jet (CAPJ) [2], an electrospinning technique to acquire anti-infective terephthalate nanofibers loaded with silver nanoparticles [3], or the use of similar silver nanoparticles on the surface of titanium alloy implants, discussing nanotechnology and the antimicrobial effect of biomaterials [4]. Another report evaluated the effect of autoclaving sterilization in several parameters (such as morphology or biocompatibility) of implants modified by nanocomposite coatings [5], and, finally, a report focused on the efficacy of echinocandins (first-line antifungal drugs) for the treatment of systemic fungal infections derived exclusively from biofilm cells (mimicking a catheter-derived biofilm infection). Regarding reviews, two papers were published. The first one discussed the occurrence of candidiasis infections in diabetes mellitus (DM) and its complications (such as species, hospitalization, organs involved), and the second one discussed the management of *Streptococcus mutans–Candida* spp. oral biofilms' infections, and the latest chemical and natural drugs used for this. These papers, which address the medical implications of the topics covered, will be summarized in the following lines.

Piszczek et al. [1] concluded that surface-modified titanium alloy implants present the most suitable physicochemical and biological properties for a potential orthopedic application, with the important advantage of not having long-term release of mutagenic substances. Other work explains that CAPJ can destroy the *Escherichia coli* cell wall and damage its DNA structure, offering effective antimicrobial activity and being a new and significant approach to fight bacterial infections [2]. Likewise, terephthalate nanofibers loaded with silver nanoparticles have been indicated as a possible new approach in anti-infective therapy against Gram-positive and Gram-negative bacteria and fungi for wound dressings or implant coatings. The silver-decorated fibers revealed low cytotoxicity and inflammatory effects and, importantly, increased antibiofilm activity, stressing the anticipation of the use of these systems with antimicrobial activity [3]. A method for assembling two different systems of dispersed silver nanoparticles [4] has proved useful against Gram-positive and Gram-negative bacteria and yeasts. The results indicate high biocidal properties and biocompatibility (low toxicity) of the studied systems (particularly for one, Ti6Al4V/TNT5/0.6AgNPs). In another paper [5], the same authors describe the morphology, structure and mechanic alterations of nanotubular titania coatings, related to the autoclaving processes. They reveal that this sterilization method does not affect its morphology and structure, but it requires the elimination of adsorbed water particles from its surface, in order to avoid damage to the architecture of nanotubular coatings. The last research work is related to the efficacy of the treatment of an *in vivo* infection originated from *Candida glabrata* biofilm cells. Rodrigues et al. [6] indicated that caspofungin or micafungin does not have a significant impact on liver and kidney fungal burden or in the recruited inflammatory infiltrate (immune response). These results underline the greater virulence of biofilms cells' infections (e.g., originating from medical devices), when compared to their planktonic counterparts.

Regarding reviews, both papers were related to fungal biofilms [7,8]. The first one assessed the incidence and prevalence of several *Candida* spp. infections in DM patients. The authors show that DM clearly predisposes individuals to fungal infections, specifically related to *Candida* spp., due to the patient's general state of immunosuppression. In fact, patients have longer hospitalization periods, and candidiasis cases are commonly associated with the prolonged use of indwelling medical devices. These issues increase the disease-management-associated costs. Lastly, an article emphasized and discussed the use of new synthetic and natural drugs, besides other strategies, with promising results for both *S. mutans*–*Candida* spp. oral mixed biofilms treatment and control. These biofilms (among the most common in oral infections) have undergone several studies, including innovative drugs/therapeutic methods (e.g., photodynamic therapy, several naturally-occurring biomolecules, and chlorhexidine added to silver nanoparticles), revealing different, but promising, clinical approaches [8].

Acknowledgments: The guest editors thank all authors and anonymous reviewers for their contribution to this Special Issue, which helped us achieve this goal in great demand. C.F.R. would like to acknowledge the UID/EQU/00511/2020 Project—Laboratory of Process Engineering, Environment, Biotechnology and Energy (LEPABE), financed by national funds through FCT/MCTES (PIDDAC). N.M. would like to thank the Portuguese Foundation for Science and Technology (FCT-Portugal) for the Strategic project ref. UID/BIM/04293/2013 and "NORTE2020—Northern Regional Operational Program" (NORTE-01-0145-FEDER-000012).

Conflicts of Interest: The authors declare no conflict of interest.

References

1. Piszczek, P.; Radtke, A.; Ehlert, M.; Jędrzejewski, T.; Sznarkowska, A.; Sadowska, B.; Bartmański, M.; Erdoğan, Y.K.; Ercan, B.; Jedrzejczyk, W. Comprehensive Evaluation of the Biological Properties of Surface-Modified Titanium Alloy Implants. *J. Clin. Med.* **2020**, *9*, 342. [CrossRef] [PubMed]
2. Lou, B.-S.; Lai, C.-H.; Chu, T.-P.; Hsieh, J.-H.; Chen, C.-M.; Su, Y.-M.; Hou, C.-W.; Chou, P.-Y.; Lee, J.-W. Parameters Affecting the Antimicrobial Properties of Cold Atmospheric Plasma Jet. *J. Clin. Med.* **2019**, *8*, 1930. [CrossRef] [PubMed]
3. Grumezescu, A.M.; Stoica, A.E.; Dima-Bălcescu, M.-Ș.; Chircov, C.; Gharbia, S.; Baltă, C.; Roșu, M.; Herman, H.; Holban, A.M.; Ficai, A.; et al. Electrospun Polyethylene Terephthalate Nanofibers Loaded with Silver Nanoparticles: Novel Approach in Anti-Infective Therapy. *J. Clin. Med.* **2019**, *8*, 1039. [CrossRef] [PubMed]

4. Radtke, A.; Grodzicka, M.; Ehlert, M.; Jędrzejewski, T.; Wypij, M.; Golińska, P. "To Be Microbiocidal and Not to Be Cytotoxic at the Same Time . . . "—Silver Nanoparticles and Their Main Role on the Surface of Titanium Alloy Implants. *J. Clin. Med.* **2019**, *8*, 334. [CrossRef] [PubMed]
5. Radtke, A.; Ehlert, M.; Jędrzejewski, T.; Bartmański, M. The Morphology, Structure, Mechanical Properties and Biocompatibility of Nanotubular Titania Coatings before and after Autoclaving Process. *J. Clin. Med.* **2019**, *8*, 272. [CrossRef] [PubMed]
6. Rodrigues, C.F.; Correia, A.; Vilanova, M.; Henriques, M.; Rodrigues, C.F.; Correia, A.; Vilanova, M.; Henriques, M. Inflammatory Cell Recruitment in Candida glabrata Biofilm Cell-Infected Mice Receiving Antifungal Chemotherapy. *J. Clin. Med.* **2019**, *8*, 142. [CrossRef] [PubMed]
7. Rodrigues, C.F.; Rodrigues, M.; Henriques, M. Candida sp. Infections in Patients with Diabetes Mellitus. *J. Clin. Med.* **2019**, *8*, 76. [CrossRef] [PubMed]
8. Salehi, B.; Kregiel, D.; Mahady, G.; Sharifi-Rad, J.; Martins, N.; Rodrigues, C.F. Management of Streptococcus mutans-Candida spp. Oral Biofilms' Infections: Paving the Way for Effective Clinical Interventions. *J. Clin. Med.* **2020**, *9*, 517. [CrossRef] [PubMed]

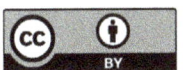

© 2020 by the authors. Licensee MDPI, Basel, Switzerland. This article is an open access article distributed under the terms and conditions of the Creative Commons Attribution (CC BY) license (http://creativecommons.org/licenses/by/4.0/).

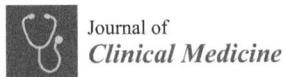

Article

Comprehensive Evaluation of the Biological Properties of Surface-Modified Titanium Alloy Implants

Piotr Piszczek [1,2,*], Aleksandra Radtke [1,2,*], Michalina Ehlert [1,2], Tomasz Jędrzejewski [3], Alicja Sznarkowska [4], Beata Sadowska [5], Michał Bartmański [6], Yaşar Kemal Erdoğan [7], Batur Ercan [7,8,9] and Waldemar Jędrzejczyk [2]

1. Faculty of Chemistry, Nicolaus Copernicus University in Toruń, Gagarina 7, Toruń 87-100, Poland; m.ehlert@doktorant.umk.pl
2. Nano-implant Ltd. Gagarina 5/102, Toruń 87-100, Poland; waldek.torun@gmail.com
3. Faculty of Biological and Veterinary Science, Nicolaus Copernicus University in Toruń, Lwowska 1, Toruń 87-100, Poland; tomaszj@umk.pl
4. International Centre for Cancer Vaccine Science, University of Gdańsk, Wita Stwosza 63, Gdańsk 80-308, Poland; alicja.sznarkowska@ug.edu.pl
5. Faculty of Biology and Environmental Protection, University of Łódź, Banacha 12/16, Łódź 90-237, Poland; beata.sadowska@biol.uni.lodz.pl
6. Faculty of Mechanical Engineering, Gdańsk University of Technology, Gabriela Narutowicza 11/12, Gdańsk 80-233, Poland; michal.bartmanski@pg.edu.pl
7. Biomedical Engineering Program, Middle East Technical University, Ankara 06800, Turkey; yasarer@metu.edu.tr (Y.K.E.); baercan@metu.edu.tr (B.E.)
8. Department of Metallurgical and Materials Engineering, Middle East Technical University, Cankaya, Ankara 06800, Turkey
9. BIOMATEN, Metu Center of Excellence in Biomaterials and Tissue Engineering, Ankara 06800, Turkey
* Correspondence: piszczek@umk.pl (P.P.); aradtke@umk.pl (A.R.); Tel.: +48-607-883-357 (P.P.); +48-600-321-294 (A.R.)

Received: 13 December 2019; Accepted: 22 January 2020; Published: 25 January 2020

Abstract: An increasing interest in the fabrication of implants made of titanium and its alloys results from their capacity to be integrated into the bone system. This integration is facilitated by different modifications of the implant surface. Here, we assessed the bioactivity of amorphous titania nanoporous and nanotubular coatings (TNTs), produced by electrochemical oxidation of Ti6Al4V orthopedic implants' surface. The chemical composition and microstructure of TNT layers was analyzed by X-ray photoelectron spectroscopy (XPS) and X-ray diffraction (XRD). To increase their antimicrobial activity, TNT coatings were enriched with silver nanoparticles (AgNPs) with the chemical vapor deposition (CVD) method and tested against various bacterial and fungal strains for their ability to form a biofilm. The biointegrity and anti-inflammatory properties of these layers were assessed with the use of fibroblast, osteoblast, and macrophage cell lines. To assess and exclude potential genotoxicity issues of the fabricated systems, a mutation reversal test was performed (Ames Assay MPF, OECD TG 471), showing that none of the TNT coatings released mutagenic substances in long-term incubation experiments. The thorough analysis performed in this study indicates that the TNT5 and TNT5/AgNPs coatings (TNT5—the layer obtained upon applying a 5 V potential) present the most suitable physicochemical and biological properties for their potential use in the fabrication of implants for orthopedics. For this reason, their mechanical properties were measured to obtain full system characteristics.

Keywords: Ti6Al4V implants; anodization process; XPS; antimicrobial activity; genotoxicity assessment; anti-inflammatory properties; mechanical properties

1. Introduction

The design and manufacture of implants, which are safe and highly accepted as being biocompatible with the human body, is a priority of modern medicine [1,2]. Works aimed at solving this issue are supported by the intense investigations on novel biomaterials and the development of modern technologies. The application of additive technologies (e.g., selective laser sintering, selective laser melting, commonly called 3D printing), which, allow for bone implant fabrication with anatomical accuracy, and lead to the shortening of the surgery duration and postoperative recovery, is a good example [3–5]. Titanium and titanium alloy powders are materials widely used in the aforementioned above-mentioned additive technologies due to the fact that implants fabricated using these powders show desirable mechanical properties, allowing them to transfer large loads. Therefore, these materials offer great potential for applications in orthopedics, dentistry, and spine surgery [6–8]. The advantage of the additive technology is its ability to fabricate porous systems, which can increase the ingrowth of bone and the anchorage of the implants [8,9]. However, low osteoconduction and integration of titanium-based implants with the bone for long-term survival, their weak anti-inflammatory properties, and the possibility of toxic components releasing into the human body requires surface modification and the formation of a layer, which significantly eliminates these above-mentioned adverse factors. These surface modifications can be carried out into two ways: (a) The roughness and wettability changes of the titanium implants' surface, which can stimulate a durable connection between the implant and the bone [9–11]; and (b) the formation of bioactive coatings, which accelerate bone formation (e.g., hydroxyapatite layers [12,13]) or increase their biocidal activity (e.g., bio-functional magnesium coating, as well as silver nanoparticles [14–16]). The formation of an oxide layer (passivation layer) on the surface of titanium/titanium alloy implants, which is practically insoluble and largely responsible for their high corrosion resistance and biocompatibility, is an important way to approach implants' surface modification [17]. The implants' surface oxidation process control lead to the fabrication of titania coatings of defined architecture, porosity, and microstructure, on titanium-based implants' surface, which may contribute to an improvement of their mechanical properties and to their bioactivity increase [18–21].

From a practical point of view, the anodic oxidation of titanium-based implants' surface in the HF solution, leading to the formation of first-generation TiO_2 (TNT) nanotube coating, seems to be particularly interesting [22–25]. Depending on the value of the applied potential [U], this method allows the following to be obtained: (a) Ordered porous layers (U = 3–10 V), consisting of nanotubes with common walls; (b) ordered tube layers (U = 10–30 V), composed of separated titania nanotubes; and (c) oxide coatings with a sponge-like structure (above U = 30 V) [24,26]. Produced TNT coatings, as obtained, are amorphous and form a uniform oxide layer of a thickness c.a. 150 nm on the entire surface of the substrate. The type of produced coating has a direct impact on the surface wettability, its porosity, and roughness, as well as on the mechanical properties. Moreover, it was found that the substrates covered with the TNT layer are characterized by more vigorous cell growth (fibroblasts) and better integration of bone with the implant surfaces [20,25,26]. The enrichment of TNT coatings with silver nanoparticles (AgNPs) using chemical vapor deposition (CVD) and atomic layer deposition (ALD) techniques, allowing control of their size and dispersion, was another direction of our works [27–30]. Forming a TNT/AgNPs system, we exploited the antimicrobial properties of silver nanoparticles without exceeding the potentially acceptable and safe dose of silver ions [16,28–30]. The composite systems produced in this way could prevent the formation of bacterial biofilms that form on the implant surface, thus being difficult to eradicate.

Our previous research [20,21,24–31] focused on the development of technology to produce the bioactive coatings on the surface of Ti6Al4V alloy substrates, i.e., widely used material in the construction of orthopedic implants. However, in order to implement the developed nanocoatings into implant fabrication, it is necessary to estimate their bioactivity in detail. Therefore, we focused on the wide-ranging immunological studies on selected coatings, i.e., TNT5 (porous one produced at U = 5 V), TNT15 (tubular one produced at U = 15 V), TNT5/AgNPs, and TNT15/AgNPs (TNT5 and TNT15 coatings enriched with silver nanoparticles), as well as on studies intended to exclude their potential genotoxicity. Studies on the antimicrobial potential of produced coatings that counteract the colonization and biofilm formation by selected bacterial and fungal strains on TNT- and TNT/AgNPs-modified Ti6Al4V surfaces were especially important for us. The results of all of these investigations are presented and discussed in this paper.

2. Materials and Methods

2.1. The Modification of the Ti6Al4V Implant Surface and the Characterization of Titania Coatings

The studied Ti6Al4V implants were modified by the fabrication of titania coatings on their surface using the anodization oxidation method, in accordance with a previously described procedure [25]. The implants were produced by 3D technology using selective laser sintering (SLS; EOS M 100; EOS GmbH Electro Optical Systems, Krailling, Germany) of Ti6Al4V powder, the chemical composition of which was consistent with ASTM F136-02a (ELI Grade 23) [32]. The crystallographic structure of the produced implants was confirmed by the XRD diffraction pattern (Figure S1) [33]. The anodization of the implants' surface was carried out at room temperature using 0.3 wt% aqueous HF solution as an electrolyte, the anodization time t = 30 min, and potentials of $U = 5$ V (TNT5) and 15 V (TNT15). After the anodization, the samples of the Ti6Al4V/TNT5 and Ti6Al4V/TNT15 systems were dried in a stream of argon at room temperature (RT), and additionally immersed in acetone and dried at 396 K for 1 h. Half of the TNT5 and TNT15 samples were enriched with silver nanoparticles using the CVD technique (metallic silver precursor—$[Ag_5(O_2CC_2F_5)_5(H_2O)_3]$) under earlier described conditions [27,30]. The morphology of the produced coatings was studied using quanta field-emission gun scanning electron microscope (SEM; Quanta 3D FEG; Carl Zeiss, Göttingen, Germany). A 30.0 kV accelerating voltage was chosen for SEM analysis and the micrographs were recorded under high vacuum using a secondary electron detector (SE). The structure of the produced oxide layers was analyzed using X-ray diffraction (XRD; PANalytical X'Pert Pro MPD X-ray diffractometer, PANalytical B.V., Almelo, The Netherlands, using Cu-Kα radiation; the incidence angle was equal to 1 deg) and raman spectroscopy (RamanMicro 200 PerkinElmer, PerkinElmer Inc., Waltham, MA, USA). X-ray photoelectron spectroscopy (XPS) spectra of the investigated samples were obtained with monochromatized Al Kα-radiation (1486.6 eV) at room temperature using an X-ray photoelectron spectrometer (PHI 5000 Versaprobe, Physical Electronics, Inc., Chanhassen, MN, USA). The sample surface was sputtered using an Ar+ ion beam for 3 times. Energy of 2.5 keV was used for each sputter and the duration of each sputter was 2 min. All surface-modified implants (named for the publication needs as TNT5, TNT15, TNT5/AgNPs, and TNT15/AgNPs) as well as non-modified Ti6Al4V and silver-enriched Ti6Al4V/AgNPs were cut into 8 × 8 × 2 and 10 × 10 × 2 mm pieces and used in all biological experiments.

2.2. Wettability and Surface Free Energy of Biomaterials

The wettability and surface free energy of the produced titania-based nanocoatings were determined using earlier described methods [25,34,35]. The contact angle was measured using a goniometer with drop shape analysis software (DSA 10 Krüss GmbH, Hamburg, Germany). Each measurement was repeated three times.

2.3. Immunological Assessment

2.3.1. Cell Culture

Human osteoblast-like MG 63 cells (European Collection of Cell Cultures, Salisbury, UK, cat. no. 86051601) were cultured at 310 K in 5% CO_2 and 95% humidity in Eagle's minimum essential medium (EMEM) containing 2 mM L-glutamine, 1 mM sodium pyruvate, MEM non-essential amino acid, heat-inactivated 10% fetal bovine serum (FBS), 100 µg/mL streptomycin, and 100 IU/mL penicillin (all compounds from Sigma-Aldrich, Darmstadt, Germany). The culture medium was changed every

2–3 days. The cells were passaged using 0.25% trypsin- ethylenediaminetetraacetic acid (EDTA) solution (Sigma-Aldrich Darmstadt, Germany). The murine macrophage cell line RAW 264.7 was obtained from European Collection of Cell Cultures (Salisbury, UK, cat. no. 91062702). The cells were cultured in Dulbecco's modified Eagle's medium supplemented with 10% Fetal Bovine *Serum* (FBS), 100 µg/mL streptomycin, and 100 IU/mL penicillin (all compounds from Sigma-Aldrich). Macrophages were maintained at 310 K in a 5% CO_2/95% humidified atmosphere, subjected to no more than 15 cell passages and utilized for experimentation at approximately 70%–80% confluency. L929 murine fibroblast cells (American Type Culture Collection, Manassas, VA, USA) were cultured at 310 K in a humidified atmosphere with 5% CO_2. The culture medium consisted of RPMI 1640 medium containing 2 mM L-glutamine (Sigma-Aldrich, Darmstadt, Germany), 10% heat-inactivated fetal bovine serum (FBS), 100 IU/mL penicillin, and 100 µg/mL streptomycin (PAA Laboratories GmbH, Cölbe, Germany). L929 cells were passaged using a cell scraper.

2.3.2. Cell Proliferation Assays

The effect of the tested specimens on the cell proliferation (measured after 24, 72, and 120 h) was studied using the MTT (3-(4,5-dimethylthiazole-2-yl)-2,5-diphenyl tetrazolium bromide; Sigma Aldrich, Darmstadt, Germany) assay. MG-63 osteoblasts and L929 fibroblasts were seeded onto the autoclaved tested nanolayers placed in a 24-well culture plate (Corning, NY, USA) at a density of 1×10^4 cells/well and cultured for 24, 72, and 120 h. RAW 264.7 macrophages were seeded onto the substrates at a density of 25×10^4 cells/well and cultivated for 24 and 48 h. Moreover, the proliferation rate of the RAW 264.7 cell line was assessed for the cells stimulated with lipopolysaccharide (LPS; derived from *Escherichia coli*; 0111:B4, Sigma Chemicals, St. Louis, MO, USA) at a dose of 10 ng/mL, which was added to the cell growth medium to create the pro-inflammatory environment. The control cells were incubated on the test samples without the presence of LPS. After the respective incubation time, the substrates were rinsed with phosphate-buffered saline (PBS, pH 7.4; 1 × working concentration, contains 155.2 mM NaCl, 2.97 mM $Na_2HPO_4 \times 7H_2O$ and 1.06 mM KH_2PO_4) and transferred to a new 24-well culture plate. The MTT (5 mg/mL; Sigma-Aldrich) solution in a respective culture medium without phenol red was added to each well and the plates were incubated for 3 h. Then, the MTT solution was aspirated and 500 µL of dimethyl sulfoxide (DMSO; 100% v/v; Sigma Aldrich, Darmstadt, Germany) was added to each well. Finally, the plates were shaken for 10 min. The absorbance was measured at the wavelength of 570 nm with the subtraction of the 630 nm background, using a microplate reader (Synergy HT; BioTek, Winooski, VT, USA). The blank groups (the plates incubated without the cells) were treated with the same procedures as the experimental groups. All measurements were done in duplicate in five independent experiments.

2.3.3. MG-63 Osteoblasts Morphology Observed by SEM

The analysis of the morphology changes and number of MG-63 osteoblasts growing on the surface of TNT coatings and Ti6Al4V orthopedic implants, which were produced using selective laser sintering 3D technology, was performed using scanning electron microscopy (SEM; Quanta 3D FEG; Carl Zeiss, Göttingen, Germany). In the case of the TNT coatings, the cells were seeded onto the specimens placed in the 24-well plate at a density of 1×10^4 cells/well, whereas the osteoblasts growing on the surface of the Ti6Al4V orthopedic implant placed in the 6-well plates were seeded at a density of 1×10^4 cells/cm². After the selected incubation time, the nanolayers were rinsed with PBS to remove non-adherent cells and fixed in 2.5% v/v glutaraldehyde (Sigma Aldrich, Darmstadt, Germany) for a minimum of 4 h (maximum 1 week). Then, the samples were washed again with PBS and dehydrated in a graded series of ethanol concentration (50%, 75%, 90%, and 100%) for 10 min. Finally, the specimens were dried in vacuum-assisted desiccators overnight and stored at room temperature until the SEM analysis was performed.

2.3.4. Alkaline Phosphatase Activity Assay

MG-63 osteoblasts were seeded onto the tested nanolayers placed in a 24-well culture plate at a density of 1×10^4 cells/well and cultured for 24, 72, and 120 h. Then, the samples were washed with PBS and lysed in 0.2% (v/v) Triton X-100 (Sigma Aldrich, Darmstadt, Germany), with the lysate centrifuged at 14.000× g for 5 min. The clear supernatants were used to measure the alkaline phosphatase (ALP) activity, which was determined using the ALP assay kit from Abcam (London, UK, cat. no. ab83369) according to the manufacturer's instructions. The intracellular total nuclear protein concentration in the final supernatants was determined using the Pierce™ BCA Protein Assay Kit (Thermo Fisher Scientific, Waltham, MA, USA) and the ALP activity was normalized to it.

2.3.5. ELISA Quantification of Cytokines and Nitric Oxide

Murine macrophage cell line RAW 264.7 were seeded in triplicate onto the tested specimens placed in 24-well tissue culture plates (Corning, NY, USA) at a density of 25×10^4 cells/well and cultured for 24 and 48 h. The pro-inflammatory environment was created by adding 10 ng/mL of LPS to the cell growth media. The control cells were incubated on the tested substrates without the presence of LPS. Protein levels of the pro-inflammatory cytokines, interleukin (IL) 1β, IL-6, and tumor necrosis factor (TNF) α; anti-inflammatory cytokine, IL-10; and total nitric oxide, secreted into the cell culture media were measured with sandwich enzyme-linked immunosorbent assays (ELISA) kits from R & D Systems (Minneapolis, MN, USA; cat. no. MLB00C, M6000B, MTA00B, M1000B and KGE001, respectively), according to the manufacturer's instructions. Colorimetric changes in the assays were detected using a Synergy HT Multi-Mode Microplate Reader. The sensitivity of the 1β, IL-6, TNF-α, IL-10, and total NO (nitric oxide) kits were less than 4.8, 1.8, 7.21, 5.22, and 0.78 μmol/L, respectively. To eliminate variation due to differences in the cell density among the samples, the cytokines and NO production were normalized to a number of 10^5 cells.

2.4. Genotoxicity Assessment

The genotoxicity of implant coatings was assessed with the use of the bacterial-reverse mutation test (Ames test) according to the OECD (Organization for Economic Co-operation and Development) guideline 471 for testing chemicals [www.oecd.org]. First, $10 \times 10 \times 2$ mm pieces of unmodified and modified implants were incubated in 0.5 mL of PBS in 310 K for 28 days, after which the solution was screened for mutagenicity in four *Salmonella typphimurium* strains: TA98, TA100, TA1535, TA1537, and one *Escherichia coli* uvrA (pKM101) strain with the use of Ames MPF™ Penta 2 Microplate Format Mutagenicity Assay (Xenometrics, Netherlands). The number of revertant colonies corresponds to the mutagenicity potential of each condition. 2-nitrofluorene (2-NF), 4-Nitroquinoline 1-oxide (4-NQO), N4-Aminocytidine (N4-ACT), and 9-Acridinamine Hydrochloride Hydrate (9-AAC) were mutagens used as strain-specific positive controls (according to the manufacturer's protocol) [34].

2.5. Microbiological Assessment

2.5.1. Microbial Strains and Growth Conditions

Bacterial reference strains: *Staphylococcus aureus* ATCC 43300 (MRSA, methicillin-resistant *S. aureus*), *Staphylococcus aureus* ATCC 29213 (MSSA, methicillin-susceptible *S. aureus*), *Escherichia coli* ATCC 25922, *Streptococcus gordonii* ATCC 10558, and *Streptococcus mutans* ATCC 25175; and fungal reference strains: *Candida albicans* ATCC 10231 and *Candida glabrata* ATCC 90030 were used in the study. Bacteria were cultured on tryptic soy agar (TSA; BTL, Warsaw, Poland) or tryptic soy broth (TSB; BTL, Poland) containing 0.25% glucose (TSB/Glu). Fungi were culture on Sabouraud Agar (SDA; BTL, Warsaw, Poland) or Roswell Park Memorial Institute (RPMI) without phenol red (Sigma, Indianapolis, USA) containing 0.25% glucose (RPMI/Glu).

2.5.2. Anti-Adhesive and Anti-Biofilm Properties of Titanium Surfaces Tested

Microbial strains were grown on appropriate liquid media for 24 h at 310 K. Then, microbial suspensions in TSB/Glu (bacteria) or RPMI/Glu (fungi) at the optical density of $OD_{535} = 0.6$ (nephelometer type Densilameter II, Brno, Czech Republic) were prepared. Biomaterial samples were added to 1 mL of microbial suspensions into the wells of 24-well tissue culture polystyrene plates (Nunc S/A, Roskilde, Denmark) and incubated for 24 h at 310 K in stable conditions to form a microbial biofilm. Microbial suspensions alone (without biomaterial) and liquid media only were used as a microbial growth control and negative control, respectively. Alamar Blue (AB; BioSource, CA, San Diego, USA) staining for bacteria and fluorescein diacetate (FDA; Sigma Aldrich Inc., MO, St. Louis, USA) staining for fungi were used to assess microbial colonization and biofilm formation on the tested biomaterials. First, the biomaterials were dipped in PBS (Biowest, MO, Riverside, USA) to gently remove microbial cells weakly bound to their surface. Then, the pieces of titanium biomaterials tested were sonicated (5 min, room temperature) in TSB or RPMI (for bacteria or fungi, respectively) to reclaim the cells forming the biofilm. The obtained microbial suspensions or medium (negative control) were added (100 µL) in quadruplicate to the tissue culture 96-well microplates (Nunc, Roskilde, Denmark) in case of bacteria and to the black 96-well microplates (Greiner Bio-One, Frickenhausen, Germany) in case of fungi. Microbial cell staining was performed as recommended by the manufacturer of AB and FDA. Finally, the fluorescence of AB at λex 550 nm/em, 585 nm, and FDA fluorescence at λex 485 nm/em, 520 nm was measured at Spectra Max i3 (Molecular Devices, CA, San Jose, USA) in the Laboratory of Microscopic Imaging and Specialized Biological Techniques at the Faculty of Biology and Environmental Protection University of Łódź. Based on fluorescence units (FUs), a percentage of metabolically active microbial cells in the biofilms formed on modified titanium samples tested in comparison to microbial biofilm on reference Ti6Al4V, considered as 100% was calculated.

2.5.3. Antimicrobial Activity of the Titanium Sample-Derived Supernatants

All titanium alloy implant samples tested were incubated separately in 1 mL of PBS without Ca^{2+} and Mg^{2+} (Biowest, MO, Riverside, USA) at 310 K for 24 h, 2 weeks, and 4 weeks. Then, biomaterial samples were removed, and to these obtained supernatants, 100 µL of microbial suspensions in TSB/Glu (bacteria) or RPMI/Glu (fungi) at the optical density of $OD_{535} = 0.6$ were added for 24 h of incubation at 310 K. Microbial suspensions (100 µL) in PBS (1 mL) were used as microbial growth controls. After incubation, microbial cultures were diluted from 10-1 to 10-6 in PBS preceded by intensive vortexing. Then, 100 µL of the suspensions (10-4-10-6) were cultured on TSA (bacteria) or SDA (fungi) and colony-forming units (CFU) were counted after 24 h of incubation at 310 K. The density of microbial suspensions after culture in the presence of titanium sample-derived supernatants was calculated using the average value of CFU counts. The experiment was performed twice, and each microbial culture was prepared in duplicate.

2.6. AFM Topography and Mechanical Properties Studies

The topography studies of implants TNT5 and TNT5/AgNPs were performed using atomic force microscopy (AFM, NaniteAFM, Nanosurf AG, Liestal, Switzerland). The measurements were performed in the non-contact mode at 55 mN force on an area 50 × 50 µm. The Sa parameters (area roughness) were calculated using the integrated software. The nanomechanical properties and nanoscratch-tests of implants TNT5 and TNT5/AgNPs were performed using Nanoindenter NanoTest Vantage (Micro Materials Ltd., Wrexham, UK). To determine the nanomechanical properties, 50 independent measurements in two different areas of the implants (2 × 25 mm) of indentation were performed on each tested implant. The 3-side diamond Berkovich indenter with an angle of 124.4° was used. The maximum force was 10 mN; 15, 5, and 10 s of loading; and dwell with maximum force and unloading, respectively. The distance between the indentations in one section (tested area) was 20 µm in both axes. The nanomechanical properties were determined using the Oliver and Pharr method [36].

To calculate Young's modulus from the reduced Young's modulus, the Poisson's ratio value of 0.25 was used. Nanoscratch tests were performed on 500 µm with a maximum applied force of 500 mN and rate loading force of 3.3 mN/s. The 3-side diamond Berkovich indenter with an angle of 124.4° was used and 5 independent measurements were performed for each tested implant. The adhesion of the coatings was assessed based on the observation of an abrupt change in the frictional force during the test.

2.7. Statistical Analysis in the Biological Assays

All values are reported as means ± standard error of the means (SEM) and they were analyzed using the nonparametric Kruskal–Wallis one-way ANOVA test, with the level of significance set at $p < 0.05$. Statistical analyses were performed for immunological assays with GraphPad Prism 7.0 (La Jolla, CA, USA) and for microbiological and genotoxicity tests with the program Statistica 12.0 (Stat Soft Inc., Tulsa Shock, OK, USA).

3. Results

3.1. Ti6Al4V Implants Modified by Titania Nanotube Coatings

The implants used in our investigations were produced by the selective laser sintering method, using Ti6Al4V ELI powder (Figure 1a). Analysis of SEM images of the implant, as obtained, revealed the presence of the non-melted or partially melted powder grains (Figure 1b). Therefore, before electrochemical modification, the surfaces of the implants were mechanically ground and sandblasted (Figure 1c). The anodization of Ti6Al4V alloy substrates using 0.3 wt% aqueous HF solution as an electrolyte enabled the production of uniform amorphous titanium dioxide layers (Figure 1d) on their surface. The electrolytic processes were performed using potentials of 5 and 15 V, which allowed the formation of nanoporous (TNT5) and nanotubular (TNT15) coatings (Figure 1e,f). Based on the SEM image analysis, the *pore diameters of TNT5 coatings* were c.a. 21 ± 4 nm and the tube diameters of TNT15 were c.a. 51 ± 9 nm. The thickness of the walls in both cases was c.a. 8 ± 1.5 nm. The part of the above-mentioned coatings was enriched with AgNPs using the CVD technique [27–30]. According to the results of our previous works, the AgNPs filled the interiors of the TNT5 nanoporous layer (Figure 1g) while in the case of TNT15, the spherical nanoparticles of diameters c.a. 10 ± 2.0 nm were located mainly on the surface of the separated nanotube walls (Figure 1h).

Analysis of the XPS depth profiles of the Ti6Al4V/TNT5 and Ti6Al4V/TNT15 systems allowed changes in the titanium oxidation states between the TNT surface layer and substrate for nano-porous and nano-tubular coatings to be traced (Tables 1 and 2, Figure S2). According to these data, the surface of the TNT5 nano-porous layer consists entirely of oxides in which the Ti oxidation state is +4, which was confirmed by the presence of peaks $2p_{3/2}$ at the binding energy (BE) at c.a. 458.9 eV and $2p_{1/2}$ at c.a. 464.6 eV (Figure S2). Simultaneously, peaks of O1s at 530.2 and 531.9 eV were assigned to the O^{2-} of Ti–O and OH^- groups, respectively. The high-resolution XPS spectra registered after the first, second, and third sputtering revealed the splitting of the Ti $2p_{3/2}$ and $2p_{1/2}$ peaks, which shows the presence of Ti components for the different valence states. To confirm the valence state of Ti in the titanium oxides (Ti^{2+}, Ti^{3+}, or Ti^{4+}), the differences in the BE (Δ(O–Ti)) of lines assigned to the oxygen (O1s) and $Ti2p_{3/2}$ component were determined. Atuchin et al. [37] and Chinh et al. [38] showed that values of the Δ(O–Ti) criterion in the Ti^{2+}, Ti^{3+}, and Ti^{4+} valence state amount to 75.0–76.7, 72.9–73.1, and 71.4–71.6 eV, respectively. According to these data, Δ(O–Ti), which for TNT5 is equal 71.3 eV, corresponds to Ti^{4+} and suggests that TiO_2 is the main component of this surface layer. The sputtering of the TNT5 sample revealed the presence of nonstoichiometric titanium oxides: After the first sputter, the layer consisted of Ti^{4+} (58%), Ti^{3+} (24%), and Ti^{2+} (18%); after the second, Ti^{2+} (12% + 55%) and Ti^0 (33%); and after the third, Ti^{2+} (35%) and Ti^0 (65%) (Tables 1 and 2).

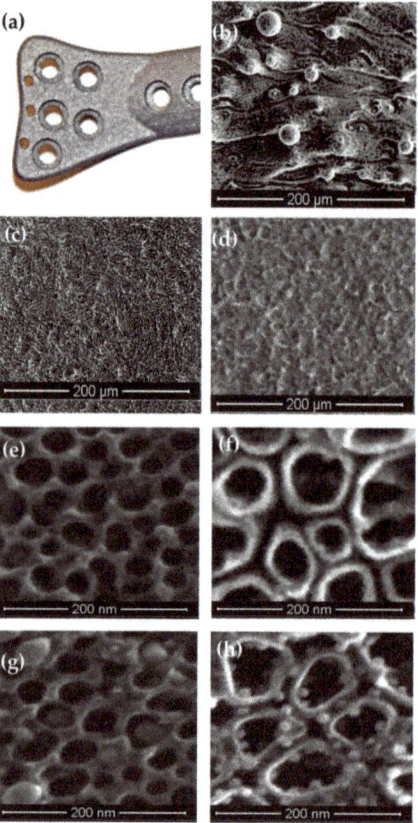

Figure 1. (a) Photography of the orthopedic implant produced using selective laser sintering of Ti6Al4V powder, SEM images of (b) the implant surface obtained, (c) implant surface after grinding and polishing, (d) surface modification of the implant by anodic oxidation using a 5 V potential, (e) the morphology of the TNT5 coating, (f) the morphology of the TNT15 coating, (g) the morphology of the TNT5/AgNPs coating, and (h) the morphology of the TNT5/AgNPs coating.

The calculated values of Δ(O–Ti) after the second sputtering were 75.3 and 76.6 eV, which, according to Atuchin et al. [37], confirm the presence of the titanium on the second oxidation state. Therefore, in Tables 1 and 2, both values are presented as Ti2+. The XPS studies of the non-sputtered layer, which consists of separated tubes (TNT 15), revealed the presence of dual $2p_{3/2}$ and $2p_{1/2}$ peaks at a binding energy (BE) of c.a. 459.0 and 457.8, and 464.7 and 463.4 eV, respectively (Figure S2). The calculated Δ(O–Ti) values of 71.2 and 72.2 eV, respectively, indicate the formation of oxides, in which titanium occurs at the +4 (86%) and +3 (14%) oxidation state. After the third sputtering of TNT15, it is possible to see the layer consisting of Ti^{4+} (30%), Ti^{3+} (23%), and Ti^{2+} (37%) oxides, and Ti^0 (10%) (Tables 1 and 2, Figure S2).

Table 1. Changes in the position of O1s and Ti2p core levels in TNT5 and TNT15 coatings (BE, binding energy) and values of the spectral energy differences between oxygen bonded to Ti^{2+}, Ti^{3+}, and Ti^{4+} ions (Δ(O–Ti) = O1s–Ti2p$_{3/2}$) during Ar^+ sputtering.

	TNT5							
	O^{2-}	Ti^{4+}		Ti^{3+}		Ti^{2+}		Ti^0
	O1s BE (eV)	2p$_{3/2}$ BE (eV)	Δ(O–Ti) (eV)	2p$_{3/2}$ BE (eV)	Δ(O–Ti) (eV)	2p$_{3/2}$ BE (eV)	Δ(O–Ti) (eV)	2p$_{3/2}$ BE (eV)
Non-sputtered	530.2	458.9	71.3	–	–	–	–	–
First Sputter	530.5	458.8	71.7	457.1	73.4	455.2	75.3	–
Second Sputter	530.6	–	–	–	–	455.2, 454.0	75.4, 76.6	453.5
Third Sputter	530.7	–	–	–	–	453.9	76.8	453.4
	TNT15							
	O^{2-}	Ti^{4+}		Ti^{3+}		Ti^{2+}		Ti^0
	O1s BE (eV)	2p$_{3/2}$ BE (eV)	Δ(O–Ti) (eV)	2p$_{3/2}$ BE (eV)	Δ(O–Ti) (eV)	2p$_{3/2}$ BE (eV)	Δ(O–Ti) (eV)	2p$_{3/2}$ BE (eV)
Non-sputtered	530.2	459.0	71.2	457.8	72.4	–	–	–
First Sputter	530.4	458.9	71.5	457.3	73.1	455.0	75.4	–
Second Sputter	530.5	458.9	71.6	457.1	73.4	454.8	75.7	–
Third Sputter	530.5	458.6	71.9	456.8	73.7	454.8	75.7	453.5

Table 2. XPS depth profile of TNT5 and TNT15.

	TNT5				TNT15			
	Ti^{4+}	Ti^{3+}	Ti^{2+}	Ti^0	Ti^{4+}	Ti^{+3}	Ti^{2+}	Ti^0
	%							
Non-sputtered	100	–	–	–	86	14	–	–
First Sputter	58	24	18	–	37	45	18	–
Second Sputter	–	–	12, 55	33	35	34	31	–
Third Sputter	–	–	35	65	30	23	37	10

3.2. Wettability and Surface Free Energy of Biomaterials

The wettability of TNT and TNT/AgNPs sample surfaces was studied by measuring the contact angles of water (polar liquid) and diiodomethane (dispersion liquid) and the surface free energy values (SFEs) were calculated (Table 3). According to these data, the surfaces of Ti6Al4V implants after sintering and machining are hydrophobic while the anodization of titanium alloy leads to an increase of its hydrophilic character. It should be noted that the type of the TNT layer (i.e., nanoporous (TNT5) and nanotubular (TNT15) is an important factor influencing the wettability of the studied coatings. The enrichment of the studied layers by AgNPs was associated with increases of the hydrophobic character of the TNT/AgNPs surfaces.

Table 3. Results of the wetting angle measurements and results of the surface free energy (SFE) measurements of the materials.

	Average Contact Angle [°] ± Standard Deviation		SFE [mJ/m^2]
	Measuring Liquid		
	Water	Diodomethane	
Ti6Al4V	108.3 ± 0.1	37.0 ± 0.2	45.4 ± 0.1
TNT5	76.4 ± 1.3	43.2 ± 2.2	39.1 ± 0.7
TNT15	62.4 ± 0.8	46.1 ± 0.7	44.08 ± 0.4
TNT5/AgNPs	131.9 ± 0.1	44.8 ± 1.6	52.8 ± 0.6
TNT15/AgNPs	124.2 ± 0.1	67.3 ± 1.0	29.1 ± 0.2

3.3. Immunological Assessment

3.3.1. Cell Proliferation Detected by the MTT Assay

The proliferation of MG-63 osteoblasts, L929 fibroblasts, and RAW 264.7 macrophages on the surface of the tested specimens was evaluated with the MTT assay (Figure 2A). MG-63 cells proliferated on all tested specimens, except for the TNT5/Ag samples. It was also noted that only TNT5 specimens promoted proliferation when referring to the reference samples (Ti6Al4V foil) after 72 and 120 h. On the other hand, the slowest cell proliferation was observed on TNT5 coatings enriched with silver nanoparticles. TNT15 specimens both with and without silver nanograins inhibited cell proliferation compared with the reference samples. Among all the investigated coatings, only TNT5 increased L929 fibroblast proliferation after 24, 72, and 120 h (Figure 2B). Moreover, TNT15 nanolayers also induced L929 cell proliferation after 120 h. Importantly, in contrast to MG-63 osteoblasts, with an increase in the incubation time, more L929 cells proliferated on all tested specimens, and none of the tested coatings caused a decrease in the level of L929 cell proliferation. The RAW 264.7 cell proliferation results after 24 and 48 h of incubation are plotted in Figure 2C. Macrophages were cultured in the pro-inflammatory environment created by adding LPS to the cell growth media or in the absence of LPS. As can be seen, with an increase of the incubation period, more cells proliferated on all tested substrates. Importantly, LPS did not affect the level of cell proliferation. After 24 h, macrophages that grew on Ti6Al4V/Ag, TNT5, and TNT5/Ag showed a greater proliferation rate than cells growing on Ti6Al4V reference alloys. After 48 h, all modified implant surfaces showed an increased proliferation rate apart from Ti6Al4V/Ag.

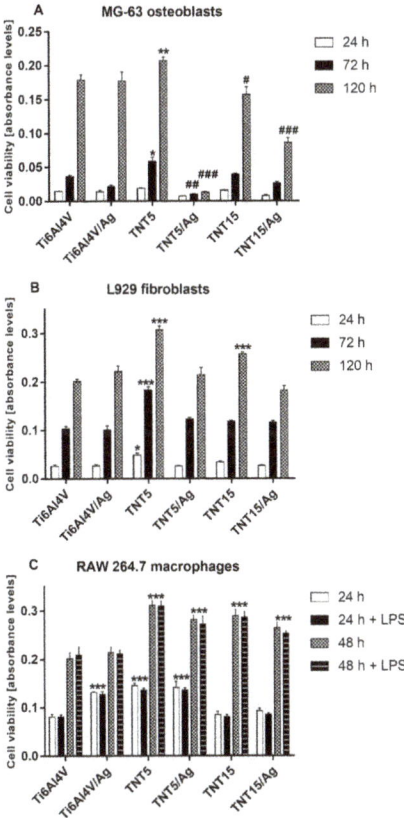

Figure 2. Proliferation of human osteoblast-like MG 63 cells (**A**), L929 murine fibroblast cells (**B**), and murine macrophage cell line RAW 264.7 (**C**) on the surface of TiO$_2$ nanotube coatings analyzed by the MTT assay (a colorimetric assay for assessing cell metabolic activity). MG-63 osteoblasts and L929 fibroblasts were cultured on the specimens for 24, 72, and 120 h, whereas RAW 264.7 macrophages were cultivated for 24 and 48 h in the presence or absence of LPS (Lipopolysaccharide). The absorbance values are expressed as means ±SEM of five independent experiments. Asterisks indicate significant differences comparing to the reference Ti6Al4V alloy foils (Ti6Al4V) (*** $p < 0.001$, * $p < 0.05$). Hash marks denote significant differences when the level of cell proliferation was lower in comparison with the reference Ti6Al4V alloy foils (### $p < 0.001$, ## $p < 0.01$, # $p < 0.05$).

3.3.2. Morphology and Proliferation Rate of MG-63 Osteoblasts Observed by Scanning Electron Microscopy

Biointegration of the TiO$_2$ nanotube coating was also evaluated with SEM micrographs. Comparative SEM images show the morphology and proliferation level of the MG-63 osteoblasts in Figure 3. These data support the MTT results and clearly demonstrate that the highest biocompatibility was observed for TNT5 samples, which is mainly related to the increase in the cell proliferation level over time (compare the micrographs presented in Figure 3c,i,o). Importantly, as can be seen in Figure 3o, MG-63 osteoblasts started to grow in layers on top of each other, which was observed after 120 h of incubation. This phenomenon was not noticed for the TNT5 samples enriched with silver nanoparticles (Figure 3p). SEM images also showed that MG-63 osteoblasts have an elongated shape and form numerous filopodia, which strongly attach the cells to the nanocoatings' surface (arrows in Figure 3g–r). These thin actin-rich plasma membrane protrusions were also generated between the cells (arrows in

Figure 3l). Finally, SEM micrographs were also used to evaluate the biointegration level of Ti6Al4V orthopedic implants, which were produced using selective laser sintering 3D technology. As can be seen in Figure 3m,n, MG-63 osteoblasts effectively attached to the implant's surface. Moreover, with an increase of the incubation time, the number of cells and their density increased.

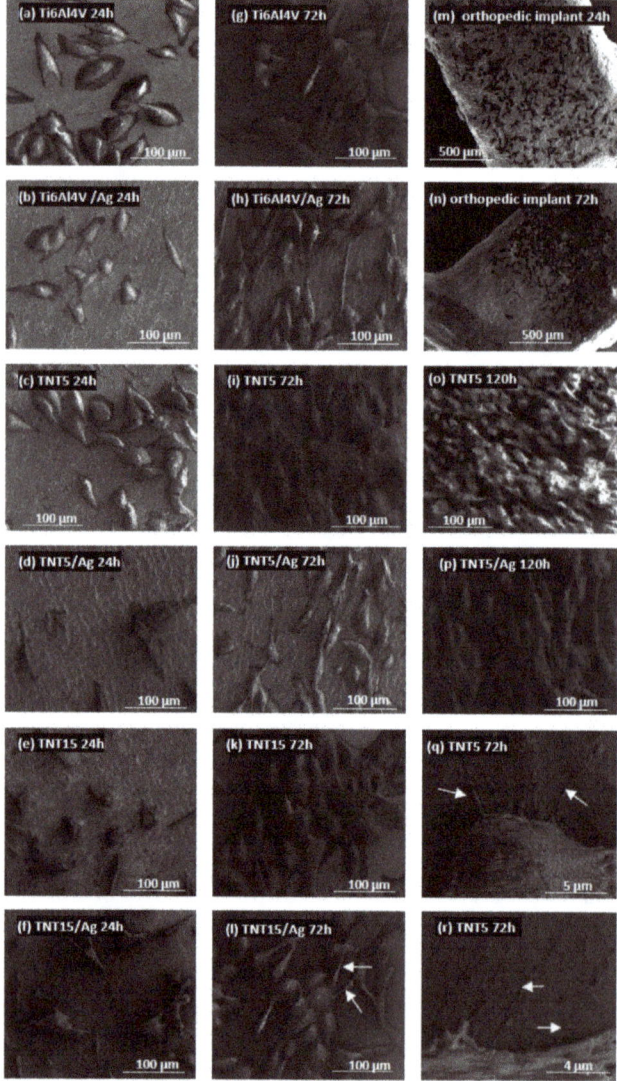

Figure 3. Scanning electron microscopy (SEM) images showing human osteoblast-like MG-63 cells that grow on the surface of the tested titania coatings and the reference Ti6Al4V alloy foils enriched or not with silver nanograins. Micrographs (**m,n**) present the cells grown on the surface of Ti6Al4V orthopedic implants, which were produced using selective laser sintering 3D technology. Arrows in image (l) indicate filopodia spread between cells and those in image (**q,r**) present filopodia penetrating deep into the samples and attaching the cells to the surface. The type of sample, cell incubation time, and scale of the images are shown in the figures as indicated.

3.3.3. Alkaline Phosphatase Activity of MG-63 Cells

Osteoblastic cell differentiation was assessed by measuring ALP activity, normalized to the total protein content after 24, 72, and 120 h of culture. Figure 4 shows the comparison of the ALP activity of MG-63 cells cultured on the tested specimens with reference Ti6Al4V alloy foils. The ALP activity of MG-63 cells grown on the all tested specimens increased over time. However, MG-63 cells cultured on the substrates enriched with silver nanograins had significantly lower ALP activity than those cultured on the reference Ti6Al4V alloy foils at the respective incubation time. In contrast, among all of the tested samples, only the TNT5 specimens induced higher ALP activity in comparison with the reference Ti6Al4V samples at a given incubation time. This phenomenon was also observed for TNT15 substrates but only after 24 h of culture.

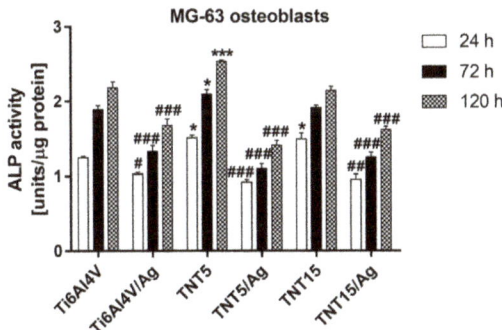

Figure 4. Alkaline phosphatase activity (ALP) of MG-63 osteoblasts growing on TiO_2 nanotube coatings produced by electrochemical anodic oxidation at potentials of 5 (TNT5) or 15 V (TNT15) and enriched with silver nanoparticles in comparison with the reference Ti6Al4V alloy foils and enriched or not with silver nanograins. The cells were cultured on the surface of the tested specimens for 24, 72, and 120 h. ALP activity [units] was calculated per μg of protein and it is expressed as the means ± SEM of five independent experiments. Asterisks indicate significant differences at the appropriate incubation time when the ALP activity of the cells growing on the tested specimens was higher compared to the reference Ti6Al4V alloy foils (Ti6Al4V) (*** $p < 0.001$, * $p < 0.05$). Hash marks denote significant differences at the appropriate incubation time when the ALP activity of osteoblasts cultivated on the tested samples was lower in comparison with the reference Ti6Al4V alloy foils (### $p < 0.001$, ## $p < 0.01$, # $p < 0.05$).

3.3.4. Secretion of Cytokines and Nitric Oxide by RAW 264.7 Macrophages

The time-course of the protein release of pro-inflammatory cytokines (IL-1β, IL-6, and TNF-α), anti-inflammatory cytokines (IL-10), and NO (nitric oxide) was assessed in 24 to 48 h of incubation by performing ELISA assays. Data show that RAW 264.7 macrophages stimulated with LPS released higher amounts of cytokines and NO over time for all tested substrates (Figure 5). However, TiO_2 nanotube coatings produced by electrochemical anodic oxidation at potentials of 5 (TNT5) and 15 V (TNT15), enriched or not with silver nanoparticles, displayed a different production of cytokines and NO. Generally, the TNT5 and TNT5/Ag samples inhibited the LPS-induced release of pro-inflammatory cytokines and NO in comparison with the reference Ti6Al4V alloy foils, whereas TNT15 and TNT15/Ag specimens enhanced the production of IL-1β, IL-6, TNF-α, and NO. Moreover, cells that grew on the surface of TNT15 substrates released significant amounts of these cytokines and NO without LPS stimulation (Figure 5E). In contrast, in the absence of LPS, the amounts of IL-1β and IL-6 measured from cells cultured on TNT5, TNT5/Ag, and Ti6Al4V/Ag specimens were below the assay detection limits, at both analyzed time points. Importantly, the presence of silver nanoparticles on the surface of all tested coatings (Ti6Al4V, TNT5, and TNT15) inhibited pro-inflammatory cytokine production in comparison with the same respective layers not enriched with silver nanograins. The level of anti-inflammatory cytokine (IL-10) was also measured. As can be seen in Figure 5D, the biggest amount of IL-10 was released by the LPS-stimulated cells growing on the surface of TNT5 and TNT5/Ag samples. On the other hand, the levels of IL-10 from cells growing on the TNT15 and TNT15/Ag specimens were lower in comparison with the reference Ti6Al4V alloy foils.

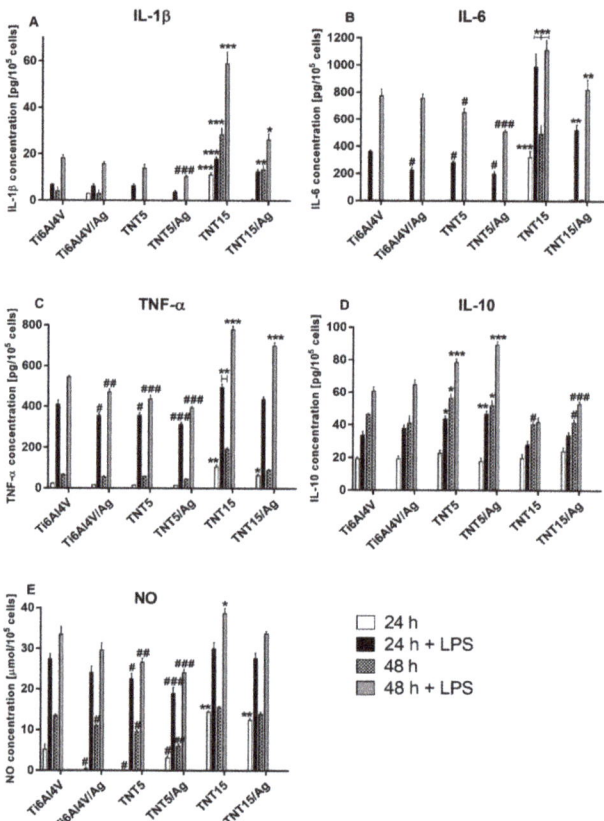

Figure 5. Secretion of pro-inflammatory (**A**–**C**) and anti-inflammatory (**D**) cytokines or total nitric oxide (**E**) by RAW 264.7 macrophages in the standard and LPS-stimulated conditions. The cells were cultured on the tested specimens for 24 and 48 h. Cytokine and nitric oxide (NO) production was normalized to a number of 105 cells. Data are expressed as mean ± SE ($n = 3$). Asterisks indicate significant differences at the appropriate incubation time when the amounts of cytokines and NO produced by the cells growing on the tested specimens were higher in comparison with the reference Ti6Al4V alloy foils (Ti6Al4V) (*** $p < 0.001$, ** $p < 0.01$, * $p < 0.05$). Hash marks denote significant differences at the appropriate incubation time when the levels of cytokines and NO secreted by the cells cultivated on the tested samples were lower in comparison with the reference Ti6Al4V alloy foils (### $p < 0.001$, ## $p < 0.01$, # $p < 0.05$).

3.4. Genotoxicity Assessment

To estimate the genotoxicity of substances released from the surface of studied implants during the 28-day incubation in PBS, the Ames assay was carried out. It was especially important to assess if silver release from TNT/AgNPs coatings could be mutagenic. This issue is associated with an increasing number of reports warning about the genotoxicity of silver nanoparticles [39,40]. The assay was performed in five genetically modified bacteria strains according to OECD guidelines TG471 (http://www.oecd.org), allowing detection of deletion, base substitution, or frameshift mutations, depending on the tester strain's engineered genotype. The number of revertant bacterial colonies corresponds to the mutagenic potential of the analyzed agents (Figure 6). None of the implant coatings demonstrated genotoxic potential in any of the bacteria strains in this assay.

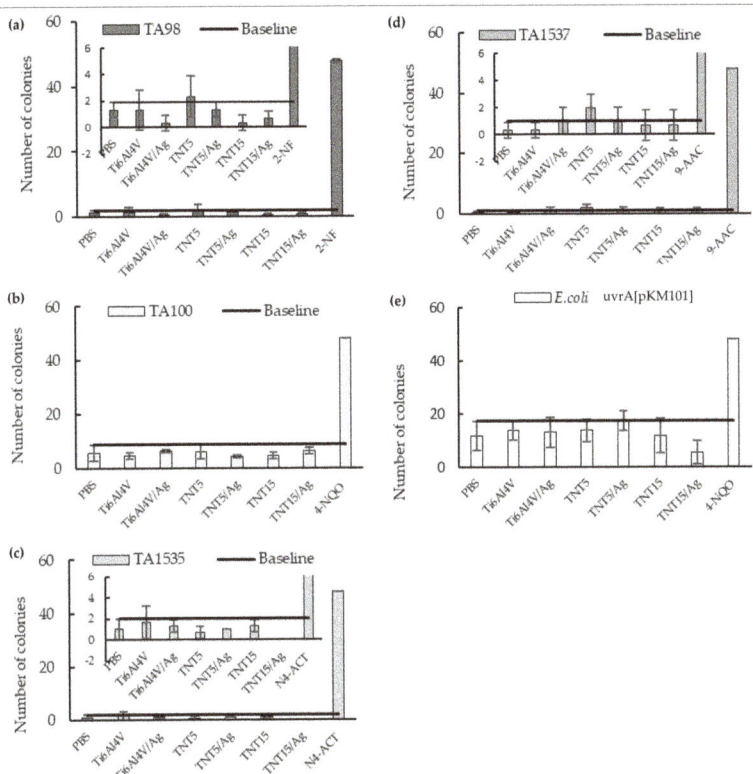

Figure 6. Assessment of implants' genotoxicity by the Ames assay performed in five genetically modified bacteria strains: (a) TA98, (b) TA100, (c) TA1535, (d) TA1537, and (e) *E.coli*; to improve the readability of Ames assay results of TA98 (a), TA1535 (c), and TA1537 (d), their enlarged versions are added.

3.5. Microbiological Assessment

The ability of implants modified with TNT and TNT/AgNPs layers to inhibit microbial colonization and biofilm formation was tested in comparison to an unmodified Ti6Al4V surface (control biomaterial) with the use of Gram-positive (*S. aureus, S. gordonii, S. mutans*) and Gram-negative (*E. coli*) bacteria, as well as fungi (*C. albicans, C. glabrata*). The metabolic activity of the microorganisms attached to the surfaces after 24 h of exposure to the microbial suspensions was measured using Alamar Blue. The results are presented in Figures 7 and 8 (for bacteria and fungi, respectively) as a percentage of the metabolic active microbes recovered from the biofilms formed on the tested surfaces in comparison to the biofilms formed on unmodified control biomaterial (Ti6Al4V) being considered as 100%. All tested modified titanium alloy implant surfaces were able to inhibit microbial colonization and biofilm formation; however, in the case of bacteria, the observed effect strongly depended on the strain used. Generally, well-defined anti-biofilm activity on the tested TNT and TNT/AgNPs layers was demonstrated against *S. aureus* ATCC 29213 and *E. coli* ATCC 25922 (Figure 8). The average percentage of biofilm inhibition, compared to the control biofilm developed on unmodified Ti6Al4V, achieved the range from 41.1 ± 3.0% ($p = 0.034$) to 49.7 ± 1.5% ($p = 0.034$) for *S. aureus* ATCC 29213 and from 33.2 ± 10.7% ($p = 0.034$) to 76.3 ± 1.5% ($p = 0.034$) for *E. coli* ATCC 25922. The weakest inhibitory effect was observed for *S. gordonii* ATCC 10558 (biofilm reduction of up to 9.0% on TNT5/AgNPs and TNT15/AgNPs, $p = 0.028$ and $p = 0.0082$, respectively). The surfaces expressed no significant or moderate activity against *S. aureus* ATCC 43300 and *S. mutans* ATCC 25175, with the exception of TNT5/AgNPs, which inhibited biofilm formation by these second bacteria of 80.9 ± 1.2% ($p = 0.021$). In the case of fungi, the inhibitory effect of the surfaces tested was similar for both strains (*C. albicans* and *C. glabrata*), achieving the level of 13.3 ± 1.6% to 33.7 ± 8.5% (Figure 8, all results were statistically significant). Interestingly, there was no great distinction in the reduction of the microbial biofilm caused by TNT surfaces and corresponding them to the TNT/AgNPs layers.

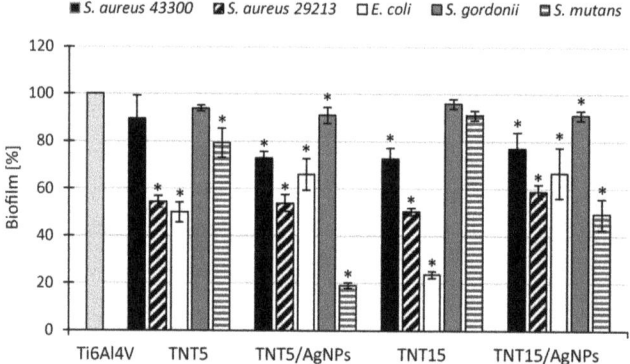

Figure 7. Bacterial biofilm on TNT- and TNT/AgNPs-modified Ti6Al4V surfaces assessed using Alamar Blue staining. The results are presented as the mean percentage ± standard deviation (SD) of the bacterial biofilm formed on the tested layers compared to a control biofilm formed on the reference biomaterial (Ti6Al4V) considered as 100%. Statistical analysis was estimated with nonparametric Kruskal–Wallis one-way ANOVA test (* significant differences, $p < 0.05$).

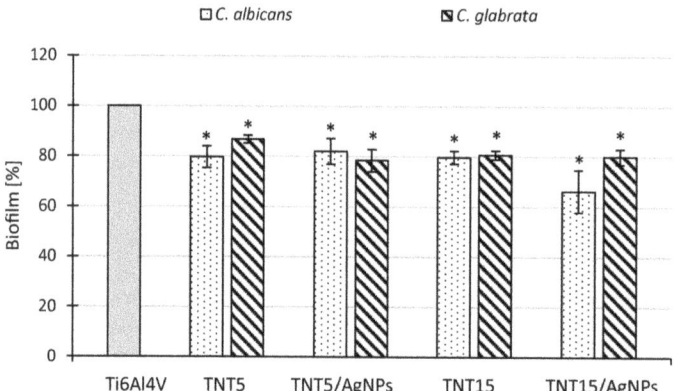

Figure 8. Fungal biofilm on TNT- and TNT/AgNPs-modified Ti6Al4V surfaces assessed using FDA (fluorescein diacetate) staining. The results are presented as the mean percentage ± standard deviation (SD) of the fungal biofilm formed on the tested layers compared to a control biofilm formed on the reference biomaterial (Ti6Al4V) considered as 100%. Statistical analysis was estimated with nonparametric Kruskal–Wallis one-way ANOVA test (* significant differences, $p < 0.05$).

Since biologically active (biostatic/biocidal) substances can be released from modified titanium surfaces when implants are in the host tissue, we also tested the antimicrobial effect of the supernatants obtained after short- (24 h) and long-term (2 and 4 weeks) biomaterial incubation in PBS to simulate such conditions. Four microbial strains were used for these studies (*S. aureus* ATCC 43300, *S. aureus* ATCC 29213, *E. coli* ATCC 25922, and *C. albicans* ATCC 10231) and the results are presented in Figure 9a–c as the mean density of microbial suspensions cultured for 24 h in the presence of biomaterial-derived supernatants (s). As expected, the type of titanium surfaces and the time of their incubation in PBS were the most important factors determining the release of biologically active substances from biomaterial samples and thus the antimicrobial activity of the supernatants tested. After a short (24 h) incubation, the supernatants showed almost no activity against bacterial strains (Figure 9a).

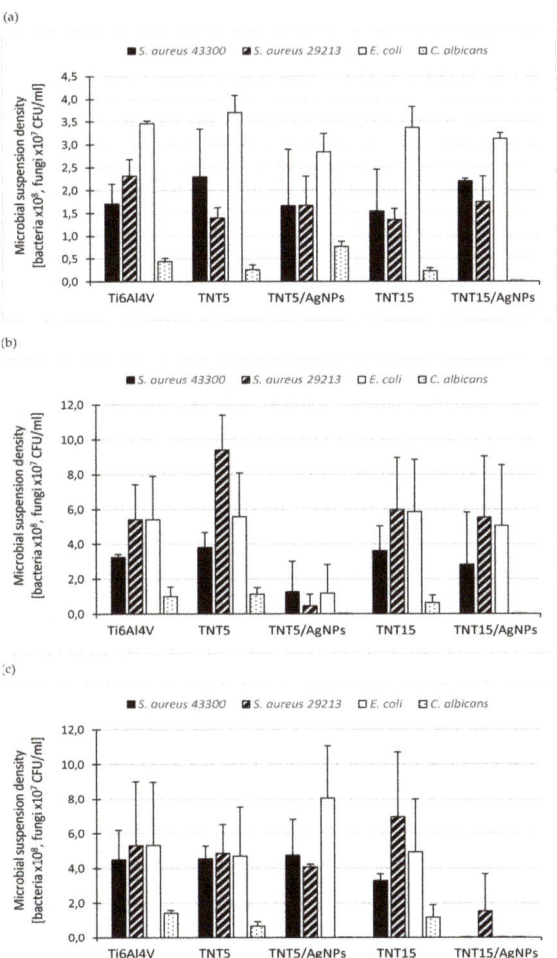

Figure 9. Antimicrobial effect of the supernatants obtained after 24 h (**a**), 2 weeks (**b**), and 4 weeks of (**c**) TNT- and TNT/AgNPs-modified Ti6Al4V surfaces' incubation in PBS, tested using the culture method and colony forming unit (CFU) counting. The results are presented as the mean microbial suspension density [CFU/mL] ± standard deviation (SD) after 24 h of culture in the presence of the tested supernatants.

The number of bacteria in the presence of the compounds released from AgNP-modified layers was reduced in the range 2.6%–27.9% for the TNT5/AgNPs supernatant and 0%–24.6% for the TNT15/AgNPs supernatant, in comparison to the number of the bacteria exposed on the control Ti6Al4V-derived supernatant. Whereas, *C. albicans* cells proved to be the most sensitive to the antimicrobial activity of the compounds released from the modified biomaterial samples. The reduction of the yeast cell number caused by the TNT15/AgNPs 24-h supernatant reached 99.9% (Figure 9a), which means it has strong biocidal activity against fungi. By extending the incubation time of the biomaterial samples, the bactericidal properties of the supernatants obtained from AgNP-containing layers increased significantly. However, the compounds released from TNT5/AgNPs demonstrated the strongest antibacterial activity after two weeks (Figure 9b) while those from TNT15/AgNPs after four weeks (Figure 9c). The two-week supernatant of TNT5/AgNPs significantly reduced the number of all tested microbial strains (both bacteria and fungi), with the reduction levels reaching 61.5%, 91.4%, 78.3%, and 99.9% for *S. aureus* ATCC 43300, *S. aureus* ATCC 29213, *E. coli*, and *C. albicans*, respectively (Figure 9b). The two-week TNT15/AgNPs-derived supernatant activity was similar only against *C. albicans* (99.8% reduction of fungal viability; Figure 9b). However, during 4 weeks of biomaterial incubation in PBS, the antimicrobial potential of the TNT15/AgNPs-derived supernatant increased significantly, causing complete elimination of most of the tested microorganisms. The reduction of the *S. aureus* ATCC 43300, *E. coli*, and *C. albicans* populations exceeded 99.9% after exposition of this supernatant (Figure 9c). The effect on *S. aureus* ATCC 29213 was a little bit weaker (71.3% of eradication) but still very strong (Figure 9c) while the supernatants derived from the TNT5 and TNT15 samples (both 2 and 4 weeks) did not exhibit killing activity against the microorganisms tested (Figure 9b,c).

3.6. AFM Topography and Nanomechanical Properties Studies

The topography images and the Sa parameter values of TNT5 and TNT5/AgNPs samples (systems whose surface shows the best biological properties) using atomic force microscopy (AFM) are presented in Figure 10. Analysis of these data showed that the implant surface has a much more extensive surface topography before the AgNP deposition process. The roughness parameters, Sa, decrease about 57% from 0.89 for TNT5 before silver deposition to 0.39 for implant TNT5/AgNPs with nanosilver on the surface. A significant decrease in the roughness value was probably caused by the deposition of silver nanoparticles in the surface cavities, which led to their smoothing.

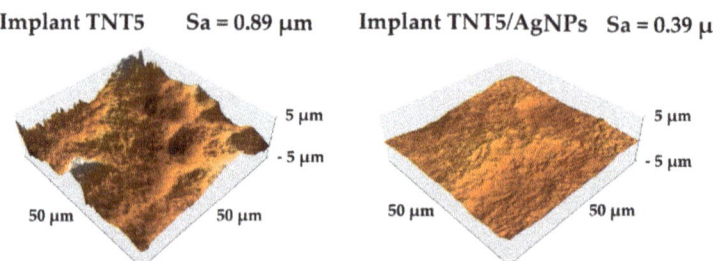

Figure 10. The topography of TNT5 and TNT5/Ag implants with Sa (Average Roughness) parameter values, which was determined using atomic force microscope (AFM).

The nanomechanical and nanoindentation properties of the tested implants (TNT5 and TNT5/AgNPs) for the two tested areas of each surface are presented in Table 4. In the case of the TNT5, no such significant differences in the mechanical properties (nanohardness and Young's modulus) were observed between the tested area surfaces (I and II) as in the case of the tested areas (I and II) of the implant TNT5/AgNPs. The presence of silver nanoparticles resulted in an increase of the nanohardness and Young's modulus and as a consequence, as increase of parameter H/E (Hardness to

Young's Modulus ratio), which determines the resistance to wear of the tested specimens. The relation between parameter H/E and wear resistance were reported [35]. The significant standard deviation values confirm the credibility and diligence of the presented results and their value in studies on the nanoindentation on titanium dioxide nanotube layer were reported previously by Jemat et al. [41] and Rayon et al. [42]. Moreover, using small values of force (10 mN) on surfaces with a high surface roughness causes significant differences between individual measurements. The 3D distribution of nanomechanical properties, such as the nanohardness and Young's modulus, for TNT5/AgNPs (tested area II) are presented in Figure 11. The presented results confirm the value of the standard deviation presented in Table 4. The presented results show the heterogeneity of the distribution of the mechanical properties and the relationship between the hardness and Young's modulus because the distributions are similar to each other.

Table 4. Nanomechanical and nanoindentation properties of the tested implant samples.

	Position of Indentation	Hardness H (GPa)	Young's Modulus E (GPa)	H/E (-)
TNT5	Area I	0.048 ± 0.079	22.49 ± 64.95	0.0044 ± 0.0024
	Area II	0.058 ± 0.105	8.12 ± 9.66	0.0063 ± 0.0049
	Area I+II	0.053 ± 0.092	17.00 ± 61.02	0.0054 ± 0.0039
TNT5/AgNPs	Area I	0.751 ± 1.145	37.99 ± 48.74	0.0114 ± 0.0077
	Area II	5.835 ± 5.720	168.57 ± 121.25	0.0266 ± 0.0135
	Area I + II	3.293 ± 4.862	103.28 ± 112.75	0.0190 ± 0.0133

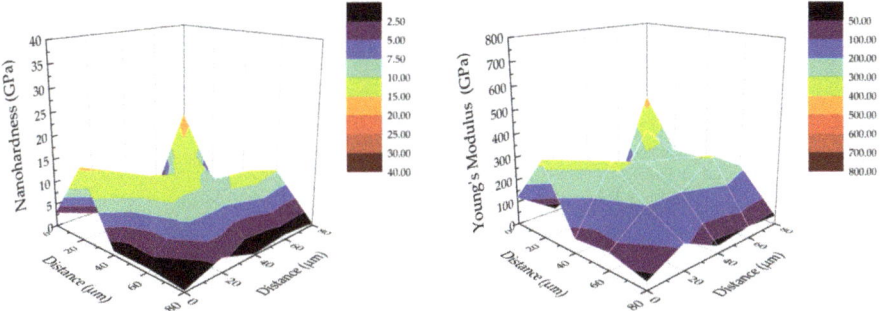

Figure 11. The nanomechanical properties (nanohardness and Young's modulus) of TNT5/Ag implant in the studied area II.

The nanoscratch test results for TNT5 and TNT5/AgNPs are presented in Table 5. Nowadays, the nanoscratch test method is a dedicated method to assess the adhesion of thin coatings or layers, as in the case of the presented tests. In Table 5, two different types of force obtained during nanoscratch test measuring for the tested coatings are presented. The critical force is the maximum applied force between the coating and the indenter during full delamination of the coating from the metallic substrate (Ti6Al4V) and the critical friction force is the maximum friction force registered during full delamination of the coating. The presence of silver nanoparticles in the composite coating (TNT5/AgNPs) caused an increased critical force (from 79.70 to 173.40 mN) and critical friction force (from 130.77 to 212.34 mN). The results obtained from nanoindentation tests determined the wear resistance of the tested surfaces (H/E ratio) correlated with the nanoscratch test results. The H/E parameter for the TNT5/AgNPs surface was significantly higher than for the TNT5 surface. The same trend was reported in the nanoscratch tests results.

Table 5. Adhesion properties of the titanium dioxide nanocoatings to the titanium alloy surfaces.

	Nanoscratch Test Properties	
	Critical Force (mN)	Critical Friction Force (mN)
TNT5	79.70 ± 33.73	130.77 ± 31.09
TNT5/AgNPs	173.40 ± 41.97	212.34 ± 66.84

4. Discussion

On the basis of our earlier works, we chose the anodic oxidation method as a surface modification of implants produced in 3D technology (SLS of Ti6Al4V ELI Grade 23 powder) [25]. Two types of amorphous coatings, which revealed suitable biointegration and antibacterial properties in preliminary studies, were selected for more comprehensive investigations, i.e., TNT5 (the ordered nanoporous) and TNT15 (the ordered nanotubular) [25,26]. Thanks to the anodic oxidation method, the TNT5 and TNT15 coatings covered the whole implant surface without cracks and gaps. This surface modification decreased the implants' hydrophobicity, whereas the enrichment with AgNPs caused the reverse effect (Table 3). Analysis of the XPS data confirmed that the surface of the TNT5 coating formed by a layer of titanium oxide, in which the titanium oxidation state is +4 (TiO_2—100%). Meanwhile, the surface TNT15 layer should be treated as a mixture, which consists of Ti^{4+} (TiO_2—86%) and Ti^{3+} (Ti_2O_3—14%) oxides (Tables 1 and 2, Figure S1) [43]. However, considering the earlier reports, we can assume that in water solutions, unstable oxides of titanium on the lower oxidation states will be oxidized up to TiO_2 [44], and therefore in all biological experiments TNT15 can also be treated as a TiO_2 layer.

The evaluation of biointegration properties of studied implants indicated that TNT5 nanoporous coating had the highest biointegration potential. TNT5 surface modification promoted proliferation of all tested cell lines while enrichment with silver nanoparticles inhibited proliferation of osteoblasts but not of fibroblasts cell lines. These results correspond to our previous findings, were we also noticed that TNT5 coatings enriched with AgNPs decreased proliferation of the MG-63 osteoblasts [30]. We have also observed that an increased nanotubes diameter (TNT15 coating) weakened the biointegration potential of the implant. Earlier works also showed that TiO_2 nanoporous coatings with smaller pores diameter promoted osteoblast vitality and differentiation [45–47]. Moreover, cell growth on nanotubes of diameter larger than 50 nm was severely impaired due to the reduced cellular activity and an extensive programmed cell death [46]. As we have demonstrated, the presence of nanosilver on the surface of nanotubes has greater cytotoxic effect on osteoblasts than the diameter of the nanotubes themselves. Our results are in line with the findings of other authors, which indicate that nanosilver is toxic for osteoblasts and osteoclasts [48,49]. On the other hand, some experimental evidence show that TiO_2 nanotubes coated with nanosilver are compatible to mammalian cells including osteoblasts [50,51]. The differences in the biocompatibility of biomaterials coated with nanosilver probably depend on the concentration and mode of AgNPs deployment on the surface of produced TNT coatings, and the rate of silver ion release to the body fluid environment [52]. An important part of our research was the determination of the inflammatory response elicited by the macrophage RAW 264.7 cell line cultured on the surface of modified implants in an inflammatory environment simulated with LPS. LPS is an outer membrane component of Gram-negative bacteria, recognized by the innate immune system as a sign of infection [53,54]. RAW 264.7 cells are widely used for inflammation studies due to the highly reproducible response to LPS derived from *Escherichia coli*, mimicking bacterial infection [55]. Our results clearly indicate that neither the investigated biomaterials nor the used dose of LPS (10 ng/ml) had any toxic effect on the RAW 264.7 macrophages. Moreover, all surface modification, besides AgNPs enrichment, promoted macrophages proliferation comparing to Ti6Al4V reference alloys. These findings are in line with Neacsu et al. [55], who also showed an increased macrophage proliferation on the nanotubes comparing to the unmodified titanium foils. Since macrophages play a key role in modulating early events in wound healing and interaction of macrophages with dental implant surfaces can be an important determinant of success of osseointegration [56,57], our results indicate the biocompatibility of the tested nanomaterials. In the next experiments, we assessed the levels of pro and anti-inflammatory cytokines, released by macrophages growing on different implant surfaces. The pro-inflammatory IL-1β, IL-6 and TNF-α are produced predominantly by activated macrophages and are involved in the up-regulation of inflammatory reactions [58]. Similarly, NO is a prominent indicator of pro-inflammatory signal transduction in inflammatory response and antimicrobial defense [59]. In contrast, one of the major anti-inflammatory cytokines is IL-10, which inhibits the production of pro-inflammatory cytokines and mediators from macrophages and dendritic cells [60]. Our results showed that TNT5 and TNT5/AgNPs samples inhibited the LPS-induced release of pro-inflammatory cytokines and NO in comparison with the references Ti6Al4V alloy foils. In contrast, TNT15 and TNT15/AgNPs enhanced production of these mediators. Moreover, presence of AgNPs on the surface of nanotubes potentiated the anti-inflammatory activities of all tested specimens According to previous reports, silver nanoparticles show the potent anti-inflammatory effect and accelerate wound healing, however the possible cytotoxic effect on mammalian cells was also observed [49,61]. These results indicate that TNT5 coatings are good candidates for manufacture of implants with anti-inflammatory properties, since inflammation has been associated with both delayed bone healing and pathogenic bone loss [62].

The assessment of the genotoxicity of implants, which surface has been modified by producing TNT5 and TNT15 coatings, as well as their subsequent enrichment with AgNPs, was an important part of our studies. Genotoxicity is an ability of the agent to directly or indirectly induce DNA damage. If not repaired by DNA repair system or eliminated by cell death, the damage might be retained in genetic material as a mutation and passed on to next generations. Accumulation of the mutations is causatively linked to many chronic diseases including cancer [63]. One of the severe mutagens are heavy metals, which can damage DNA directly by formation of adducts and intra- and inter- strand and DNA-protein crosslinks or indirectly through induction of massive oxidative stress. Therefore implants, especially long-term implants which remaining in the body cavity for long periods, i.e. months or years, should be scrutinized in terms of genotoxicity. Widely used in implantology titanium alloy (Ti6Al4V), a reference implant in our studies, was shown not to induce DNA damage [64]. However surface modifications of this alloy, especially with silver nanoparticles, are the source of potential DNA damaging molecules released from the implant coating, which was widely discussed in earlier reports [39,65,66]. For this reason, the biological systems enriched with AgNPs should be given special attention [40,66]. The molecular mechanism behind the genotoxic properties of AgNPs is still unsolved but involves the direct production of hydroxyl radicals and induction of oxidative stress resulting in DNA damage [66]. In the *in vivo* studies in mice the AgNPs could reach bone marrow and liver, and generate cytotoxicity to the reticulocytes and oxidative DNA damage to the liver [39]. The DNA damaging effect of NPs depends on their size, concentration and time of exposure [66,67]. Therefore it is important to analyze if silver released in a long term from the implant surface could induce DNA damage and result in mutations. In this study we took advantage of the first line in vitro gene mutation study recommended by OECD (TG 471) – bacterial reverse mutation test (Ames test), adjusted to verify mutagenicity of molecules released from the differently modified implant surfaces during 28 days incubation in PBS. Five tester strains were used to detect deletion, base substitution or frame shift mutations, depending on the tester strain's engineered genotype. None of the implant coatings tested, regardless of surface modification or AgNPs enrichment, released substances of mutagenic properties in any of the strains analyzed. This is a good prognosis for the investigated implant/TNT coating modifications discussed in this study. Their nanoporous (TNT5) and nanotubular (TNT15) morphology promotes implant biointegration and allows for controlled release of silver sufficient to kill bacteria and fungi and at the same time not inducing DNA damage.

The new generation of implants should not only facilitate their tissue integration but also prevent microbial colonization and biofilm formation. Serious medical problems associated with the introduction of implants to the human body are infections, which can lead to increased patients failure and mortality [68–71]. To solve this problem, the implant surface is modified by the formation of bioactive nanostructures (e.g., TiO$_2$ nanotubes, nanofibers) and/or their enrichment with metal nanoparticles (mainly silver and copper) [20,27,28,72–74]. In our previous study it has been shown that TiO$_2$ nanotubes formed on titanium alloy (Ti6Al4V), in particular the coatings obtained using low-potential anodic oxidation, possessed in vitro anti-biofilm activity tested on *S. aureus* model [25]. In the present work both amorphous titania layers (TNT5 and TNT15) and silver nanoparticles (AgNPs) were used to modify titanium alloy surface. Their antimicrobial potential against broad range of Gram-positive and Gram-negative bacteria, as well as fungi, was tested during direct contact of the microorganisms with biomaterial samples (anti-adhesive and anti-biofilm effect). Moreover, their exposition of analyzed microbials on the supernatants probably containing the components released from biomaterial samples (biocidal effect) has been evaluated. We demonstrated that all tested modified titanium surfaces were able to inhibit microbial colonization and biofilm formation in comparison to control Ti6Al4V. Similar to our previous study [28] anti-biofilm effect strongly depended on bacterial strain used. For instance, *S. aureus* ATCC 29213 (methicillin-susceptible *S. aureus* strain, MSSA) was more sensitive to direct contact with tested biomaterials less effectively colonizing modified surfaces than *S. aureus* ATCC 43300 (methicillin-resistant *S. aureus* strain, MRSA). Previously, inhibitory effect of TiO$_2$ nanotubes and Ag grains on *S. aureus* ATCC 29213 biofilm was demonstrated, while biofilm formation by *S. aureus* H9 MRSA clinical strain was not affected in the same conditions [28]. Interestingly, we did not observe differences in anti-adhesive/anti-biofilm activity of TNT enriched and not enriched with AgNPs. Nanostructural modification of implant surfaces was suggested to limit direct microbial cell contact with such layer, which determine the ability of nanostructures to inhibit microbial colonization and biofilm formation [73,75–77]. The mechanisms of AgNPs antimicrobial activity are more complex and multidirectional, resulting from many targets in microbial cells for Ag+ activity, such as cell wall synthesis, membrane transport, including electron transport in respiratory chain, protein functions, as well as DNA transcription and translation [73,78,79]. Thus we could have expected that modification of titanium surface by both TNT and AgNPs would potentiate antimicrobial effect of such biomaterials. Especially since the antibacterial activity of AgNPs-enriched titanium coatings was demonstrated [28,75,80]. However, for the antimicrobial activity, Ag+ should be released from the nanoparticles in the nearest proximity of the microbes. As seen in SEM images, majority of AgNPs were inside or entrapped between TiO$_2$ nanotubes, which limited the direct contact with the microorganisms during short-time studies. Therefore, demonstrated anti-adhesive and anti-biofilm activities of both TNT- and TNT/AgNPs layers were similar in short time. However, in long lasting experiments, the TNT/AgNPs biocidal activity was higher than Ti6Al4V and TNT-modified surfaces. TNT5/AgNPs-derived supernatant exhibited bactericidal activity after 2 weeks incubation and TNT15/AgNPs-derived one after 4 weeks, suggesting that the morphology of these layers can influence the release of Ag+ and thus their concentrations in the surrounding physiological fluids and tissues. Godoy-Gallardo et al. [81] assessed antibacterial effect of Ti dental implants modified by Ag (electrodeposition) *in vivo* using dog model of ligature-induced peri-implantitis. During long-lasting experiment (peri-implantitis was initiated 2 months after implantation and the effects were observed up to next 4 months) Ag$^+$ release and their accumulation in the tissues around dental implants were demonstrated, which probably contributed to the reduced bacteria colonization of the implant surface. Moreover, a decreased bone resorption in Ag modified impants was shown, representing yet another positive effect of an antimicrobial modification [81]. These results confirm our assumption that after implantation Ag ions release occurs *in vivo* and may modify the conditions in micro-niche influencing microbial growth, colonization, biofilm formation, and thus limiting inflammation. Interestingly, in our in vitro study fungicidal activity of TNT/AgNPs-derived supernatants was constantly very strong (almost 100% of *C. albicans* mortality), regardless the nanotubes type (TNT5/15) or incubation time (2/4 weeks), suggesting higher sensitivity of *Candida* cells to Ag+ than bacterial cells. Besinis et al. [75] also showed highly antibacterial activity of silver plated Ti6Al4V discs coated with nano-hydroxyapatite (Ag-nHA) and silver plated Ti6Al4V discs coated with micro-hydroxyapatite (Ag-mHA), causing 100% mortality of bacteria in surrounded media, which was attributed to a small but effective slow release of Ag from the layers. Similar to our results, Besinis et al. [75] in the study on colonization of modified titanium discs layers by oral streptococci also did not observe anti-biofilm activity against *Streptococcus sanguis*. However, the enrichment with Ag strengthened anti-biofilm activity. In our studies TNT/AgNPs samples also significantly reduced *S. gordonii* and *S. mutans* adhesion and biofilm formation (although not so spectacularly). Summarizing, the enrichment with AgNPs results in anti-adhesive and anti-biofilm properties of the titanium implants against microbial strains.

The results of biological studies indicate that Ti6Al4V implants with TNT5 or TNT5/AgNPs surface modifications exhibit most suitable properties (biocompatibility, immunological activity, lack of genotoxicity, and antimicrobial activity) for their use in the construction of implants, e.g. for the orthopedy. Therefore, these systems were chosen for surface roughness parameters (Sa) and mechanical properties determination. Sa parameter of the coatings used for implants is important in the case of human cells and tissue adhesion, cells proliferation and time of healing [76]. The high level of roughness ensures better tissue adhesion and primary stability between the implant and bone. It has also been proven that surfaces with higher roughness have a positive effect on the time of healing after implantation [77,78]. On the other hand, the increased roughness results in an increased surface area, which can encourage bacterial adhesion (such as *S. aureus*) and increase peri-implantitis occurrence [79]. Therefore, when designing the new generation of implants it is important to enrich their surface with the antibacterial protection, which in our case consisted from AgNPs. The deposition of silver nanoparticles on the surface of TNT5 layers led to smoothing of the surface and roughness reduction. A similar effect was noticed by Bahadur et al. for TiO_2 layers doped by Ag nanoparticles [80]. In order to determine the biomechanical compatibility of biomaterials used in the construction of implants, especially long-term ones, it is important to determine Young's Modulus [26,42,82,83]. The results of earlier works revealed the influence of this factor on the surrounding living tissue, such as bone [84–87]. The significant difference in Young's Modulus between implants and human bone (especially cortical human bone ~ 20 GPa) can induce bone loosening and reduced bone quality in the implant surrounding and in consequence loosening of the implant in the bone [88,89]. Considering obtained results, the lower value of Young's Modulus of the implant/TNT5 coating system, the more biocompatible it is. On the other hand higher nanohardness value obtained for Implant TNT5/AgNPs was similar for results reported for TiO_2 [82,90]. Analysis of the distribution of nanomechanical property (nanohardness and Young's Modulus) confirmed the uneven distribution of the tested properties on the surface of the implants (Figure 11). The same effect was reported by Rayón et al. [42]. Obtaining a homogeneous distribution of nanomechanical properties was impossible due to the roughness of the samples and the geometry and structure of the nanotube. The results obtained confirm that the increase in the nanohardness value causes an increase in the Young's modulus. Increase of the nanomechanical properties values (H and E) increased H/E ratio, which describes the resistance to wear. The relationship between wear resistance and value of H/E ratio was reported [35]. Moreover, an increase in fracture toughness is attributed to higher values of Young's Modulus (E) and nanohardness (H) [91]. The obtained H/E ratio value correlated with nanoscratch-test results. The nanoscratch-test technique was used to study the adhesion properties of thin coatings or layers [42,82,92]. The forces used during implantation procedure may provoke the coating full delamination; therefore the coatings should have proper adhesion to the metallic substrate. Higher adhesion was obtained for the TNT5/AgNPs, which is attributed to the stronger metallic bonds, which occur. An important aspect in the context of implant modification is the determination of their compression resistance, but unfortunately conventional tests do not include nano-scale modification tests. The following parameters can indirectly indicate the strength of the coating: H/E, H^3/E^2. Both parameters can be determined indirectly from the results obtained during nanoindentation measurements. The first parameter allows determining the wear resistance, while the second parameter allows determining the material's ability to propagate energy at plastic deformation during loading [93]. For the studied modifications, the value of the H/E parameter was 0.0054 ± 0.0039 and 0.0190 ± 0.0133, respectively for TNT5 and TNT5/AgNPs and H^3/E^2 ~ 4.71 Pa and 4768.97 Pa for TNT5 and TNT5/AgNPs, respectively. These results indicate and confirm that the presence of silver nanoparticles on the surface of TiO$_2$ nanotubes significantly affects both the wear resistance as well as the material's ability to propagate energy at plastic deformation during loading which suggests better tribological and strength properties of the tested surface.

5. Conclusions

According to the results presented here, the most suitable physicochemical, mechanical, and biological properties were presented by Ti6Al4V implants fabricated by selective laser sintering technology, the surface of which was modified by anodization at the 5 V potential, resulting in TNT5 nanoporous coating production. The use of Ti6Al4V/TNT5 and Ti6Al4V/TNT5/AgNPs systems seem to be a promising approach to manufacture implants with anti-inflammatory properties. Both TNT5 and TNT5/AgNPs did not release substances demonstrating mutagenic properties, which is important for the practical use of these materials in implantology. TNT5/AgNPs surfaces also demonstrated the strongest bactericidal and fungicidal activity, most probably thanks to the release of active Ag ions during long-lasting contact with the fluids. It is highly beneficial for implant recipients (i.e. patients) to maintain sterile conditions in the surrounding physiological fluids or tissues after implantation. Finally, mechanical studies proved that both a suitable wear resistance and the ability to propagate energy at plastic deformation during loading characterize this system.

Supplementary Materials: The following are available online at http://www.mdpi.com/2077-0383/9/2/342/s1, Figure S1: X-ray diffraction patterns for both sizes of studied Ti6Al4V implants produced using SLS technique, Figure S2: High resolution XPS spectra of TNT5 and TNT15 samples non sputtered and after third sputter.

Author Contributions: Conceptualization, P.P. and A.R.; methodology, P.P., A.R., W.J.; formal analysis, P.P., A.R., T.J., M.B., B.S., A.S., Y.K.E.; investigation, P.P., A.R., M.E., T.J., M.B., B.S., B.E., and A.S.; data curation, P.P.; writing—original draft preparation, P.P., A.R., T.J., M.B., B.S., M.W., and A.S.; writing—review and editing, P.P. and A.R.; supervision, P.P.; project administration, P.P. and A.R.; funding acquisition, A.R. and P.P. All authors have read and agreed to the published version of the manuscript.

Funding: This research was funded by the Regional Operational Program of the Kuyavian-Pomeranian Voivodeship (1.3.1. Support for research and development processes in academic enterprises), within the grant obtained by Nano-implant Ltd. The APC was funded by Nano-implant Ltd.

Acknowledgments: The authors would like to acknowledge networking support by the COST Action CA16122. The authors would like to thank M.Sc. Marlena Grodzicka for help in carrying out works on the production of TNT/AgNPs systems, Marzena Więckowska-Szakiel for help in carrying out microbiological studies and Jakub Piotrowski for help in carrying out immunological tests.

Conflicts of Interest: The authors declare no conflict of interest.

References

1. Buser, D.; Sennerby, L.; De Bruyn, H. Modern implant dentistry based on osseointegration: 50 years of progress, current trends and open questions. *Periodontology 2000* **2017**, *73*, 7–21. [CrossRef]
2. Scholz, M.-S.; Blanchfield, J.P.; Bloom, L.D.; Coburn, B.H.; Elkington, M.; Fuller, J.D.; Gilbert, M.E.; Muflahi, S.A.; Pernice, M.F.; Rae, S.I.; et al. The use of composite materials in modern orthopaedic medicine and prosthetic devices: A review. *Compos. Sci. Technol.* **2011**, *71*, 1791–1803. [CrossRef]
3. Cronskär, M.; Lars-Erik Rännar, L.-E.; Bäckström, M. Implementation of Digital Design and Solid Free-Form Fabrication for Customization of Implants in Trauma Orthopaedics. *J. Med. Biol. Eng.* **2010**, *32*, 91–96. [CrossRef]
4. Lim, K.M.; Park, J.W.; Park, S.J.; Kang, H.K. 3D-Printed Personalized Titanium Implant Design,Manufacturing and Verification for Bone Tumor Surgery of Forearm. *Biomed. J. Sci. Tech.* **2018**, *10*. [CrossRef]
5. Manić, M.; Stamenković, Z.; Mitković, M.; Stojković, M.; Shepherd, D.E.T. Design of 3D Model of Customized Anatomically Adjusted Implants. *Facta Univ. Ser. Mech. Eng.* **2015**, *13*, 269–282.
6. Pilliar, R.M. Metallic Biomaterials. In *Biomedical Materials*; Narayan, R.C., Ed.; Springer Science+Business Media, LLC: Berlin/Heidelberg, Germany, 2009; Volume 2, pp. 41–81. [CrossRef]
7. Wang, D.; Wang, Y.; Wu, S.; Lin, H.; Yang, Y.; Fan, S.; Gu, C.; Wang, J.; Song, C. Customized a Ti6Al4V Bone Plate for Complex Pelvic Fracture by Selective Laser Melting. *Materials* **2017**, *10*, 35. [CrossRef]

8. Moiduddin, K.; Mian, S.H.; Umer, U.; Alkhalefah, H. Fabrication and Analysis of a Ti6Al4V Implant for Cranial Restoration. *Appl. Sci.* **2019**, *9*, 2513. [CrossRef]
9. Xue, W.; Krishna, B.V.; Bandyopadhyay, A.; Bose, S. Processing and biocompatibility evaluation of laser proceeded porous titanium. *Acta Biomater.* **2007**, *3*, 1007–1018. [CrossRef]
10. Sarker, A.; Tran, N.; Rifai, A.; Brandt, M.; Tran, P.A.; Leary, M.; Fox, K.; Williams, R. Rational design of additively manufactured Ti6Al4V implants to control *Staphylococcus aureus* biofilm formation. *Materialia* **2019**, *5*, 100250. [CrossRef]
11. Chu, T.G.; Khouja, N.; Chahine, G.; Kovacevic, R.; Koike, M.; Okabe, T. *In vivo* Evaluation of a Novel Custom-Made press-Fit Dental Implant Through Electron Beam Melting® (EBM®). *Int. J. Dent. Oral Sci.* **2016**, *3*, 358–365.
12. Minagar, S.; Wang, J.; Bernt, C.C.; Ivanova, E.P.; Wen, C. Cell response of anodized nanotubes on titanium and titanium alloys. *J. Biomed. Mater. Res. A* **2013**, *101A*, 2726–2739. [CrossRef]
13. Radtke, A. Photocatalytic Activity of Titania Nanotube Coatings Enriched With Nanohydroxyapatite. *Biomed. J. Sci. Tech. Res.* **2019**, *15*. [CrossRef]
14. Li, X.; Gao, P.; Wan, P.; Pei, Y.; Shi, L.; Fan, B.; Shen, C.; Xiao, X.; Yang, K.; Guo, Z. Novel Bio-functional Magnesium Coating on Porous Ti6Al4V Orthopaedic Implants: *In vitro* and *In vivo* Study. *Sci. Rep.* **2017**, *7*, 40755. [CrossRef] [PubMed]
15. Godoy-Gallardo, M.; Rodríguez-Hernández, A.G.; Delgado, L.M.; Manero, J.M.; Gil, F.J.; Rodríguez, D. Silver deposition on titanium surface by electrochemical anodizing process reduces bacterial adhesion of *Streptococcus sanguinis* and *Lactabacillus salivarius*. *Clin. Oral Impl. Res.* **2015**, *26*, 1170–1179. [CrossRef] [PubMed]
16. Piszczek, P.; Radtke, A. Silver Nanoparticles Fabricated Using Chemical Vapor Deposition and Atomic Layer Deposition Techniques: Properties, Applications and Perspectives: Review. In *Noble and Precious Metals*; Seehra, M.S., Bristow, A.D., Eds.; IntechOpen: London, UK, 2018; pp. 187–213.
17. Kasemo, B.; Lausmaa, J. Biomaterial and implant surfaces: A surface science approach. *Int. J. Oral Maxillofac. Implant.* **1988**, *3*, 247–259.
18. Takebe, J.; Itoh, S.; Okada, J.; Ishibashi, K. Anodic oxidation and hydrothermal treatment of titanium results in a surface that causes increased attachment and altered cytoskeletal morphology of rat bone marrow stromal cells in vitro. *J. Biomed. Mater. Res.* **2000**, *51*, 398–407. [CrossRef]
19. Dzhurinskiy, D. Bioactive antimicrobial coatings for implantable medical devices formed by plasma electrolytic oxidation. *Met. Form.* **2018**, *29*, 65–76.
20. Radtke, A.; Topolski, A.; Jedrzejewski, T.; Kozak, W.; Sadowska, B.; Wieckowska-Szakiel, M.; Piszczek, P. Bioactivity Studies on Titania Coatings and the Estimation of Their Usefulness in the Modification of Implant Surfaces. *Nanomaterials* **2017**, *4*, 90. [CrossRef]
21. Radtke, A.; Bal, M.; Jędrzejewski, T. Novel titania nanocoatings produced by the anodic anodization with the use of the cyclically changing potential; their photocatalytic activity and biocompability. *Nanomaterials* **2018**, *8*, 712. [CrossRef]
22. Gong, D.; Grimes, C.A.; Varghese, O.K.; Hu, W.; Singh, R.S.; Chen, Z.; Dickey, E.C. Titanium oxide nanotube arrays prepared by anodic oxidation. *J. Mater. Res.* **2001**, *16*, 3331–3334. [CrossRef]
23. Macak, J.M.; Tsuchiya, H.; Ghicov, A.; Yasuda, K.; Hahn, R.; Bauer, S.; Schmuki, P. TiO_2 nanotubes: Self-organized electrochemical formation, properties and applications. *Curr. Opin. Solid State Mater. Sci.* **2007**, *11*, 3–18. [CrossRef]
24. Lewandowska, Ż.; Piszczek, P.; Radtke, A.; Jędrzejewski, T.; Kozak, W.; Sadowska, B. The Evaluation of the Impact of Titania Nanotube Covers Morphology and Crystal Phase on Their Biological Properties. *J. Mater. Sci. Mater. Med.* **2015**, *26*, 163. [CrossRef] [PubMed]
25. Radtke, A.; Topolski, A.; Jędrzejewski, T.; Sadowska, B.; Więckowska-Szakiel, M.; Szubka, M.; Talik, E.; Nielsen, L.P.; Piszczek, P. Studies on the bioactivity and photocatalytic properties of titania nanotube coatings produced with the use of the low potential anodization of Ti6Al4V alloy surface. *Nanomaterials* **2017**, *7*, 197. [CrossRef]
26. Radtke, A.; Ehlert, M.; Bartmański, M.; Jędrzejewski, T. The morphology, structure, mechanical properties and biocompatibility of nanotubular titania coatings before and after autoclaving process. *J. Clin. Med.* **2019**, *8*, 272. [CrossRef]

27. Radtke, A.; Jędrzejewski, T.; Kozak, W.; Sadowska, B.; Więckowska-Szakiel, M.; Talik, E.; Mäkelä, M.; Leskelä, M.; Piszczek, P. Optimization of the silver clusters PEALD process on the surface of 1-D titania coatings. *Nanomaterials* **2017**, *7*, 193. [CrossRef] [PubMed]
28. Piszczek, P.; Lewandowska, Ż.; Radtke, A.; Jędrzejewski, T.; Kozak, W.; Sadowska, B.; Szubka, M.; Talik, E.; Fiori, F. Biocompatibility of Titania Nanotube Coatings Enriched with Silver Nanograins by Chemical Vapor Depositiom. *Nanomaterials* **2017**, *7*, 274. [CrossRef] [PubMed]
29. Radtke, A.; Grodzicka, M.; Ehlert, M.; Muzioł, T.; Szkodo, M.; Bartmański, M.; Piszczek, P. Studies on silver ions releasing processes and mechanical properties of surface-modified titanium alloy implants, International Journal of Molecular Science. *Int. J. Mol. Sci.* **2018**, *19*, 3962. [CrossRef]
30. Radtke, A.; Grodzicka, M.; Ehlert, M.; Jędrzejewski, T.; Wypij, M.; Golińska, P. "To Be Microbiocidal and Not to be Cytotoxic at the Same Time."-Silver Nanoparticles in Their Main Role on the Surface of the Titania Alloy Implant. *J. Clin. Med.* **2019**, *8*, 334. [CrossRef]
31. Radtke, A. 1D Titania Nanoarchitecture as Bioactive and Photoactive Coatingas for Modern Implants: A Review. In *Application of Titanium Dioxide*; Janus, M., Ed.; InTech: Croatia, 2017; pp. 73–102.
32. Sonntag, R.; Reinders, J.; Gibmeier, J.; Kretzer, J.P. Fatigue Performance of Medical Ti6Al4V Alloy after Mechanical Surface Treatments. *PLoS ONE* **2015**, *10*, e0121963. [CrossRef]
33. Yuan, Y.; Lee, T.R. Chapter 1 Contact Angle and Wetting Properties. In *Surface Science Techniques, Springer Series in Surface Sciences*; Bracco, G., Holst, B., Eds.; Springer: Berlin/Heidelberg, Germany, 2013; pp. 3–34. [CrossRef]
34. Flückiger-Isler, S.; Kamber, M. Direct comparison of the Ames microplate format (MPF) test in liquid medium with the standard Ames pre-incubation assay on agar plates by use of equivocal to weakly positive test compounds. *Mutat. Res. Toxicol. Environ. Mutagen* **2012**, *747*, 36–45. [CrossRef]
35. Leyland, A.; Matthews, A. Design criteria for wear-resistant nanostructured and glassy-metal coatings. *Surf. Coat. Technol.* **2004**, *177–178*, 317–324. [CrossRef]
36. Oliver, W.C.; Pharr, G.M. An improved technique for determining hardness and elastic modulus using load and displacement sensing indentation experiments. *J. Mater. Res.* **1992**, *7*, 1564–1583. [CrossRef]
37. Atuchin, V.V.; Kesler, V.G.; Pervukhina, N.V.; Zhang, Z. Ti 2p and O 1s core levels and chemical bonding in titanium-bearing oxides. *J. Electron Spectrosc. Relat. Phenom.* **2006**, *152*, 18–24. [CrossRef]
38. Chinh, V.D.; Broggi, A.; Di Palma, L.; Scarsella, M.; Sperenza, G.; Vilardi, G.; Thang, P.N. XPS Spectra Analysis of Ti^{2+}, Ti^{3+} Ions and Dye Photodegradation Evaluation of Titania-Silica Mixed Oxide Nanoparticles. *J. Phys. D Appl. Phys.* **2017**, *10*. [CrossRef]
39. Wen, H.; Dan, M.; Yang, Y.; Lyu, J.; Shao, A.; Cheng, X.; Chen, L.; Xu, L. Acute toxicity and genotoxicity of silver nanoparticle in rats. *PLoS ONE* **2017**, *12*, e0185554. [CrossRef] [PubMed]
40. Li, Y.; Qin, T.; Ingle, T.; Yan, J.; He, W.; Yin, J.J.; Chen, T. Differential genotoxicity mechanisms of silver nanoparticles and silver ions. *Arch Toxicol.* **2017**, *91*, 509–519. [CrossRef] [PubMed]
41. Jemat, A.; Ghazali, M.J.; Razali, M.; Otsuka, Y.; Rajabi, A. Effects of TiO_2 on microstructural, mechanical properties and in-vitro bioactivity of plasma sprayed yttria stabilised zirconia coatings for dental application. *Ceram. Int.* **2017**, *44*, 4271–4281. [CrossRef]
42. Rayón, E.; Bonache, V.; Salvador, M.D.; Bannier, E.; Sánchez, E.; Denoirjean, A.; Ageorges, H. Nanoindentation study of the mechanical and damage behaviour of suspension plasma sprayed TiO_2 coatings. *Surf. Coat. Technol.* **2012**, *206*, 2655–2660. [CrossRef]
43. Wysocki, B.; Maj, P.; Sitek, R.; Buhagiar, J.; Kurzydłowski, K.J.; Święszkowski, W. Laser and Electron Beam Additive Manufacturing Methods of Fabricating Titanium Bone Implants. *Appl. Sci.* **2017**, *7*, 657. [CrossRef]
44. Hiromoto, S.; Hanawa, T.; Asami, K. Composition of surface oxide film of titanium with culturing Marine fibroblast L929. *Biomaterials* **2004**, *25*, 979–986. [CrossRef]
45. Brammer, K.S.; Oh, S.; Cobb, C.J.; Bjursten, L.M.; van der Heyde, H.; Jin, S. Improved bone-forming functionality on diameter-controlled TiO_2 nanotube surface. *Acta Biomater.* **2009**, *5*, 3215–3223. [CrossRef] [PubMed]
46. Park, J.; Bauer, S.; von der Mark, K.; Schmuki, P. Nanosize and vitality: TiO_2 nanotube diameter directs cell fate. *Nano Lett.* **2007**, *7*, 1686–1691. [CrossRef] [PubMed]
47. Park, J.; Bauer, S.; Schlegel, K.A.; Neukam, F.W.; von der Mark, K.; Schmuki, P. TiO_2 nanotube surfaces: 15 nm–an optimal length scale of surface topography for cell adhesion and differentiation. *Small* **2009**, *5*, 666–671. [CrossRef]

48. Albers, C.E.; Hofstetter, W.; Siebenrock, K.A.; Landmann, R.; Klenke, F.M. In vitro cytotoxicity of silver nanoparticles on osteoblasts and osteoclasts at antibacterial concentrations. *Nanotoxicology* **2013**, *7*, 30–36. [CrossRef] [PubMed]
49. Castiglioni, S.; Cazzaniga, A.; Locatelli, L.; Maier, J.A.M. Silver Nanoparticles in Orthopedic Applications: New Insights on Their Effects on Osteogenic Cells. *Nanomaterials (Basel)* **2017**, *7*, 124. [CrossRef] [PubMed]
50. Shivaram, A.; Bose, S.; Bandyopadhyay, A. Mechanical degradation of TiO_2 nanotubes with and without nanoparticulate silver coating. *J. Mech. Behav. Biomed. Mater.* **2016**, *59*, 508–518. [CrossRef] [PubMed]
51. Zhao, L.; Wang, H.; Huo, K.; Cui, L.; Zhang, W.; Ni, H.; Zhang, Y.; Wu, Z.; Chu, P.K. Antibacterial nano-structured titania coating incorporated with silver nanoparticles. *Biomaterials* **2011**, *32*, 5706–5716. [CrossRef]
52. Esfandiari, N.; Simchi, A.; Bagheri, R. Size tuning of Ag-decorated TiO_2 nanotube arrays for improved bactericidal capacity of orthopedic implants. *J. Biomed. Mater. Res. A.* **2014**, *102*, 2625–2635. [CrossRef]
53. Fenton, M.J.; Golenbock, D.T. LPS-binding proteins and receptors. *J. Leuk. Biol.* **1998**, *64*, 25–32. [CrossRef]
54. Netea, M.G.; Kullberg, B.J.; van der Meer, J.W. Circulating cytokines as mediators of fever. *Clin. Infect. Dis.* **2000**, *31*, S178–S184:. [CrossRef]
55. Neacsu, P.; Mazare, A.; Cimpean, A.; Park, J.; Costache, M.; Schmuki, P.; Demetrescu, I. Reduced inflammatory activity of RAW 264.7 macrophages on titania nanotube modified Ti surface. *Int. J. Biochem. Cell. Biol.* **2014**, *55*, 187–195. [CrossRef] [PubMed]
56. Furuhashi, A.; Ayukawa, Y.; Atsuta, I.; Okawachi, H.; Koyano, K. The difference of fibroblast behavior on titanium substrata with different surface characteristics. *Odontology* **2012**, *100*, 199–205. [CrossRef] [PubMed]
57. Tan, K.S.; Qian, L.; Rosado, R.; Flood, P.M.; Cooper, L.F. The role of titanium surface topography on J774A.1 macrophage inflammatory cytokines and nitric oxide production. *Biomaterials* **2006**, *27*, 5170–5177. [CrossRef] [PubMed]
58. Dinarello, C.A. Proinflammatory cytokines. *Chest* **2000**, *118*, 503–508. [CrossRef]
59. Radi, R. Nitric oxide, oxidants, and protein tyrosine nitration. *Proc. Natl. Acad. Sci. USA* **2004**, *101*, 4003–4008. [CrossRef]
60. Mosser, D.M.; Zhang, X. Interleukin-10: new perspectives on an old cytokine. *Immunol. Rev.* **2008**, *226*, 205–218. [CrossRef]
61. Ullah Khan, S.; Saleh, T.A.; Wahab, A.; Khan, M.H.U.; Khan, D.; Ullah Khan, W.; Rahim, A.; Kamal, S.; Fahad, S. Nanosilver: new ageless and versatile biomedical therapeutic scaffold. *Int. J. Nanomedicine.* **2018**, *13*, 733–762. [CrossRef]
62. Goodman, S.B.; Ma, T. Cellular chemotaxis induced by wear particles from joint replacements. *Biomaterials* **2010**, *31*, 5045–5050. [CrossRef]
63. Swift, L.H.; Golsteyn, R.M. Genotoxic anti-cancer agents and their relationship to DNA damage, mitosis, and checkpoint adaptation in proliferating cancer cells. *Int. J. Mol. Sci.* **2014**, *15*, 3403–3431. [CrossRef]
64. Velasco-Ortega, E.; Jos, A.; Cameán, A.M.; Pato-Mourelo, J.; Segura-Egea, J.J. In vitro evaluation of cytotoxicity and genotoxicity of a commercial titanium alloy for dental implantology. *Mutation Res. Genetic Toxicol. Environ. Mutag.* **2010**, *702*, 17–22. [CrossRef]
65. Ghosh, M.J.M.; Sinha, S.; Chakraborty, A.; Mallick, S.K.; Bandyopadhyay, M.; Mukherjee, A. In vitro and in vivo genotoxicity of silver nanoparticles. *Mut. Res./Genet. Toxicol. Environ. Mutagen.* **2012**, *749*, 60–69. [CrossRef]
66. Li, Y.; Bhalli, J.A.; Ding, W.; Yan, J.; Pearce, M.G.; Sadiq, R.; Cunningham, C.K.; Jones, M.Y.; Monroe, W.A.; Howard, P.C.; et al. Cytotoxicity and genotoxicity assessment of silver nanoparticles in mouse. *Nanotoxicology* **2014**, *8*, 36–45. [CrossRef]
67. Lebedová, J.; Hedberg, Y.S.; Odnevall Wallinder, I.; Karlsson, H.L. Size-dependent genotoxicity of silver, gold and platinum nanoparticles studied using the mini-gel comet assay and micronucleus scoring with flow cytometry. *Mutagenesis* **2018**, *33*, 77–85. [CrossRef] [PubMed]
68. Burmølle, M.; Thomsen, T.R.; Fazli, M.; Dige, I.; Christensen, L.; Homøe, P.; Tvede, M.; Nyvad, B.; Tolker-Nielsen, T.; Givskov, M.; et al. Biofilms in chronic infections - a matter of opportunity - monospecies biofilms in multispecies infections. *FEMS Immunol. Med. Microbiol.* **2010**, *59*, 324–336. [CrossRef]
69. Høiby, N.; Bjarnsholt, T.; Givskov, M.; Molin, S.; Ciofu, O. Antibiotic resistance of bacterial biofilms. *Intern. J. Antim. Agents* **2010**, *35*, 322–332. [CrossRef]

70. Leid, J.G.; Cope, E. Population level virulence in polymicrobial communities associated with chronic disease. *Front. Biol.* **2011**, *6*, 435–445. [CrossRef]
71. Mottola, C.; Matias, C.S.; Mendes, J.J.; Melo-Cristino, J.; Tavares, L.; Cavaco-Silva, P.; Oliveira, M. Susceptibility patterns of *Staphylococcus aureus* biofilms in diabetic foot infections. *BMC Microbiol.* **2016**, *16*, 1–9. [CrossRef]
72. Jin, J.; Zhang, L.; Shi, M.; Zhang, Y.; Wang, Q. Ti-GO-Ag nanocomposite: the effect of content level on the antimicrobial activity and cytotoxicity. *Int. J. Nanomed.* **2017**, *12*, 4209–4224. [CrossRef]
73. Lan, M.-Y.; Liu, C.-P.; Huang, H.-H.; Lee, S.-W. Both enhanced biocompatibility and antibacterial activity in Ag-decorated TiO2 nanotubes. *PLoS ONE* **2013**, *8*, 1–8. [CrossRef]
74. Liu, R.; Memarzadeh, K.; Chang, B.; Zhang, Y.; Ma, Z.; Allaker, R.P.; Ren, L.; Yang, K. Antibacterial effect of copper-bearing titanium alloy (Ti-Cu) against. *Strept. Mutans Porphyrom. Gingival. Scientific Rep.* **2016**, *6*, 29985. [CrossRef]
75. Besinis, A.; Hadi, S.D.; Le, H.R.; Tredwin, C.; Handy, R.D. Antibacterial activity and biofilm inhibition by surface modified titanium alloy medical implants following application of silver, titanium dioxide and hydroxyapatite nanocoatings. *Nanotoxicology* **2017**, *11*, 327–338. [CrossRef] [PubMed]
76. Dudek, K.; Dulski, M.; Goryczka, T.; Gerle, A. Structural changes of hydroxyapatite coating electrophoretically deposited on NiTi shape memory alloy. *Ceram. Int.* **2018**, *44*, 11292–11300. [CrossRef]
77. He, J.; Zhou, W.; Zhou, X.; Zhong, X.; Zhang, X.; Wan, P.; Zhu, B.; Chen, W. The anatase phase of nanotopography titania plays an important role on osteoblast cell morphology and proliferation. *J. Mater. Sci. Mater. Med.* **2008**, *19*, 3465–3472. [CrossRef] [PubMed]
78. Ferreira Soares, P.B.; Moura, C.C.G.; Claudino, M.; Carvalho, V.F.; Rocha, F.S.; Zanetta-Barbosa, D. Influence of implant surfaces on osseointegration: A histomorphometric and implant stability study in rabbits. *Braz. Dent. J.* **2015**, *26*, 451–457. [CrossRef] [PubMed]
79. Wang, X.; Wang, G.; Liang, J.; Cheng, J.; Ma, W.; Zhao, Y. Staphylococcus aureus adhesion to different implant surface coatings: An in vitro study. *Surf. Coatings Technol.* **2009**, *203*, 3454–3458. [CrossRef]
80. Bahadur, J.; Agrawal, S.; Panwar, V.; Parveen, A.; Pal, K. Antibacterial properties of silver doped TiO_2 nanoparticles synthesized via sol-gel technique. *Macromol. Res.* **2016**, *24*, 488–493. [CrossRef]
81. Godoy-Gallardo, M.; Manzanares-Céspedes, M.C.; Sevilla, P.; Nart, J.; Manzanares, N.; Manero, J.M.; Gil, F.J.; Boyd, S.K.; Rodríguez, D. Evaluation of bone loss in antibacterial coated dental implants: An experimental study in dogs. *Mater. Sci. Eng. C Mater. Biol. Appl.* **2016**, *1*, 538–545. [CrossRef]
82. Wang, W.K.; Wen, H.C.; Cheng, C.H.; Hung, C.H.; Chou, W.C.; Yau, W.H.; Yang, P.F.; Lai, Y.S. Nanotribological properties of ALD-processed bilayer TiO_2/ZnO films. *Microelectron. Reliab.* **2014**, *54*, 2754–2759. [CrossRef]
83. Bartmanski, M.; Zielinski, A.; Majkowska-Marzec, B.; Strugala, G. Effects of solution composition and electrophoretic deposition voltage on various properties of nanohydroxyapatite coatings on the Ti13Zr13Nb alloy. *Ceram. Int.* **2018**, 19236–19246. [CrossRef]
84. Sumner, D.R.; Galante, J.O. Determinants of stress shielding: Design versus materials versus interface. *Clin. Orthop. Relat. Res.* **1992**, *274*, 202–212. [CrossRef]
85. Ridzwan, M.I.Z.; Shuib, S.; Hassan, A.Y.; Shokri, A.A.; Mohammad Ibrahim, M.N. Problem of stress shielding and improvement to the hip implant designs: A review. *J. Med. Sci.* **2007**, *7*, 460–467. [CrossRef]
86. Huiskes, R.; Weinans, H.; Van Rietbergen, B. The relationship between stress shielding and bone resorption around total hip stems and the effects of flexible materials. *Clin. Orthop. Relat. Res.* **1992**, 124–134. [CrossRef]
87. Asgharzadeh Shirazi, H.; Ayatollahi, M.R.; Asnafi, A. To reduce the maximum stress and the stress shielding effect around a dental implant–bone interface using radial functionally graded biomaterials. *Comput. Methods Biomech. Biomed. Engin.* **2017**, *20*, 750–759. [CrossRef] [PubMed]
88. Noyama, Y.; Miura, T.; Ishimoto, T.; Itaya, T.; Niinomi, M.; Nakano, T. Bone loss and reduced bone quality of the human femur after total hip arthroplasty under stress-shielding effects by titanium-based implant. *Mater. Trans.* **2012**, *53*, 565–570. [CrossRef]
89. Drevet, R.; Ben Jaber, N.; Fauré, J.; Tara, A.; Ben Cheikh Larbi, A.; Benhayoune, H. Electrophoretic deposition (EPD) of nano-hydroxyapatite coatings with improved mechanical properties on prosthetic Ti6Al4V substrates. *Surf. Coatings Technol.* **2015**, *301*, 94–99. [CrossRef]
90. Charles, A.H. *Handbook of Ceramics, Glasses, and Diamonds*, Charles, A.H., Ed.; The McGraw-Hill Companies Inc.: New York, NY, USA, 2001. [CrossRef]

91. Manoj Kumar, R.; Kuntal, K.K.; Singh, S.; Gupta, P.; Bhushan, B.; Gopinath, P.; Lahiri, D. Electrophoretic deposition of hydroxyapatite coating on Mg-3Zn alloy for orthopaedic application. *Surf. Coatings Technol.* **2016**, *287*, 82–92. [CrossRef]
92. Bartmański, M.; Cieślik, B.; Głodowska, J.; Kalka, P. Electrophoretic deposition (EPD) of nanohydroxyapatite - nanosilver coatings on Ti13Zr13Nb alloy. *Ceram. Int.* **2017**, *43*, 11820–11829. [CrossRef]
93. Chernozem, R.V.; Surmeneva, M.A.; Krause, B.; Baumbach, T.; Ignatov, V.P.; Tyurin, A.I.; Loza, K.; Epple, M.; Surmenev, R.A. Hybrid biocomposites based on titania nanotubes and a hydroxyapatite coating deposited by RF-magnetron sputtering: Surface topography, structure, and mechanical properties. *Appl. Surf. Sci.* **2017**, *426*, 229–237. [CrossRef]

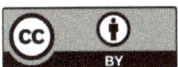

© 2020 by the authors. Licensee MDPI, Basel, Switzerland. This article is an open access article distributed under the terms and conditions of the Creative Commons Attribution (CC BY) license (http://creativecommons.org/licenses/by/4.0/).

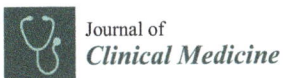

Article

Parameters Affecting the Antimicrobial Properties of Cold Atmospheric Plasma Jet

Bih-Show Lou [1,2], Chih-Ho Lai [3,4,5,6], Teng-Ping Chu [7], Jang-Hsing Hsieh [7,8], Chun-Ming Chen [7], Yu-Ming Su [7], Chun-Wei Hou [1], Pang-Yun Chou [9] and Jyh-Wei Lee [7,8,9,10,*]

- [1] Chemistry Division, Center for General Education, Chang Gung University, Taoyuan 33302, Taiwan; blou@mail.cgu.edu.tw (B.-S.L.); romeomonkey@msn.com (C.-W.H.)
- [2] Department of Nuclear Medicine and Molecular Imaging Center, Chang Gung Memorial Hospital, Taoyuan 33305, Taiwan
- [3] Department of Microbiology & Immunology, Chang Gung University, Taoyuan 33302, Taiwan; chlai@mail.cgu.edu.tw
- [4] Molecular Infectious Disease Research Center, Chang Gung Memorial Hospital, Taoyuan 33305, Taiwan
- [5] School of Medicine, China Medical University and Hospital, Taichung 40402, Taiwan
- [6] Department of Urology, University of Texas Southwestern Medical Center, Dallas, TX 75390, USA
- [7] Center for Plasma and Thin Film Technologies, Ming Chi University of Technology, New Taipei 24301, Taiwan; bmw7458@gmail.com (T.-P.C.); jhhsieh@mail.mcut.edu.tw (J.-H.H.); cmchen@mail.mcut.edu.tw (C.-M.C.); ymsu73@gmail.com (Y.-M.S.)
- [8] Department of Materials Engineering, Ming Chi University of Technology, New Taipei 24301, Taiwan
- [9] Plastic and Reconstructive Surgery, and Craniofacial Research Center, Chang Gung Memorial Hospital, Taoyuan 33305, Taiwan; chou.asapulu@gmail.com
- [10] Department of Mechanical Engineering, Chang Gung University, Taoyuan 33302, Taiwan
- * Correspondence: jefflee@mail.mcut.edu.tw

Received: 19 October 2019; Accepted: 7 November 2019; Published: 9 November 2019

Abstract: Using the Taguchi method to narrow experimental parameters, the antimicrobial efficiency of a cold atmospheric plasma jet (CAPJ) treatment was investigated. An L9 array with four parameters of CAPJ treatments, including the application voltage, CAPJ-sample distance, argon (Ar) gas flow rate, and CAPJ treatment time, were applied to examine the antimicrobial activity against *Escherichia coli* (*E. coli*). CAPJ treatment time was found to be the most influential parameter in its antimicrobial ability by evaluation of signal to noise ratios and analysis of variance. 100% bactericidal activity was achieved under the optimal bactericidal activity parameters including the application voltage of 8.5 kV, CAPJ-sample distance of 10 mm, Ar gas flow rate of 500 sccm, and CAPJ treatment time of 300 s, which confirms the efficacy of the Taguchi method in this design. In terms of the mechanism of CAPJ's antimicrobial ability, the intensity of hydroxyl radical produced by CAPJ positively correlated to its antimicrobial efficiency. The CAPJ antimicrobial efficiency was further evaluated by both DNA double-strand breaks analysis and scanning electron microscopy examination of CAPJ treated bacteria. CAPJ destroyed the cell wall of *E. coli* and further damaged its DNA structure, thus leading to successful killing of bacteria. This study suggests that optimal conditions of CPAJ can provide effective antimicrobial activity and may be grounds for a novel approach for eradicating bacterial infections.

Keywords: Taguchi method; antimicrobial efficiency; cold atmospheric-pressure plasma jet (CAPJ); *Escherichia coli*; DNA double-strand breaks; scanning electron microscopy

1. Introduction

Cold, or non-thermal, atmospheric-pressure plasma jets (CAPJ) have gained attention in biomedical applications [1–6] due to unique characteristics, comprising of a complex plasma chemistry without the need for elevated gas temperatures as required for traditional thermal plasma [7,8]. In addition, the high energy electrons of CAPJ can produce reactive oxygen species (ROS) with slightly higher temperature than ambient environment in an open air. The ROS produced by CAPJ plays a significant role in promising inactivation of bacteria [9,10], which can be used in developing antimicrobial treatments for infectious diseases or in sterilization of reusable thermal sensitive medical devices to prevent the outbreak of antibiotic-resistant bacteria [11]. Although these properties have led to extensive use of CAPJ in material processing and biomedical applications, consistent use of CAPJ without risks remains difficult. As the performance of CAPJ is dependent on the operational parameters, understanding how each parameter impacts the plasma's properties is necessary and can allow for adjustment of the plasma for use in different applications.

E. coli is often used as an indicator of hygiene and safety in food products [12], and it is commonly found in community and hospital-acquired infections. E. coli is one of the most common and deadly pathogens causing pediatric urinary tract infection, intra-abdominal infection, or acute lung injury [13–16] and can lead to life-threatening intestinal infections in immunocompromised patients [17]. In addition, empiric antibiotic therapy may be ineffective with multidrug-resistant E. coli which will delay care and may cause further harm to the patient [18,19]. Therefore, we selected E. coli to investigate the antimicrobial efficiency of CAPJ treatment. The aim of this work is to develop the interventions by CAPJ treatment to prevent E. coli-induced diseases.

The influence of operational parameters of CAPJ, such as operation power, CAPJ-sample distance, gas mixtures composition, and treatment periods need to be determined to generate consistent results when using CAPJ. In general, a large number of experiments are required to optimize the processing parameters to improve the antimicrobial efficiency by changing one parameter value at a time. Such approach is time consuming, costly, and labor intensive. In this study, a systematic and efficient approach using the Taguchi experimental method design [20–23] is applied to the CAPJ system in determining the optimal process parameters for the highest antimicrobial efficiency. The optimal condition of CAPJ was determined experimentally and the antimicrobial mechanism of CAPJ was explored using DNA damage assay and microbial microstructure analysis.

2. Experimental Section

2.1. Plasma Experimental Setup

Figure 1 depicts the setup of the CAPJ used. A quartz tube with 4 mm inner diameter was covered with two parallel cylindrical pure copper electrodes, which were connected with a high voltage pulsed direct current (DC) power supply for generating the plasma jet [24]. The distance between two Cu electrode was 15 mm. The frequency and the duty cycle of the power supply were fixed at 10,000 Hz and 50%, respectively. In this work, the He gas flow rate was kept at 5 slm (standard liter per min), and the argon gas flow rate was changed from 0 to 500 sccm (standard cubic centimeter per min). Taguchi method with L9 experiment was applied to discover the optimal sterilization effect. The CAPJs were generated under four different processing parameters in three various conditions as listed in Table 1, including the applying voltage of 6.5, 7.5, and 8.5 kV; the distance between CAPJ downstream and sample surface of 10, 20, and 30 mm; the CAPJ treating time of 60, 180, and 300 s; and the Ar gas flow rates of 0, 200, and 500 sccm. The radical compositions at the CAPJ downstream of each experiment was detected by an optical emission spectrometer (OES, AvaSpec ULS2048L, Avantes, Louisville, CO, USA) in the wavelength ranging from 200 to 1100 nm. The integration time for the OES detection was 80 ms.

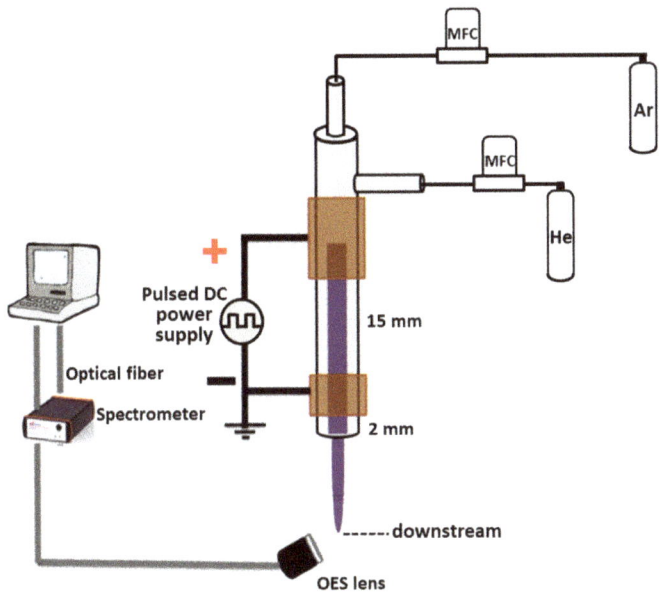

Figure 1. The setup of a cold atmospheric plasma jet (CAPJ).

Table 1. Factors and levels of CAPJ parameters for the antimicrobial of E. coli.

Symbol	Process Parameter	Level 1	Level 2	Level 3
A	Application voltage (kV)	6.5	7.5	8.5
B	CAPJ-sample distance (mm)	10	20	30
C	Ar gas flow rate (sccm)	0	200	500
D	CAPJ treatment time (s)	60	180	300

2.2. Bacterial Strain and Culture

E. coli (ATCC 25922[TM]) was used as a reference strain, which was described elsewhere [25]. The bacteria were routinely cultured in Luria–Bertani (LB) broth (Becton Dickinson, Franklin Lakes, NJ, USA) at 37 °C for 24 h to reach the logarithmic phase and performed in the following experiments.

2.3. In Vitro Growth Inhibition Assay

E. coli was cultured in LB broth at 37 °C for 24 h. The bacterial suspension was adjusted to an optical density of 1.0 at 600 nm (OD_{600}), which corresponded to 1×10^5 colony-forming units (CFUs)/mL. The bacteria were untreated by CAPJ under various combinations of experimental parameters assigned as S1–S9 revealed in Table 2. The untreated E. coli was assigned as S0 (control). The bacteria were serial diluted in phosphate buffer saline (PBS) and plated onto LB agar plates. After incubation at 37 °C for 24 h, the viable CFUs were counted. The bactericidal activity was represented as a percentage of CAPJ treated one divided by the untreated control group (S0). The results were expressed as the means of three independent experiments performed in duplicate.

$$\text{The bactericidal activity} = (N_x/N_0) \times 100\%$$

where N_0 and N_x are the number of the viable bacteria on an untreated control S0 and CAPJ treated S_x (x = 1–9) experiment after incubation at 37 °C for 24 h, respectively.

Table 2. Antimicrobial conditions of *E. coli* using the Taguchi L9 orthogonal array table. Symbols and numbers of control factors reflect the parameters and levels in Table 1.

Sample #	Control Factors			
	A	B	C	D
S1	1	1	1	1
S2	1	2	2	2
S3	1	3	3	3
S4	2	1	2	3
S5	2	2	3	1
S6	2	3	1	2
S7	3	1	3	2
S8	3	2	1	3
S9	3	3	2	1

2.4. Taguchi Method

Four control factors of the Taguchi experiment including (A) application voltage (kV), (B) CAPJ downstream-sample distance (mm), (C) Ar gas flow rate (sccm), and (D) CAPJ treatment time (s) were applied to analyze the influence of the sterilization parameters on *E. coli*. Three levels were considered for each factor and shown in Table 1. Table 2 represented the Taguchi design and structure of L9 orthogonal array reflecting the parameters and levels in Table 1. The higher the better concept was applied to estimate the significant parameters of CAPJ sterilization treatment by data analysis and signal-to-noise (S/N) ratios. The contribution percentages of individual parameters were determined by analysis of variance (ANOVA) [26]. The S/N ratio is defined as follows:

$$\frac{S}{N} = -10 \times \log\left[\frac{1}{n}\sum_{i=1}^{n}\frac{1}{y^2}\right]$$

where n is the number of experiments and y is the observed data.

A confirmation test was carried out to validate the Taguchi's optimization approach. The summary statistic S/N at optimal conditions was calculated after the sanative parameters, which can be used to determine the optimal condition.

$$(S/N)_{opt} = m + (m_x - m) + (m_y - m)$$

where m is the overall mean, and m_x and m_y are the mean effect sensitive parameters at the optimal level [19]. The L9 orthogonal array for sample designation and detailed CAPJ treated parameters was tabulated in Table 3, which was the designed L9 orthogonal array in Table 2 filled with the corresponding parameters assigned in Table 1.

Table 3. The Taguchi L9 sample designation and detailed CAPJ parameters.

Sample Designation		S1	S2	S3	S4	S5	S6	S7	S8	S9
CAPJ conditions	A (kV)	6.5	6.5	6.5	7.5	7.5	7.5	8.5	8.5	8.5
	B (mm)	10	20	30	10	20	30	10	20	30
	C (sccm)	0	200	500	200	500	0	500	0	200
	D (s)	60	180	300	300	60	180	180	300	60

2.5. Bacterial Viability Assay

The LIVE/DEAD Bacterial Viability Kit (Thermo Fisher Scientific, Camarillo, CA, USA) was subjected to analyze the viability of bacterial populations based on the membrane integrity [27]. Two nucleic acid fluorescent dyes, SYTO9 and propidium iodide (PI), were used to determine the bacterial viability. The *E. coli* bacteria suspensions, which were untreated (S0) and CAPJ treated under S10, were collected and washed with PBS. The prepared samples were stained with SYTO9 and PI, according to the manufacturer's instructions. The stained bacteria were then analyzed by a confocal laser scanning microscope (LSM 780; Carl Zeiss, Göttingen, Germany). The quantification of fluorescence intensity was performed by using a FACSCalibur flow cytometer (Becton Dickinson, San Jose, CA, USA).

2.6. DNA Damage Assay

A plasmid DNA, pGL3 (2 µg/µL) (Promega, Madison, WI, USA) was untreated (S0) or S10 CAPJ treated. Both the S0 and S10 CAPJ treated plasmids were then dissolved in DNA suspension buffer. DNA solution was loaded on 1.0% agarose gel for electrophoresis. Ethidium bromide-stained DNA was visualized under UV light. Photograph was taken by using a UV transilluminator (Azure Biosystems c400; Dublin, CA, USA).

2.7. Field Emission Scanning Electron Microscope Analysis

The morphologies of untreated S0 and S10 CAPJ treated bacteria were analyzed using a field-emission scanning electron microscope (FE-SEM, JSM 6701F, JEOL, Akishima, Japan). The bacteria samples were fixed in slides with 2% glutaraldehyde for 2 h, followed by washing with saline solution, and then exposed to 25%, 50%, and 75% of ethanol for 20 min, respectively, and finally immersed in 100% of ethanol for one hour. The slides were dried using a critical point dryer for 2 h afterwards. The bacteria samples were coated with a thin platinum layer around 5 nm thick by a sputter system (JFC 1600, JEOL, Akishima, Japan).

2.8. In Vivo Evaluation

Animal experiments were performed in accordance with the ethical standard approved by the Institutional Animal Care and Use Committee, Chang Gung University (Approval No. CGU105-032). Three male Sprague-Dawley (SD) rats with body weight range of 550 ± 30 g were study. The animals were housed under controlled conditions of temperature of 21–22 °C, relative humidity of 55% to 65%, and a 12 h light/dark cycle with artificial lighting. The animals received a standard feed and water ad libitum and were acclimatized under the aforementioned conditions before wounding experiment to create one full-thickness wounds with 17 mm in diameter on each side of rat's shoulder as described in literature [28,29]. The right-side wounds were treated with S10 CAPJ, and the left side wounds were kept untreated as control (S0). Two bacterial swabs were immediately taken from each superficial wound site right after CAPJ treatment on day 0 and day 4. Swabs were immediately immersed in 3 mL PBS and inoculated 200 µL sample on LB agar plates. After incubation at 37 °C for 24 h, the CFUs were counted.

2.9. Statistical Analysis

During the ANOVA calculation, the relation of between-group comparisons was performed using the chi-square with Fisher exact test by SPSS program (version 18.0, SPSS, Inc., Chicago, IL, USA). A *p*-value less than 0.05 was considered statistically significant.

3. Results

3.1. Plasma Characterization

The temperature of He-based CAPJ was measured at the distance of 10 mm from the nozzle, and it rose continually for the first 5 min and then kept constant for at least 30 min under pure He gas flow rate of 5 slm, as shown in Figure 2. The temperatures increased from 34.5, 35.5, 36.5 to 38.5 °C when the applying voltages were increased from 6.5, 7.5, 8.5 to 9.5 kHz, respectively.

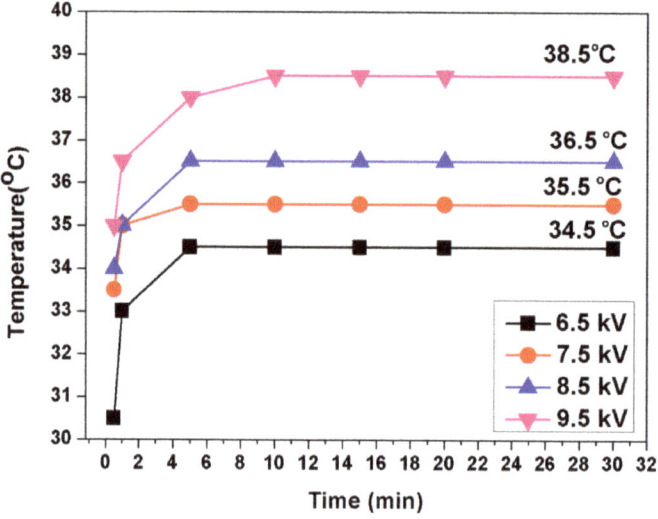

Figure 2. CAPJ temperature keeps steady for at least 30 min. Temperature changes of CAPJs operated at different applied voltages ranging from 6.5 to 9.5 kV under a fixed He gas flow rate of 5 slm. The temperature was detected at the position of 1 cm below the downstream of CAPJ.

The compositions of ROS generated by CAPJ are mainly dependent on both the working gas and the atmospheric air. The compositions, therefore, can be controlled by the working gas mixture. Figure 3a–c illustrate the excited and radiant species in optical emission spectroscopy (OES) spectra under the mixtures of various Ar gas flow rates of 0, 200, and 500 sccm into a fix He gas flow rate of 5 slm with the application voltage of 6.5 kV. The emission lines between 300 and 400 nm, 450 and 700 nm and 700 and 900 nm were dominated by the nitrogen (N), He, and Ar atoms, respectively. Both hydroxyl radical (OH) emission at 309 nm and nitrogen monoxide (NO) emission at 283 nm are of particular interest because they might play an effective role for bacterial growth inhibition [1,30,31]. The intensities of OH radicals remarkably increased with increasing Ar gas flow rate but were unaffected at various application voltages, as observed in Figure 3d. It is also important to point out that the temperature of each Ar added CAPJ test was below 38.5 °C.

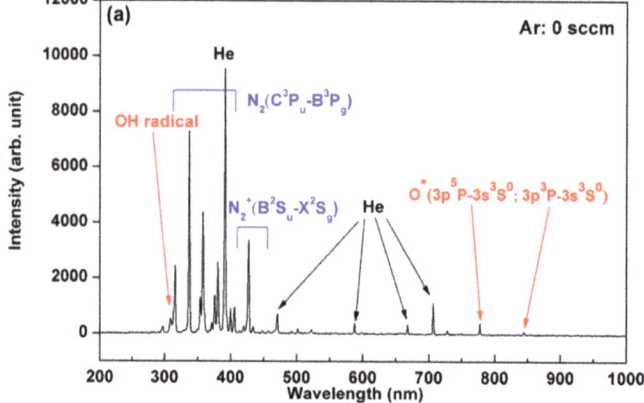

Figure 3. *Cont.*

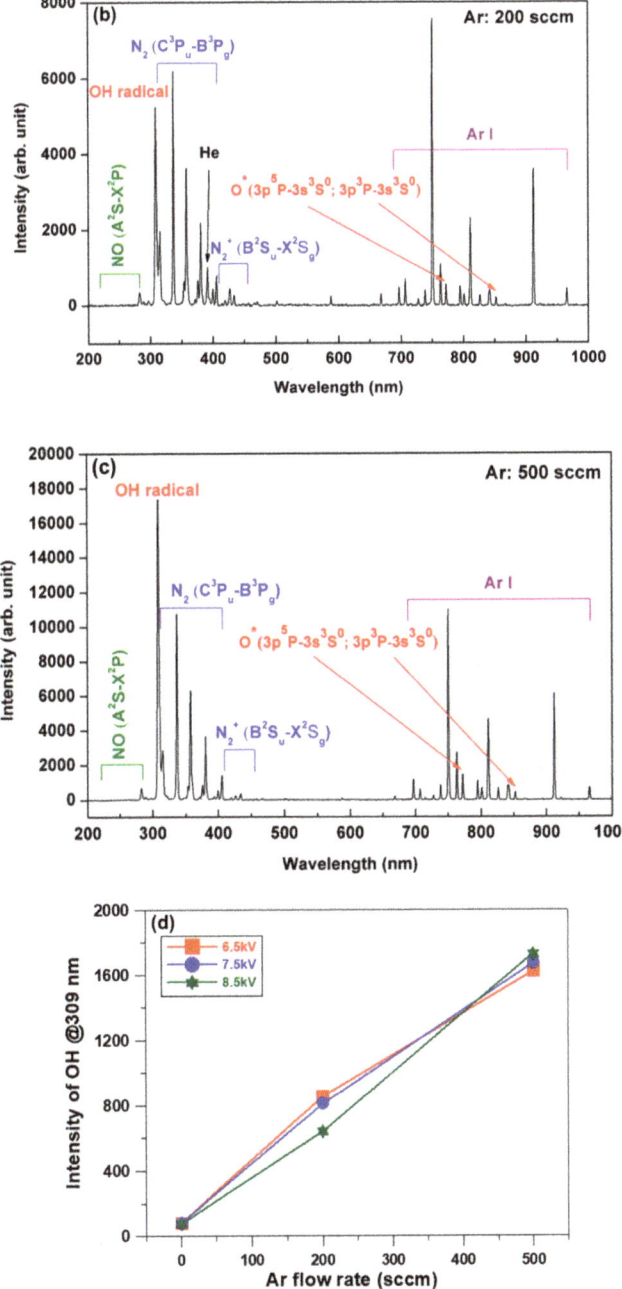

Figure 3. CAPJ plasma characterizes by OES. The OES spectra of the CAPJs operated at a fixed applied voltage of 6.5 kV and fixed He gas flow rate of 5 slm and (**a**) without Ar gas inlet, (**b**) with 200 sccm Ar gas and (**c**) with 500 sccm Ar gas, and (**d**) the dependence of Ar flow rate on the intensity of OH radicals @ 309 nm.

3.2. CAPJ Possess Bactericidal Activity

The bactericidal activity was investigated under various plasma parameters designed using the Taguchi method shown in Figure 4 and summarized in Table 4. Comparing with the untreated control sample S0, the bactericidal activities against *E coli* by CAPJ treated under S1 to S9 were 45.7%, 31.3%, 90.6%, 92.8%, 53.2%, 37.7%, 85.9%, 100%, and 22.6%, respectively.

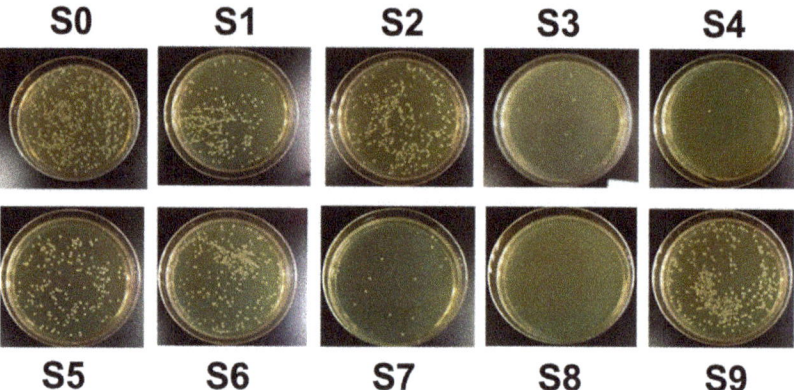

Figure 4. Bacterial colonies evaluate the bactericidal activity of CAPJ operating parameters. Photos of bacterial colonies of control S0 and CAPJ treated samples (**S1**) to (**S9**) with a combination of different Taguchi experimental parameters. The visualized colonies grew on the LB agar plates were counted and represented in CFU as tabulated in Table 4.

Table 4. The bactericidal activity of *E. coli* by nine different CAPJ treatments.

Sample Designation.	S1	S2	S3	S4	S5	S6	S7	S8	S9
Bactericidal activity (%)	45.7	31.3	90.6	92.8	53.2	37.7	85.9	100.0	22.6

3.3. Analysis of the Bactericidal Activity by Using Taguchi Method

The four important operating parameters of CAPJ to achieve desired performance considered in this study were application voltages, CAPJ-sample distance, Ar gas flow rate, and CAPJ treatment time, which are noted as A, B, C, and D, respectively, in Table 1, and each was given three levels. The greater S/N value corresponded to the better performance regardless of the category of the performance characteristics [26]. Therefore, parameters with high S/N value and the better efficiency were selected to define the optimal level of the operating parameters. The average S/N ratios for each level of each parameter, in terms of bactericidal activity, were shown in Figure 5. The horizontal red line was the overall mean of the S/N values. The best combination of process parameters corresponding to the bactericidal activity was found to be A3B2C3D3, which correlates to application voltage of 8.5 kV, CAPJ-sample distance of 10 mm, Ar gas flow rate of 500 sccm, and CAPJ treatment time of 300 s. Furthermore, the CAPJ treatment time was discovered as the most impactful factor for bactericidal activity because of the greatest range of outcomes between the three experimental levels.

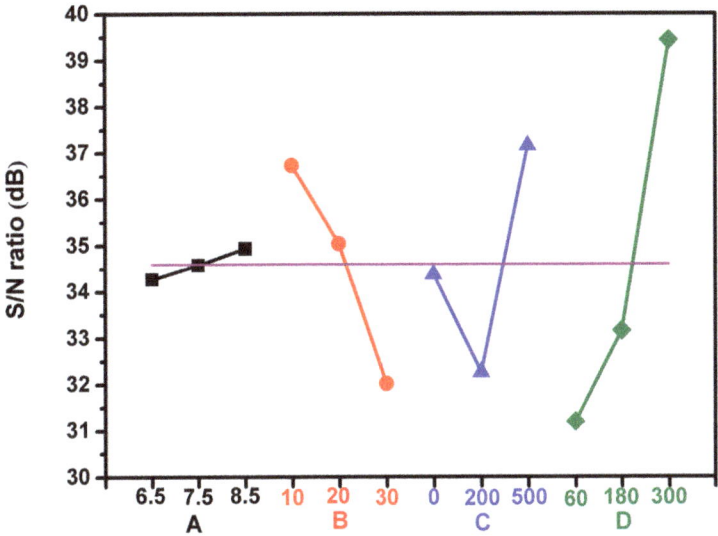

Figure 5. Taguchi analysis determines the best set of parameter combination. The effect diagrams for antimicrobial of CAPJ are based on the higher S/N and the better efficiency. Four factors include A: applying voltage (kV), B: CAPJ-sample distance (mm), C: Ar gas flow rate (sccm), and D: CAPJ treated time.

The relative significance of each parameter was investigated by ANOVA to estimate their contributions. The ANOVA results of the control factors, A, B, C, and D were calculated for the bactericidal activity and the degree of freedom, sum of squares, variance, and percentage contributions are shown in Table 5. Higher percentage contribution correlated to more significant influence of the overall process. Factor D, the CAPJ treatment time, was the most impactful with the highest variance of 4.70 and a percentage contribution of 76.5%. This was followed by factor C, Ar gas flow rate, and factor B, CAPJ-sample distance, with contributions of 12.1% and 11.2%, respectively. Meanwhile, the contributions of 0.2% for factor A, application voltage, is obtained implying its insignificant role.

Table 5. Summary of the ANOVA results for the bactericidal activity of E. coli by CAPJ.

	Source of Variance	Degree of Freedom	Sum of Square	Variance	Contribution (%)
A,	Application voltage (kV)	2	0.68	0.01	0.2
B,	CAPJ-sample distance (mm)	2	34.04	0.69	11.2
C,	Ar gas flow rate (sccm)	2	36.15	0.74	12.1
D,	CAPJ treatment time (s)	2	111.04	4.70	76.5
	Total	8	181.91	6.15	100.0

3.4. Validation of Bactericidal Activity Conferred by CAPJ Treated under S10

Based on the optimal condition deduced from the Taguchi method, the CAPJ condition with the application voltage of 8.5 kV, CAPJ-sample distance of 10 mm, He/Ar gas flow of 5 slm/500 sccm, and CAPJ treated time of 300 s was assigned as S10, and a confirmation test was performed to validate the conclusions on the previous discovery. As compared with the control S0, the bactericidal activity of S10 was up to 100% in Figure 6.

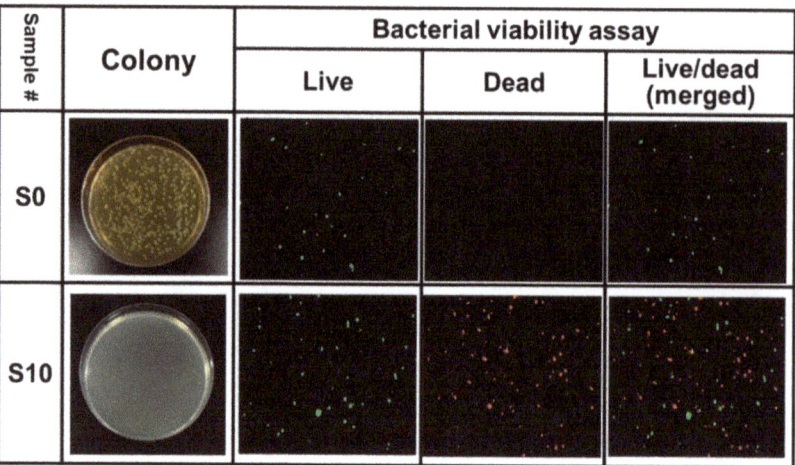

Figure 6. S10 CAPJ induces bacterial death. Photos of bacterial colonies of control S0 and confirmation test of CAPJ treated under S10, fluorescence live/dead bacterial viability assay images of *E. coli* without CAPJ (S0) and with CAPJ treated under S10.

To further verify whether the S10 CAPJ possesses potent bactericidal activity, a LIVE/DEAD Bacterial Viability assay was employed. As shown in Figure 6, dead bacteria, appearing with red fluorescence, were rarely observed in the control group, but those bacteria treated with S10 CAPJ had significantly more dead bacteria presented in the lower panel of Figure 6. These results confirmed that the S10 CAPJ had the most effective bactericidal activity in the treatment of bacterial pathogens and indicated that the Taguchi method is handy to find the optimal parameters on the bactericidal activity by CAPJ.

3.5. CAPJ Treatment Induced DNA Double-Strand Breaks (DSB) and Disruption of Cell Wall Integrity

To further explore the mechanism of the bactericidal activity by CAPJ treatment, we conducted a DNA electrophoresis assay. As shown in Figure 7, the untreated plasmid DNA (S0) was intact and exhibited the supercoiled and circular forms. In contrast, clear smear DNA fragments were shown in the plasmid DNA treated with S10 CAPJ, indicating that CAPJ contributed to induce DSB in bacteria. To strengthen our findings, the morphologies of *E. coli* were visualized by FE-SEM after bacteria was treated by S10 CAPJ. In the control group without CAPJ treatment, the bacterial shape and cell wall showed intact morphologies (Figure 8a,b). By contrast, FE-SEM images of the bacteria treated with S10 CAPJ exhibited a shriveled and burst appearance on the bacterial surface (Figure 8c,d). Taken together, these results demonstrated that CAPJ treated under S10 sustainably inhibited bacterial growth by inducing DSB and disrupting cell wall integrity.

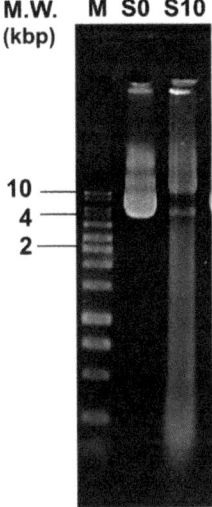

Figure 7. S10 CAPJ induces DNA double-strand breaks (DSB). The pGL3 (2 µg/µL) was untreated (S0) or treated with S10 CAPJ. The plasmid DNA was loaded on 1.0% agarose gel for electrophoresis. Ethidium bromide-stained DNA was visualized under UV light. The positions of the size markers are shown at left of the image. M, DNA marker.

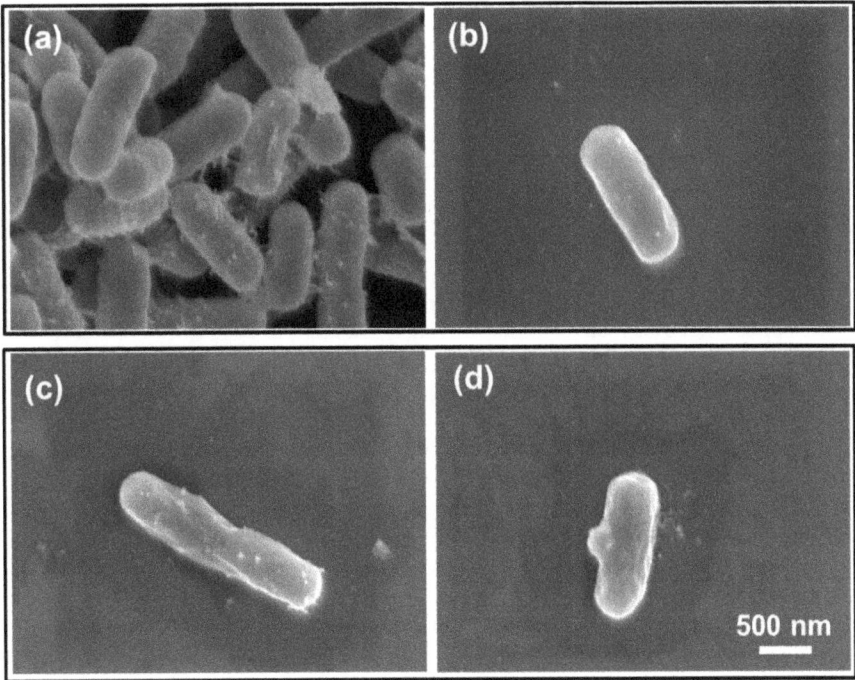

Figure 8. S10 CAPJ disrupts bacterial cell wall integrity. The FE-SEM images of the bacterial morphologies before CAPJ treatment (**a**,**b**) and after S10 CAPJ treatment (**c**,**d**).

3.6. In Vivo Evaluation

Bactericidal activity in vivo evaluation by CAPJ treatment was presented in Figure 9. SD rates were used to create wound exposure and analyze the bacterial infection as described in the Experimental Section. The wounds were either untreated (S0) or treated with S10 CAPJ, and wound exudates were collected on days 0 and 4. Our results showed that S10 CAPJ treatment remarkably decreased bacterial load on day 0 when compared to S0. Most importantly, this effect is still seen on day 4, which showed that the bacterial infection continued to be reduced in rat treated with S10 CAPJ.

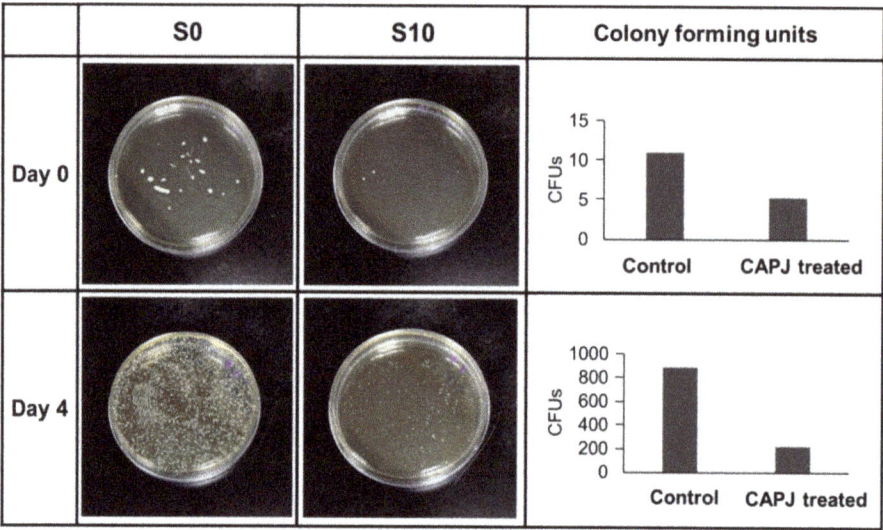

Figure 9. S10 CAPJ reduces bacterial infection in the wound. Rat wound was untreated or treated with S10 CAPJ, and the bacterial loads in the wound were counted on days 0 and 4. Viable bacteria were represented as colony forming units (CFUs).

4. Discussion

Infectious disease remains a great challenge in the field of public health as it is among the top 10 causes of death and also leads the cause of disability [32]. Inadequate antibiotic therapy worsens the control of pathogenic microbes and leads to drug resistance. The discovery of new and effective antibacterial agents or methods is quite a challenge because of its time and financially consuming nature. In addition, poor sanitation and increasing international travel have made transmission of infectious diseases easier.

This study focused on the development and optimizations of a sterilization technique using CAPJ utilizing the Taguchi method to shorten to experimental time spent on trial and error. In general, a design of orthogonal arrays of Taguchi analysis provides a maximum number of main factors to be estimated to minimize experimental trials. S/N ratios are transferred from the responses in the bactericidal activity by CAPJ treatment. ANOVA can further determine the contribution of CAPJ operating parameters on the preferable efficiency of antimicrobial condition. The effectiveness of Taguchi's optimization approach is evaluated by antimicrobial effect, where 100% was obtained with the CAPJ using parameters obtained from the Taguchi method. As determined by the Taguchi method, the optimal antimicrobial activity is achieved with CAPJ parameters of application voltage 8.5 kV, APJ-sample distance 10 mm, Ar gas flow rate 500 sccm, and treatment time 300 s. We found CAPJ treatment time affected the plasma's efficacy the most, and it required 5 min of treatment to achieve 100% bactericidal activity. By extension, the principles and concepts of Taguchi approach can also benefit industry reducing experimental trials of the performance, quality, and cost [22,33].

A number of studies represent very promising results for infection control by atmospheric pressure plasma [25]. In this work, we demonstrated that CAPJ built in our lab inhibited bacterial growth. The beneficial effects of plasma in sterilization are not yet fully understood, so we used our CAPJ to explore proposed mechanisms described in the literature. The observed temperatures of this CAPJ clearly indicated that consecutive plasma treatment by CAPJ remains below human body temperature for 30 min without causing thermal injury by utilizing the application voltage lower than 8.5 kV (Figure 2), which is an important requirement for biological applications. Previous studies reported that reactive oxygen, hydrogen peroxide, and UV photons produced by cold plasmas might target cell membrane and cell wall for antibacterial activity [34,35]. From the plasma diagnostics by OES (Figure 3), there is nearly no emission in the germicidal UV-C region around 254 nm [36]. The effect of heat and UV radiation as the main antimicrobial mechanism for plasma component, therefore, is unlikely.

On the other hand, The Ar mixed into He-based plasma described in this study contains OH and NO radicals, nitrogen and oxygen species, and metastable species of He and Ar (Figure 3), which probably interact with biological organisms to generate further reactive species [37]. Previous reports demonstrated ROS from different technologies might target different components of bacterial cells [38], which subsequently leads to the destruction of bacterial cell wall to achieve antimicrobial strategies. For example, ROS attacks the polyunsaturated fatty acids of the fatty acid membrane to initiate a self-propagating chain reaction [39], induces lipid peroxidation in Gram-negative bacteria [40], decomposes macromolecules such as DNA and protein [41], and breaks important C–O, C–N and C–C bonds of the peptidoglycan structure [42]. The distinguished emission at 309 nm in Figure 3 is a measurement for substantial amount of OH radicals, which are produced by plasma chemical reactions of dissociation and excitation of water molecules present in the air and are likely the part of plasma that is lethal toward living bacterial cells [43,44]. The intensity of OH produced by CAPJ is influenced by the feed gas mixture and increases with increasing Ar flow rate similar to a previous report [45]. The amount of OH radicals positively correlates to the antimicrobial efficiency as well. Deleterious OH radicals are the dominant reactive species and play a significant role in cell death [46,47].

It has been known that bacterial colonization of wounds exacerbated inflammation around the injury sites and slowed the skin healing. A previous study in bacteria infected skin diseases shows that *E. coli* is one of the four main Gram-negative bacteria among 90 isolated bacteria cultured from skin ulcers [48]. In the present study, we first assessed whether CAPJ possessed bactericidal effects on pathogenic *E. coli* and validated the bactericidal activity by using the animal experiment. We showed that S10 CAPJ treatment dramatically decreased bacterial load on day 4 as compared to untreated rat. However, we did not identify the bacterial species that were presented on the wounds. Our results are in line with previous in vitro studies, which showed that cold atmospheric plasma can decrease bacterial load independent of the strains [49,50]. Although CAPJ can effectively reduce bacterial loads in the animal study, further identification of bacterial species is worth studying in the future research.

According to the observation of both the DNA damage assay (Figure 7) and the morphology of bacteria after CAPJ treatment by FE-SEM (Figure 8), CAPJ disrupts bacterial cell walls and induces DNA damage to exercise its antimicrobial effect in plasma mediated reactions. Figure 10 is a schematic that suggests the antimicrobial mechanism of CAPJ treatment noted in this study.

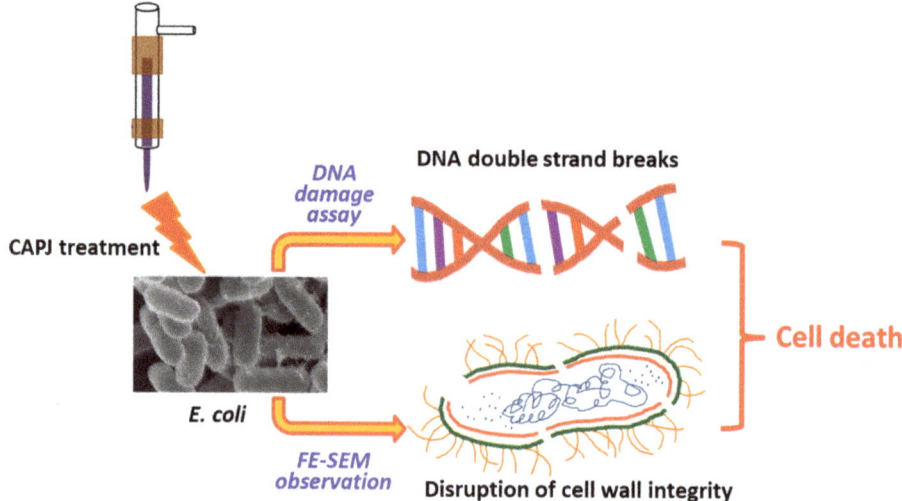

Figure 10. Antimicrobial mechanism of CAPJ treatment. The mechanism of the antimicrobial efficiency by CAPJ is suggested to kill the bacteria by destroying the cell wall of *E. coli*, damaging its DNA structure.

5. Conclusions

In this work, experimental design using the Taguchi method with a L9 orthogonal array was confirmed by S/N ratios and ANOVA, to optimize the operating parameters of CAPJ, achieving the best antimicrobial efficacy against *E. coli*. Parameters obtained via the Taguchi method were confirmed by 100% antimicrobial activity, with the final parameters of 8.5 kV CAPJ application voltage, 10 mm CAPJ-sample distance, 500 sccm Ar gas flow rate, and 300 s CAPJ treatment time. These parameters were further applied to wounds created on a rat model and showed a marked decrease in microbial load compared to an untreated wound, suggesting CPAJ have safe and effective application in vivo. As the intensity of hydroxyl radical produced by CAPJ is positively correlated to its antimicrobial efficiency, reactive species likely play a significant role for the plasma sterilization in this study. According to the observation of both the DNA damage assay and the bacterial cell wall integrity test after CAPJ treatment, the antimicrobial mechanism of CAPJ works through cell wall destruction and further DNA damage, thus ensuring antimicrobial activity. This makes CAPJ a promising and effective antimicrobial technique.

Author Contributions: B.-S.L., C.-H.L., and J.-W.L. designed the experiment, analyzed data, and wrote the paper. J.-H.H. designed CAPJ device. T.-P.C. and Y.-M.S. employed in vitro experiments. C.-M.C., C.-W.H., and P.-Y.C. performed in vivo experiment.

Funding: The authors gratefully acknowledge the financial support of the Ministry of Science and Technology, Taiwan, through contract nos. MOST 108-2218-E-030 and MOST 106-2218-E-131-003. The financial support from the Chang Gung Memorial Hospital through contract no. CMRPD5H0032 to B.S. Lou is also acknowledged.

Conflicts of Interest: The authors have no conflicts of interest relevant to this article.

References

1. Weltmann, K.D.; Von Woedtke, T. Plasma medicine-current state of research and medical application. *Plasma Phys. Control. Fusion* **2016**, *59*, 014031. [CrossRef]
2. Kong, M.G.; Kroesen, G.; Morfill, G.; Nosenko, T.; Shimizu, T.; van Dijk, J.; Zimmermann, J.L. Plasma medicine: An introductory review. *New J. Phys.* **2009**, *11*, 115012.
3. Laroussi, M. Low temperature plasma-based sterilization: Overview and state-of-the-art. *Plasma Process Polym.* **2005**, *2*, 391–400. [CrossRef]

4. Ehlbeck, J.; Schnabel, U.; Polak, M.; Winter, J.; Von Woedtke, T.; Brandenburg, R.; Von dem Hagen, T.; Weltmann, K.D. Low temperature atmospheric pressure plasma sources for microbial decontamination. *J. Phys. D Appl. Phys.* **2010**, *44*, 013002. [CrossRef]
5. Von Woedtke, T.; Reuter, S.; Masur, K.; Weltmann, K.D. Plasmas for medicine. *Phys. Rep.* **2013**, *530*, 291–320. [CrossRef]
6. Penkov, O.V.; Khadem, M.; Lim, W.S.; Kim, D.E. A review of recent applications of atmospheric pressure plasma jets for materials processing. *J. Coat. Technol. Res.* **2015**, *12*, 225–235. [CrossRef]
7. Bruggeman, P.J.; Sadeghi, N.; Schram, D.C.; Linss, V. Gas temperature determination from rotational lines in non-equilibrium plasmas: A review. *Plasma Sources Sci. Technol.* **2014**, *23*, 023001. [CrossRef]
8. Uchida, G.; Mino, Y.; Suzuki, T.; Ikeda, J.I.; Suzuki, T.; Takenaka, K.; Setsuhara, Y. Decomposition and oxidation of methionine and tryptophan following irradiation with a nonequilibrium plasma jet and applications for killing cancer cells. *Sci. Rep.* **2019**, *9*, 6625. [CrossRef]
9. Vandamme, M.; Robert, E.; Lerondel, S.; Sarron, V.; Ries, D.; Dozias, S.; Sobilo, J.; Gosset, D.; Kieda, C.; Legrain, B.; et al. ROS implication in a new antitumor strategy based on non-thermal plasma. *Int. J. Cancer* **2012**, *130*, 2185–2194. [CrossRef]
10. Homma, T.; Furuta, M.; Takemura, Y. Inactivation of Escherichia coli Using the Atmospheric Pressure Plasma Jet of Ar Gas. *Jpn. J. Appl. Phys.* **2013**, *52*, 036201. [CrossRef]
11. Klämpfl, T.G.; Isbary, G.; Shimizu, T.; Li, Y.F.; Zimmermann, J.L.; Stolz, W.; Schlegel, J.; Morfill, G.E.; Schmidt, H.U. Cold atmospheric air plasma sterilization against spores and other microorganisms of clinical interest. *Appl. Environ. Microbiol.* **2012**, *78*, 5077–5082. [CrossRef] [PubMed]
12. Choi, Y.; Lee, S.; Lee, H.; Lee, S.; Kim, S.; Lee, J.; Ha, J.; Oh, H.; Lee, Y.; Kim, Y.; et al. Rapid Detection of Escherichia coli in Fresh Foods Using a Combination of Enrichment and PCR Analysis. *Korean J. Food Sci. Anim. Resour.* **2018**, *38*, 829. [PubMed]
13. Bryce, A.; Hay, A.D.; Lane, I.F.; Thornton, H.V.; Wootton, M.; Costelloe, C. Global prevalence of antibiotic resistance in paediatric urinary tract infections caused by Escherichia coli and association with routine use of antibiotics in primary care: Systematic review and meta-analysis. *Bmj* **2016**, *352*, i939. [CrossRef]
14. Abo Basha, J.; Kiel, M.; Görlich, D.; Schütte-Nütgen, K.; Witten, A.; Pavenstädt, H.; Kahl, B.C.; Dobrindt, U.; Reuter, S. Phenotypic and Genotypic Characterization of Escherichia coli Causing Urinary Tract Infections in Kidney-Transplanted Patients. *J. Clin. Med.* **2019**, *8*, 988. [CrossRef] [PubMed]
15. Devaney, J.; Horie, S.; Masterson, C.; Elliman, E.; Barry, F.; O'Brien, T.; Curley, G.; Toole, D.; Laffey, J. Human mesenchymal stromal cells decrease the severity of acute lung injury induced by *E. coli* in the rat. *Thorax* **2015**, *70*, 625–635. [CrossRef]
16. Chen, H.C.; Lin, W.L.; Lin, C.C.; Hsieh, W.H.; Hsieh, C.H.; Wu, M.H.; Wu, J.Y.; Lee, C.C. Outcome of inadequate empirical antibiotic therapy in emergency department patients with community-onset bloodstream infections. *J. Antimicrob. Chemother.* **2013**, *68*, 947–953. [CrossRef] [PubMed]
17. Vila, J.; Sáez-López, E.; Johnson, J.R.; Römling, U.; Dobrindt, U.; Cantón, R.; Giske, C.G.; Naas, T.; Carattoli, A.; Martínez-Medina, M.; et al. Escherichia coli: An old friend with new tidings. *FEMS Microbiol. Rev.* **2016**, *40*, 437–463. [CrossRef]
18. Peralta, G.; Sanchez, M.B.; Garrido, J.C.; De Benito, I.; Cano, M.E.; Martínez-Martínez, L.; Roiz, M.P. Impact of antibiotic resistance and of adequate empirical antibiotic treatment in the prognosis of patients with Escherichia coli bacteraemia. *J. Antimicrob. Chemother.* **2007**, *60*, 855–863. [CrossRef]
19. Wang, J.L.; Lee, C.C.; Lee, C.H.; Lee, N.Y.; Hsieh, C.C.; Hung, Y.P.; Tang, H.J.; Ko, W.C. Clinical Impact of Sequence Type 131 in Adults with Community-Onset Monomicrobial Escherichia Coli Bacteremia. *J. Clin. Med.* **2018**, *7*, 508. [CrossRef]
20. Ross, P.J. *Taguchi Techniques for Quality Engineering*; McGraw-Hill International Book Company: New York, NY, USA, 1996.
21. Dhawane, S.H.; Kumar, T.; Halder, G. Biodiesel synthesis from Hevea brasiliensis oil employing carbon supported heterogeneous catalyst: Optimization by Taguchi method. *Renew. Energy* **2016**, *89*, 506–514. [CrossRef]
22. Sivasakthivel, T.; Murugesan, K.; Thomas, H.R. Optimization of operating parameters of ground source heat pump system for space heating and cooling by Taguchi method and utility concept. *Appl. Energy* **2014**, *116*, 76–85. [CrossRef]

23. Chang, C.T.; Yang, Y.C.; Lee, J.W.; Lou, B.S. The influence of deposition parameters on the structure and properties of aluminum nitride coatings deposited by high power impulse magnetron sputtering. *Thin Solid Films* **2014**, *572*, 161–168. [CrossRef]
24. Bolouki, N.; Hsieh, J.H.; Li, C.; Yang, Y.Z. Emission Spectroscopic Characterization of a Helium Atmospheric Pressure Plasma Jet with Various Mixtures of Argon Gas in the Presence and the Absence of De-Ionized Water as a Target. *Plasma* **2019**, *2*, 20. [CrossRef]
25. Mai-Prochnow, A.; Murphy, A.B.; McLean, K.M.; Kong, M.G.; Ostrikov, K.K. Atmospheric pressure plasmas: Infection control and bacterial responses. *Inter. J. Antimicrob. Agents* **2014**, *43*, 508–517. [CrossRef]
26. Kochure, P.G.; Nandurkar, K.N. Application of taguchi methodology in selection of process parameters for induction hardening of EN8 D Steel. *IJMER* **2012**, *2*, 3736–3742.
27. Boulos, L.; Prévost, M.; Barbeau, B.; Coallier, J.; Desjardins, R. LIVE/DEAD® BacLight™: Application of a new rapid staining method for direct enumeration of viable and total bacteria in drinking water. *J. Microbiol. Methods* **1999**, *37*, 77–86. [CrossRef]
28. Dunn, L.; Prosser, H.C.; Tan, J.T.; Vanags, L.Z.; Ng, M.K.; Bursill, C.A. Murine model of wound healing. *JoVE* **2013**, *75*, e50265. [CrossRef]
29. Kubinova, S.; Zaviskova, K.; Uherkova, L.; Zablotskii, V.; Churpita, O.; Lunov, O.; Dejneka, A. Non-thermal air plasma promotes the healing of acute skin wounds in rats. *Sci. Rep.* **2017**, *7*, 45183. [CrossRef]
30. Wende, K.; Williams, P.; Dalluge, J.; Van Gaens, W.; Aboubakr, H.; Bischof, J.; Von Woedtke, T.; Goyal, S.M.; Weltmann, K.D.; Bogaerts, A.; et al. Identification of the biologically active liquid chemistry induced by a nonthermal atmospheric pressure plasma jet. *Biointerphases* **2015**, *10*, 029518. [CrossRef]
31. Ahn, H.J.; Kim, K.I.; Hoan, N.N.; Kim, C.H.; Moon, E.; Choi, K.S.; Yang, S.S.; Lee, J.S. Targeting cancer cells with reactive oxygen and nitrogen species generated by atmospheric-pressure air plasma. *PLoS ONE* **2014**, *9*, e86173. [CrossRef]
32. World Health Organization. *Prioritization of Pathogens to Guide Discovery, Research and Development of New Antibiotics for Drug-Resistant Bacterial Infections, Including Tuberculosis*; World Health Organization: Geneva, Switzerland, 2017.
33. Unal, R.; Dean, E.B. Taguchi approach to design optimization for quality and cost: An overview. In Proceedings of the 13th Annual Conference of the International Society of Parametric Analysts, New Orleans, LA, USA, 21–24 May 1991.
34. Graves, D.B. The emerging role of reactive oxygen and nitrogen species in redox biology and some implications for plasma applications to medicine and biology. *J. Phys. D Appl. Phys.* **2012**, *45*, 42. [CrossRef]
35. Moisan, M.; Barbeau, J.; Crevier, M.C.; Pelletier, J.; Philip, N.; Saoudi, B. Plasma sterilization. Methods and Mechanisms. *Pure Appl. Chem.* **2002**, *74*, 349–358. [CrossRef]
36. Boudam, M.K.; Moisan, M.; Saoudi, B.; Popovici, C.; Gherardi, N.; Massines, F. Bacterial spore inactivation by atmospheric-pressure plasmas in the presence or absence of UV photons as obtained with the same gas mixture. *J. Phys. D Appl. Phys.* **2006**, *39*, 3494. [CrossRef]
37. Brun, P.; Bernabè, G.; Marchiori, C.; Scarpa, M.; Zuin, M.; Cavazzana, R.; Zaniol, B.; Martines, E. Antibacterial efficacy and mechanisms of action of low power atmospheric pressure cold plasma: Membrane permeability, biofilm penetration and antimicrobial sensitization. *J. Appl. Microbiol.* **2018**, *125*, 398–408. [CrossRef]
38. Vatansever, F.; de Melo, W.C.; Avci, P.; Vecchio, D.; Sadasivam, M.; Gupta, A.; Chandran, R.; Karimi, M.; Parizotto, N.A.; Yin, R.; et al. Antimicrobial strategies centered around reactive oxygen species–bactericidal antibiotics, photodynamic therapy, and beyond. *FEMS Microbiol. Rev.* **2013**, *37*, 955–958. [CrossRef]
39. Mylonas, C.; Kouretas, D. Lipid peroxidation and tissue damage. *In Vivo (Athens Greece)* **1999**, *13*, 295–309.
40. Joshi, S.G.; Cooper, M.; Yost, A.; Paff, M.; Ercan, U.K.; Fridman, G.; Friedman, G.; Fridman, A.; Brooks, A.D. Nonthermal dielectric-barrier discharge plasma-induced inactivation involves oxidative DNA damage and membrane lipid peroxidation in Escherichia coli. *Antimicrob. Agents Chemother.* **2011**, *55*, 1053–1062. [CrossRef]
41. Hosseinzadeh Colagar, A.; Memariani, H.; Sohbatzadeh, F.; Valinataj Omran, A. Nonthermal atmospheric argon plasma jet effects on *Escherichia coli* biomacromolecules. *Appl. Biochem. Biotechnol.* **2013**, *171*, 1617–1629. [CrossRef]
42. Yusupov, M.; Neyts, E.C.; Khalilov, U.; Snoeckx, R.; Van Duin, A.C.T.; Bogaerts, A. Atomic-scale simulations of reactive oxygen plasma species interacting with bacterial cell walls. *New J. Phys.* **2012**, *14*, 093043. [CrossRef]

43. Brandenburg, R.; Ehlbeck, J.; Stieber, M.; von Woedtke, T.; Zeymer, J.; Schlüter, O.; Weltmann, K.D. Antimicrobial treatment of heat sensitive materials by means of atmospheric pressure Rf-driven plasma jet. *Contrib. Plasma Phys.* **2007**, *47*, 72–79. [CrossRef]
44. Gaunt, L.F.; Beggs, C.B.; Georghiou, G.E. Bactericidal action of the reactive species produced by gas-discharge nonthermal plasma at atmospheric pressure: A review. *IEEE Trans. Plasma Sci.* **2006**, *34*, 1257–1269. [CrossRef]
45. Shen, J.; Cheng, C.; Fang, S.; Xie, H.; Lan, Y.; Ni, G.; Meng, Y.; Luo, J.; Wang, X. Sterilization of Bacillus subtilis spores using an atmospheric plasma jet with argon and oxygen mixture gas. *Appl. Phys. Express* **2012**, *5*, 036201. [CrossRef]
46. Kohanski, M.A.; Dwyer, D.J.; Hayete, B.; Lawrence, C.A.; Collins, J.J. A common mechanism of cellular death induced by bactericidal antibiotics. *Cell* **2007**, *130*, 797–810. [CrossRef] [PubMed]
47. Kang, S.K.; Choi, M.Y.; Koo, I.G.; Kim, P.Y.; Kim, Y.; Kim, G.J.; Mohamed, A.A.H.; Collins, G.J.; Lee, J.K. Reactive hydroxyl radical-driven oral bacterial inactivation by radio frequency atmospheric plasma. *Appl. Phys. Lett.* **2011**, *98*, 143702. [CrossRef]
48. Yang, H.; Wang, W.S.; Tan, Y.; Zhang, D.J.; Wu, J.J.; Lei, X. Investigation and analysis of the characteristics and drug sensitivity of bacteria in skin ulcer infections. *Chin. J. Traumatol.* **2017**, *20*, 194–197. [CrossRef] [PubMed]
49. Isbary, G.; Morfill, G.; Schmidt, H.U.; Georgi, M.; Ramrath, K.; Heinlin, J.; Karrer, S.; Landthaler, M.; Shimizu, T.; Steffes, B.; et al. A first prospective randomized controlled trial to decrease bacterial load using cold atmospheric argon plasma on chronic wounds in patients. *Br. J. Dermatol.* **2010**, *163*, 78–82. [CrossRef]
50. Daeschlein, G.; Napp, M.; Lutze, S.; Arnold, A.; von Podewils, S.; Guembel, D.; Jünger, M. Skin and wound decontamination of multidrug-resistant bacteria by cold atmospheric plasma coagulation. *JDDG* **2015**, *13*, 143–149. [CrossRef]

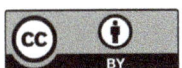

© 2019 by the authors. Licensee MDPI, Basel, Switzerland. This article is an open access article distributed under the terms and conditions of the Creative Commons Attribution (CC BY) license (http://creativecommons.org/licenses/by/4.0/).

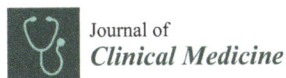

Article

Electrospun Polyethylene Terephthalate Nanofibers Loaded with Silver Nanoparticles: Novel Approach in Anti-Infective Therapy

Alexandru Mihai Grumezescu [1,2,3], Alexandra Elena Stoica [1,4], Mihnea-Ștefan Dima-Bălcescu [4], Cristina Chircov [1,4], Sami Gharbia [5], Cornel Baltă [5], Marcel Roșu [5], Hildegard Herman [5], Alina Maria Holban [1,6], Anton Ficai [1], Bogdan Stefan Vasile [1], Ecaterina Andronescu [1,*], Mariana Carmen Chifiriuc [3] and Anca Hermenean [1,7]

1. Department of Science and Engineering of Oxide Materials and Nanomaterials, Faculty of Applied Chemistry and Materials Science, University Politehnica of Bucharest, 060042 Bucharest, Romania
2. Academy of Romanian Scientists, 050094 Bucharest, Romania
3. ICUB, Research Institute of Bucharest University, University of Bucharest, 030018 Bucharest, Romania
4. Faculty of Engineering in Foreign Languages, University Politehnica of Bucharest, 060042 Bucharest, Romania
5. Institute of Life Sciences, Vasile Goldis Western University of Arad, 310414 Arad, Romania
6. Microbiology Immunology Department, Faculty of Biology, University of Bucharest, 050107 Bucharest, Romania
7. Faculty of Medicine, Vasile Goldis Western University of Arad, 310045 Arad, Romania
* Correspondence: ecaterina.andronescu@upb.ro; Tel.: +4021-402-39-97

Received: 17 May 2019; Accepted: 7 July 2019; Published: 16 July 2019

Abstract: Polyethylene terephthalate (PET) is a major pollutant polymer, due to its wide use in food packaging and fiber production industries worldwide. Currently, there is great interest for recycling the huge amount of PET-based materials, derived especially from the food and textile industries. In this study, we applied the electrospinning technique to obtain nanostructured fibrillary membranes based on PET materials. Subsequently, the recycled PET networks were decorated with silver nanoparticles through the chemical reduction method for antimicrobial applications. After the characterization of the materials in terms of crystallinity, chemical bonding, and morphology, the effect against Gram-positive and Gram-negative bacteria, as well as fungal strains, was investigated. Furthermore, in vitro and in vivo biocompatibility tests were performed in order to open up potential biomedical applications, such as wound dressings or implant coatings. Silver-decorated fibers showed lower cytotoxicity and inflammatory effects and increased antibiofilm activity, thus highlighting the potential of these systems for antimicrobial purposes.

Keywords: polyethylene terephthalate; PET; silver nanoparticles; electrospinning; nanofibers; antimicrobial agents; biocompatibility

1. Introduction

Electrospinning is a simple and versatile technique, used to fabricate continuous fibers from a large number of polymers, with diameters ranging from micrometers to several nanometers [1–3]. The resulting fibrous mats are characterized by large effective surface areas, continuously interconnected pores, high surface roughness, and usually high porosity [4,5]. It is a highly versatile technique, allowing for the development of structures with various morphologies, including core–shell, hollow, and yarn, only by varying the parameters of the electrospinning, i.e., voltage, feed rate, collector type, distance, and nozzle design [6,7].

Polyethylene terephthalate (PET) is a class of engineered polyesters broadly used in numerous industries owing to its mechanical and thermal properties. PET materials are used in a wide range of applications, such as the automotive industry, filtering membranes, biosensors, protective clothing [8–11], surgical meshes, drug delivery systems, and tissue engineering scaffolds (i.e., vascular grafts and ligament and tendon substitutes) [11–16].

Most of the annual world's consumption of PET estimated at 13 million tons comes from the packaging industry, raising great concern for environmental pollution [17], with an increasing scientific focus on developing reuse and recycling technologies of PET materials. In this regard, electrospinning is an interesting approach for the fabrication of non-woven nanofiber mats that could reduce environmental waste materials by producing recycled PET materials that could replace previously used materials [18,19]. Moreover, PET electrospun nanofibers could be further implemented in water filtration [20] and heavy-metal adsorption [21] applications. This approach has the potential to significantly decrease the amount of PET waste, by reusing this material in other non-packaging applications.

As reports show that 10% of patients entering an acute hospital develop a healthcare-associated infection, with 9% of cases being surgical wound infections, the risk of wound infections is causing great concern to healthcare professionals [22]. In this context, electrospun nanomaterials are widely investigated for their antimicrobial properties. The common strategy for developing such materials is represented by the attachment or encapsulation of antimicrobial agents, such as antibiotics, cyclodextrins, and metal or metal-oxide nanoparticles onto or into the supporting nanofibers [23]. Silver is the preferred metal oxide used as an antimicrobial agent [24–30]. Moreover, its nanosized form shows enhanced beneficial properties, owing to the small size, large specific surface area, and quantum effect [31], properties which are correlated with its low toxicity [27,32,33], allowing for the development of diverse applications focused on preventing microbial contamination in different environments or treating microbial infections [34]. There are several studies reporting the uniform incorporation of silver nanoparticles into the electrospun fibers for enhanced antimicrobial abilities [35].

The aim of this study was to obtain electrospun nanostructured fibrillary antimicrobial membranes based on PET materials and silver nanoparticles for different antimicrobial applications. Specifically, the silver nanoparticles were applied onto the surface of the PET materials in order to enrich it with large-spectrum biocidal properties. The different fibers were obtained by adjusting the flow rate of the electrospinning process, since this parameter is very important in ensuring fiber strength and it may impact the morphology and fiber size [36,37]. The in vitro and in vivo biocompatibility issues of PET containing silver nanoparticles were evaluated in order to establish their suitability for biomedical applications. Our goal was to develop a PET-based material that could be further implemented in wound dressing and biomedical coating areas (i.e., implants, medical surfaces, medical textiles), while simultaneously reducing the environmental waste produced by PET usage.

2. Experimental Section

2.1. Materials

The polyester polymer was obtained from recycled PET bottles available from a local supplier. The bottles previously contained water. Dichloromethane (molecular weight (Mw) = 84.96 g/mol) was purchased from Chimopar trading SRL. Trifluoroacetic acid (Mw = 114.02 g/mol) was obtained from Fluka Analytical. Silver nitrate, NaOH, D-glucose, and eugenol were purchased from Sigma-Aldrich. All chemicals were of analytical purity and used with no further purification.

2.2. Electrospinning Deposition of PET Nanofibers

The electrospinning method was used to obtain nanostructured membranes from recycled PET. This method is used to produce membranes made up of a fibrous network with interconnected, overlapping, and randomly distributed fibers. Firstly, the PET bottles were cut into small pieces (about

1 cm^2) and then added to a mixture of trifluoroacetic acid and dichloromethane. After the complete dissolution of the polymer, electrospinning was performed using the parameters described in Table 1 and Scheme 1.

Table 1. The parameters utilized for electrospinning. PET—polyethylene terephthalate.

Sample	Output 1 (kV)	Output 2 (kV)	Heat (KW)	Humidity (%)	Temperature (°C)	Feed Rate (mL/h)
PET_2.5_ctrl						2.5
PET_5_ctrl	−5.73	17.53	0.6	35	27	5
PET_7.5_ctrl						7.5
PET_10_ctrl						10

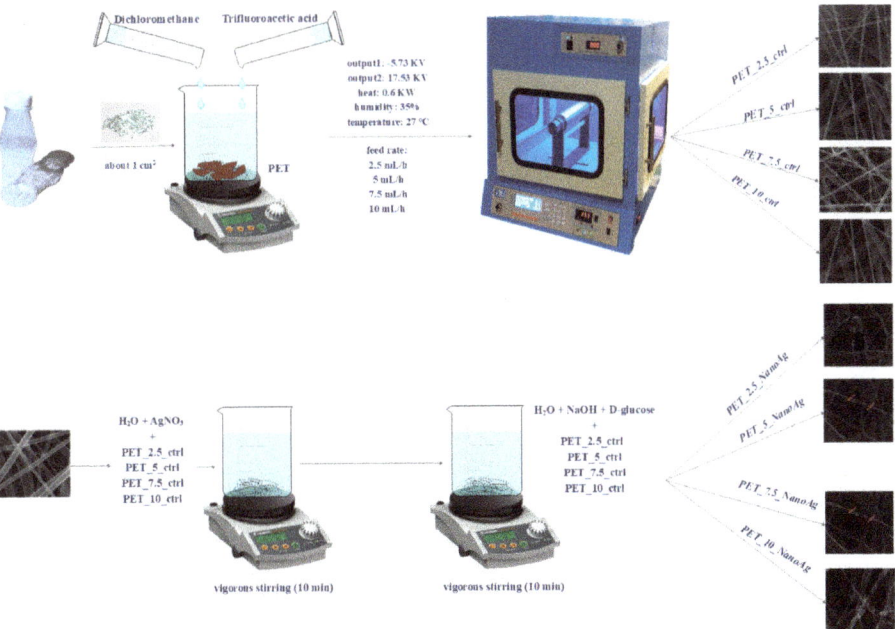

Scheme 1. Synthesis process for control and silver-loaded polyethylene terephthalate (PET_X_ctrl and PET_X_NanoAg).

2.3. Silver Nanoparticle (NanoAg) Synthesis

Silver nanoparticles were prepared by reduction. Briefly, two solutions were obtained: one containing 0.1% silver nitrate (0.1 g of AgNO$_3$ + 99.9 mL of H$_2$O) and one containing the reducing agent (300 mL of H$_2$O + 3 g of NaOH + 1 g of D-glucose + 500 uL of eugenol). Sections of the PET's fibrous networks were placed in the AgNO$_3$ solution and left for 10 min under vigorous stirring; subsequently, they were removed and immersed in the reducing agent solution for an equal amount of time. The obtained samples were washed twice with deionized water and allowed to dry at room temperature. After this, the samples were weighed by comparison with the controls in order to estimate the amount of silver nanoparticles immobilized on the fiber surface. The quantified NanoAg varied between 0.998 mg/cm^2 and 1.003 mg/cm^2, with an average of measurement ~1 mg/cm^2 in the case of all samples. Samples coated with silver nanoparticles were noted as PET_2.5_NanoAg, PET_5_NanoAg, PET_7.5_NanoAg, and PET_10_NanoAg.

2.4. Physico-Chemical Characterization

Infrared spectroscopy. Infrared (IR) spectra were obtained using a Nicolet iN10 MX Fourier-transform (FT)-IR microscope (Thermo Fischer Scientific, Waltham, MA, USA) with a liquid nitrogen-cooled mercury cadmium telluride (MCT) detector with a measurement range of 4000–700 cm^{-1}. Spectra collection was performed in reflection mode at a resolution of 4 cm^{-1}. For each spectrum, 32 scans were co-added and converted to absorbance using the OmincPicta software (Version 1, Thermo Fischer Scientific, Waltham, MA, USA).

X-ray diffraction. Grazing incidence X-ray diffraction (GIXRD) was performed with a Panalytical Empyrean diffractometer (PANalytical, Almelo, The Netherlands), using CuK radiation (1.541874 A) equipped with a 2× Ge (2 2 0) hybrid monochromator for Cu and a parallel plate collimator on the PIXcel3D. Scanning was performed on the 2θ axis in the range of 5–80°, with an incidence angle of 0.5°, a step size of 0.04°, and a time step of 3 s.

Scanning electron microscopy. In order to investigate the morphology and size of the nanostructured membranes, images produced by recording the resultant secondary electron beam with an energy of 30 keV of the samples were taken with a scanning electron microscope purchased from FEI (Hillsboro, OR, USA).

Transmission electron microscopy (TEM). Electron diffraction on selected area. In order to obtain transmission electron microscopy images, the samples were placed on a carbon-coated copper grid at room temperature. The TEM images were acquired using a high-resolution Tecnai™ G2 F30 S-TWIN transmission microscope equipped with selected area electron diffraction (SAED), purchased from FEI (Hillsboro, OR, USA). This microscope operates in transmission mode at a voltage of 300 kV, while the point and line resolution are guaranteed with values of 2 Å and 1 Å, respectively. The SAED analysis for silver nanoparticles was performed in a light field using the Tecnai™ G2 F30 S-TWIN high-resolution electronic microscope equipped with SAED, purchased from FEI (Hillsboro, OR, USA).

2.5. In Vitro Biocompatibility

2.5.1. Cell Line

Human amniotic fluid stem cells (AFSC) were used to evaluate the biocompatibility of the prepared samples. The AFSC cells were cultured in Dulbecco's modified Eagle's medium (DMEM) supplemented with 10% fetal bovine serum (FBS) and 1% antibiotics (penicillin, streptomycin/neomycin). All cells were maintained at 37 °C in a humidified incubator with 5% CO_2.

2.5.2. MTT (3-(4,5-Dimethylthiazolyl-2)-2,5-diphenyltetrazolium bromide) Assay

The evaluation of cell viability was performed by measuring the degree of reduction of a tetrazolium salt solution, MTT (3-(4,5-dimethylthiazolyl-2)-2,5-diphenyltetrazolium bromide), to insoluble purple formazan crystals by viable cells. In this purpose, the AFSC cells were seeded in 96-well plates, with a density of 3000 cells/well under different experimental conditions. Subsequently, a volume of 10 μL of 12 mM MTT was added and the cells were incubated at 37 °C for 4 h. A volume of 100 μL of SDS–HCl solution was further added, vigorously pipetted to solubilize the formazan crystals, incubated for 1 h, and read at 570 nm (TECAN spectrophotometer, Männedorf, Switzerland).

2.6. In Vitro Antibacterial Tests

2.6.1. Growth of Planktonic (Floating) Microorganisms in the Presence of Material

To test the effect of the obtained material on the growth of microorganisms in liquid medium (planktonic cultures), the obtained material was cut into 1-cm^2 samples and sterilized by exposure to ultraviolet (UV) radiation for 30 min on each side. One fragment of the sterile material was individually deposited in a well of a six-well sterile plate. Over the deposited materials, 2 mL of liquid medium and then 20 μL of 0.5 McFarland microbial suspension (bacteria—*Staphylococcus aureus* American

Type Culture Collection (ATCC) 25923 and *Pseudomonas aeruginosa* ATCC 27853) or 1McFarland (yeast—*Candida albicans* ATCC 10231) prepared in sterile physiological water, 0.9% NaCl salt, was added to the wells. The as-prepared six-well plates were incubated at 37 °C for 24 h. At the end of the incubation time, 200 µL of the obtained microbial suspension was transferred to 96 sterile plates, and the turbidity of the microbial cultures (absorbance) was spectrophotometrically measured at 600 nm.

2.6.2. Evaluation of Adhesion and Biofilm Formation

To test the effect of fibrillated materials on microbial adhesion and biofilm production, the sterile material samples treated as described above were washed with sterile saline water (SSW), and the medium was changed to allow the microbial cells—adhered onto the surface of the material samples in the first 24 h of incubation—to continue biofilm development and maturation for another 24, 48, and 72 h. After the end of each incubation period, the colonized sample was washed with AFS to remove non-adherent microorganisms and deposited in a sterile tube in 1 mL of SSW. The tube was vigorously vortexed for 30 s and sonicated for 10 s to harvest the cells from the biofilm. The obtained cell suspension was diluted, and various ten-fold serial dilutions were seeded on solid culture media plates in triplicate, to obtain and quantify the number of viable cells, expressed in colony-forming units (CFU)/mL.

2.7. In Vivo Biocompatibility Evaluation

2.7.1. Animals and Ethics

CD1 mice were housed in controlled-airflow cabinets with 12-h light cycles and constant temperature and humidity conditions. Animal experiments were performed in accordance with the guidelines of the Vasile Goldis Western University of Arad and approved by the Ethical Committee.

2.7.2. Experimental Design and Surgical Procedures

The mice were randomly assigned to 18 groups ($n = 5$): control, PET_2.5_ctrl, PET_5_ctrl, PET_7.5_ctrl, PET_10_ctrl, PET_2.5_NanoAg, PET_5_NanoAg, PET_7.5_NanoAg, and PET_10_NanoAg, for one day and seven days.

Before the experiment, the material samples (1 cm^2) were sterilized under UV light for 30 min (both faces) and implanted into a subcutaneous pocket in the dorsum of the animals. For the surgical procedure, the animals were anesthetized by intraperitoneal injection of xylazine/ketamine.

Animals were allowed to recover from anesthesia, housed in individual cages, and observed daily for evidence of wound complications, such as redness, infection, edema, abscess, hematoma, encapsulation, or skin dehiscence.

On days two and seven post-surgery, the animals were euthanatized by anesthetic overdose and the implanted materials, together with the surrounding tissues, were explanted and collected for analysis. Blood was sampled by cardiac puncture to assess acute inflammatory markers, in order to be able to exclude systemic inflammation.

2.7.3. Biochemical Analysis

Venous blood samples were centrifuged at 3500 rpm for 10 min and analyzed for C-reactive protein (CRP) levels, using the CRP FL (ChemaDiagnostica, Monsano, Italy) kit and a Mindray BS-120 Chemistry Analyzer (ShenzenMindray Bio-Medical Electronics Co., Ltd., Nanshan, Shenzhen, China).

2.7.4. Histopathological Analysis

For the histopathological study, explant samples were fixed in phosphate-buffered formaldehyde solution (4%, pH 7.2, 0.05 M), embedded in paraffin, sectioned at 5 µm, and stained with hematoxylin and eosin (H&E) and Gomori's trichrome kit (Leica Biosystems, 38016SS1, Nussloch, Germany).

Microscopic sections were analyzed with an Olympus BX43 microscope equipped with a digital camera Olympus XC30 and CellSense software and graded for the amount of tissue reaction.

Sections were scored on the degree of inflammatory infiltrate (including acute and chronic inflammatory cells), fibroblasts and neovascularization. Each histometric parameter was graded on a scale of 0–4 for the amount of tissue reaction: − (not present); sp (sporadic) to ++++ (extensive).

2.7.5. Immunohistochemistry

Immunohistochemical studies were performed on paraffin-embedded explant tissue sections of 5 nm thickness, previously deparaffinized and rehydrated using a standard technique. Rabbit polyclonal anti-tumor necrosis factor (TNF)-α diluted 1:100 (Santa Cruz, California) was used as a primary antibody.

Immunoreactions were visualized employing a Novocastra Peroxidase/DAB kit (Leica Biosystems, Nussloch, Germany), according to the manufacturer's instructions. Negative control sections were processed by the substitution of primary antibodies with irrelevant immunoglobulins of matched isotype used in the same conditions as primary antibodies. Stained slides were analyzed under bright-field microscopy.

2.8. Statistical Analysis

Experimental data were statistically evaluated using GraphPad Prism 3.03 software (GraphPad Software, Inc., La Jolla, CA, USA), and one-way analysis of variance, followed by a Bonferroni test. A p-value < 0.05 was considered to indicate a statistically significant difference.

3. Results

The electrospinning method was used to obtain nanostructured membranes from recycled PET. Different flow rates were used, and the resulted samples were noted according to each flow rate. These samples, prepared at four different flow rates, were further used in combination with silver nanoparticles in order to create alternative biomedical materials. A total of eight different samples were obtained, four with silver nanoparticles and four as controls for in vitro and in vivo tests.

3.1. Characterization of the Obtained Materials

Silver nanoparticles obtained through a silver nitrate reduction reaction were characterized by transmission electron microscopy. Figure 1 shows that the size of the obtained particles was in the nanoscale range, varying between 25 and 85 nm. The SAED pattern allowed the identification of the crystalline phases present in the sample, with NanoAg being the only crystalline phase.

Subsequently, NanoAg was characterized by X-ray diffraction. Figure 2 highlights the crystallinity of the synthesized nanoparticles, with the only identified crystalline phase being NanoAg through the four diffraction interferences characteristic of silver nanoparticles.

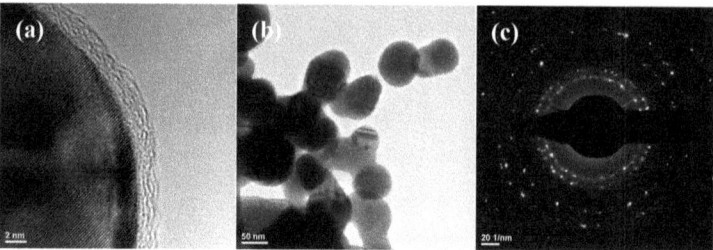

Figure 1. Transmission electron microscopy (TEM) images recorded for (**a**,**b**) silver nanoparticles (NanoAg) and selected area electron diffraction (SAED) pattern (**c**).

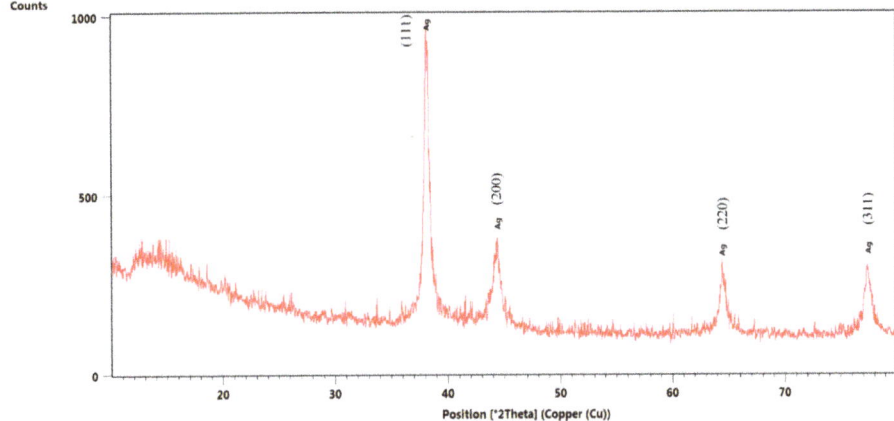

Figure 2. X-ray diffractogram recorded for NanoAg.

Infrared spectroscopy was used to evaluate the integrity of functional groups during post-processing by electrospinning. Figure 3 reveals that the four experimental variants did not show functional group degradation, absorption band movements, or significant intensity changes. The PET characteristic absorption bands can be identified as follows: 2961 cm^{-1} characteristic of the C–H bond, and 1714 cm^{-1} characteristic of the C=O group. Also, absorption bands of C–C and C–O bonds were observed in the molecular fingerprint area.

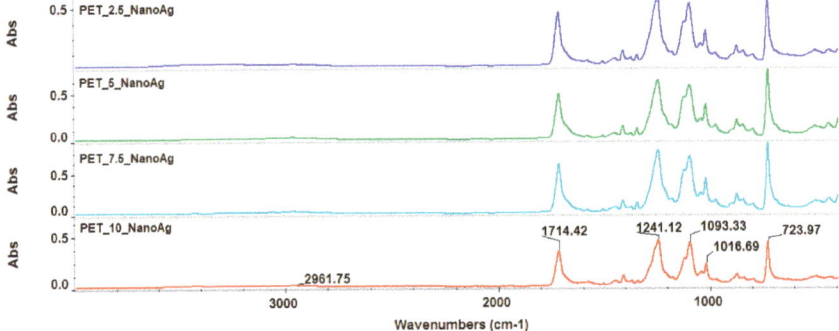

Figure 3. Fourier-transform infrared (FT-IR) spectra recorded for the silver-loaded polyethylene terephthalate (PET_X_NanoAg) samples.

Scanning electron microscopy allowed for the identification of the nanostructured membrane morphology and the presence of silver nanoparticles on the fiber surface. Figure 4 reveals the presence of an uneven deposition of silver nanoparticles on the surface of the fibrous membrane in all experimental variants. There was a general tendency of clumping at the nodes of the fibrous network, as the nodes acted as nucleation centers for nanoparticle growth.

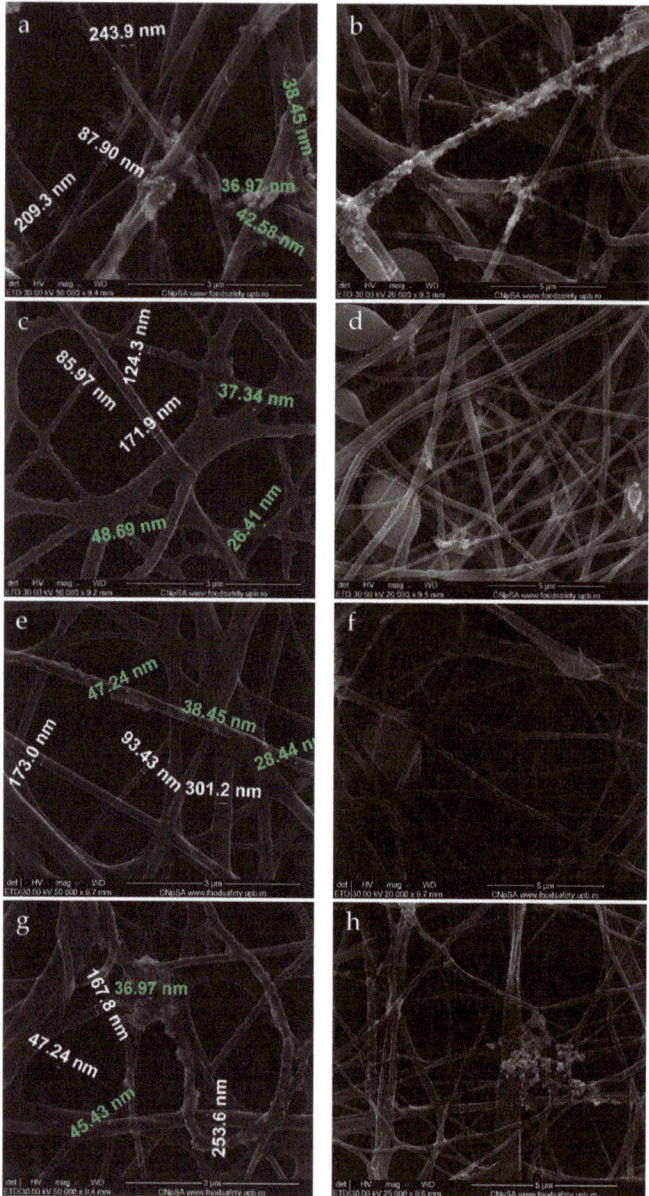

Figure 4. SEM images recorded for PET_X_NanoAg at various flows: (**a,b**) PET_2.5_NanoAg; (**c,d**) PET_5_NanoAg; (**e,f**) PET_7.5_NanoAg; (**g,h**) PET_10_NanoAg. Green text—dimensions for nanoAg; white text—dimensions for PET fibers.

The electrospun fibers had dimensions ranging between 60 and 250 nm, and the size of the silver particles on the surface of the fibers ranged between 8 and 50 nm. A more detailed representation of the PET_5_NanoAg is presented in Figure 5, highlighting the presence of silver nanoparticles agglomerating at the fiber nodes.

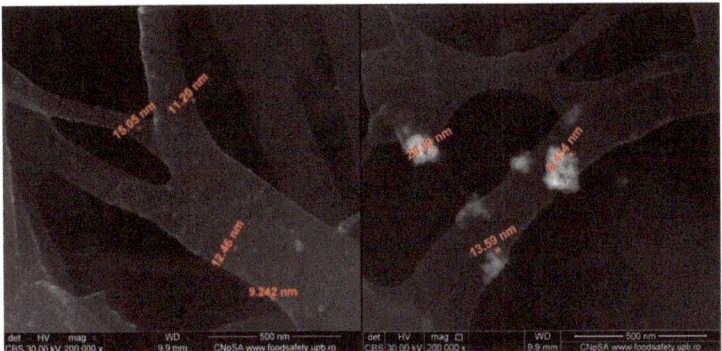

Figure 5. SEM images recorded in backscattering for PET_5_NanoAg.

The nanostructured membranes with modified surface obtained at a flow rate of 2.5 mL/h were also characterized by transmission electron microscopy (Figure 6), which highlighted the nanometric size of the silver particles and their dispersibility over the surface of the PET fibers.

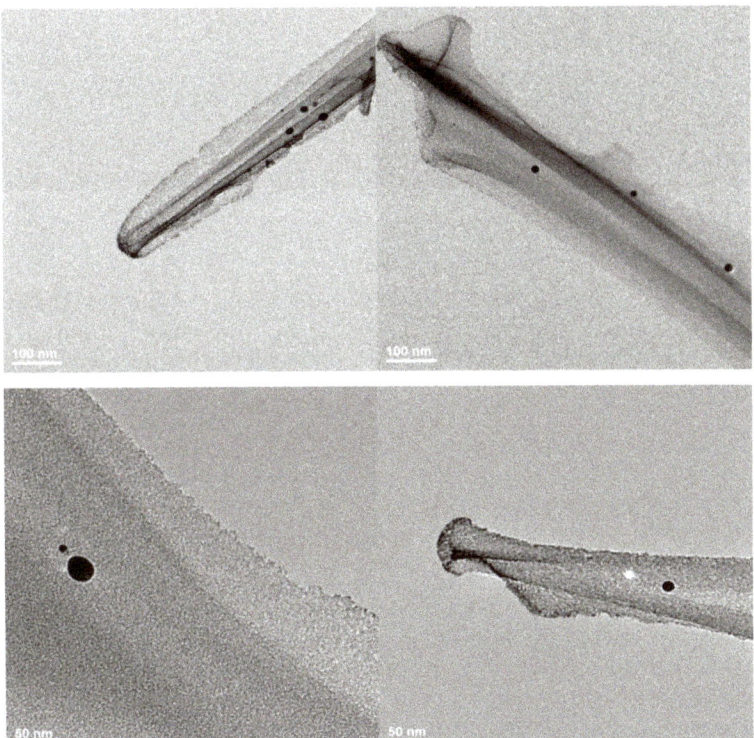

Figure 6. TEM images recorded for PET_2.5_NanoAg.

3.2. Antimicrobial Properties of the Prepared Samples

Contamination of the environment with undesired microorganisms has negative consequences in different fields, including human health. Microorganisms can grow planktonically, although a great majority of them are adherent to different interfaces and surfaces. Adherent microorganisms are more difficult to remove than microorganisms developing in the planktonic state, due to their ability to form specialized multicellular communities, called biofilms, in which cells may have a different behavior compared to planktonic ones, biochemically and genetically, rendering them more resilient to different stressors. Currently, alternative methods for limiting microbial colonization of raw materials and industrial installations, as well as of biomaterials intended for medical applications, are being studied [38].

In the majority of the experimental variants (except the assays on *C. albicans*), it can be seen that the highest inhibitory activities were obtained in PET samples for which the deposition of fibers by electrospinning was achieved at a flow rate of 10 or 7.5 mL/h (*p*-values ranged from 0–0.05 for *S. aureus* and *P. aeruginosa*).

From the three tested microbial strains, the recycled PET containing NanoAg nanoparticles proved to exhibit the best inhibitory effect on the planktonic growth of *S. aureus* (*p*-value was lower than 0.001), followed by *P. aeruginosa* (*p*-value was lower than 0.05), as compared with the NanoAg free controls (Figure 7).

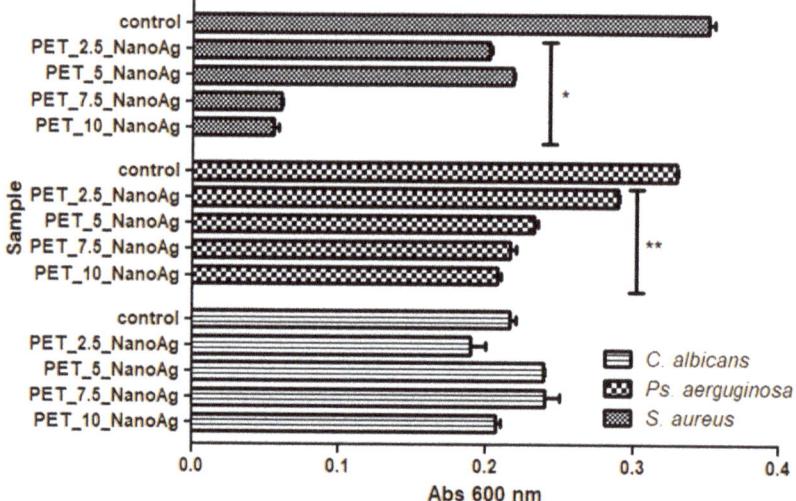

Figure 7. Graphic representation of the recorded absorbance values of *Staphylococcus aureus*, *Pseudomonas aeruginosa*, and *Candida albicans* cultures, expressing the multiplication capacity of these cells after cultivation for 24 h in the presence of recycled PET_X_NanoAg materials. * $p \leq 0.001$, ** $p \leq 0.05$ after the comparison of control with NanoAg-containing PET fibers obtained by applying various flow rates).

In the case of the *C. albicans* yeast strain, the inhibitory effect of the planktonic cultures was relatively low, in contrast with the antibacterial one; surprisingly, the most obvious inhibitory effect was observed for PET_2.5_NanoAg, but the result was not statistically significant.

In the case of the assessment of biofilm formation capacity, the results proved to be similar with the data obtained on planktonic cultures, with few variables.

The inhibition effect of *S. aureus* biofilm development was observed at all stages of biofilm development, starting with initial adherence (up to 24 h), continuing with biofilm maturation (up to 48 h) until dispersion (when cells or cell aggregates detach from the biofilm to colonize new surfaces) (Figure 8). The anti-biofilm effect was due to the decrease of viable cells embedded in the biofilm, by 1 to 4 logs, with these data being statistically significant (*p*-values ranged from 0.001–0.05). Similar to the results obtained on planktonic cells, the PET_7.5_NanoAg and PET_10_NanoAg samples also proved to be the most efficient in biofilm inhibition. It can be observed that the anti-biofilm efficiency decreases over the course of biofilm development. This inverse relationship is seen for all four samples, although it is more evident for PET_2.5_NanoAg and PET_5_NanoAg samples (Figure 8).

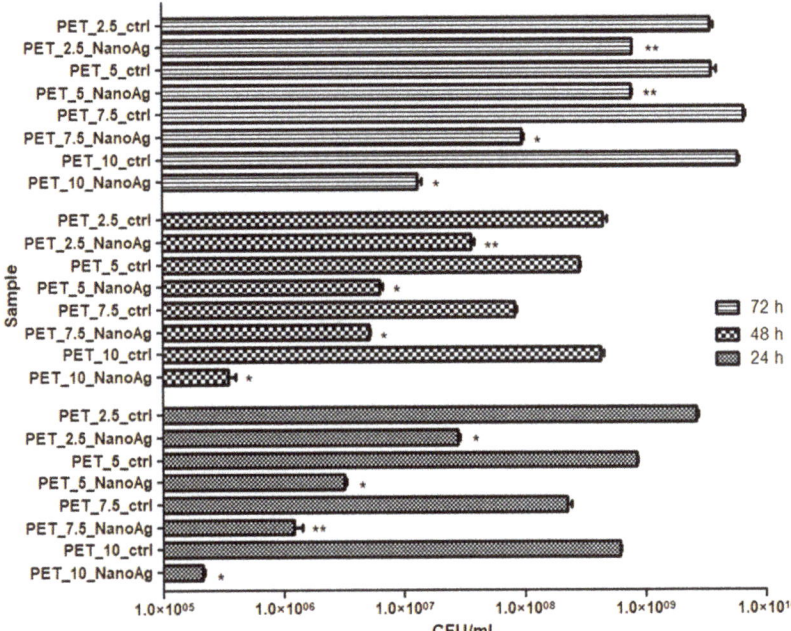

Figure 8. Graphic representation of colony-forming units (CFU)/mL representing the number of *S. aureus* viable cells included in the monospecific biofilms developed on the surface of the materials, quantified after 24 h, 48 h, and 72 h at 37 °C. * $p \leq 0.001$, ** $p \leq 0.05$ comparing control PET and NanoAg PET obtained at the same flow rate.

P. aeruginosa is a microorganism with multiple natural resistance mechanisms, making it an opportunistic pathogen that can colonize with maximum efficiency a great number of environments. Biofilms produced by this opportunistic microorganism are very difficult to eradicate with current antimicrobial substances [39]. The results obtained in this study showed that *P. aeruginosa* has a limited capacity to form biofilms on the obtained nanostructured membranes (Figure 9).

It must be noted that the PET_7.5_NanoAg and PET_10_NanoAg samples proved to be slightly more active against the biofilm formation in *P. aeruginosa*, as compared with the other tested variants. As revealed by Figure 9, the biofilm inhibition capacity of the obtained fibers was maintained relatively constant in all tested time conditions.

A poor capacity to form biofilms in the presence of the developed nanostructured membranes was observed not only for the bacterial strains, but also for the fungal *C. albicans* strain. In the case of the fungal strain, a dynamic of biofilm growth similar to that observed in case of the Gram-positive *S. aureus* strain was recorded, with an inverse relationship between the age of the biofilm and the intensity of the anti-biofilm effect. However, the efficiency of different tested samples was completely different from that obtained against the two bacterial strains, in the following order: PET_2.5_NanoAg > PET_5_NanoAg > PET_7.5_NanoAg > PET_10_NanoAg (Figure 10).

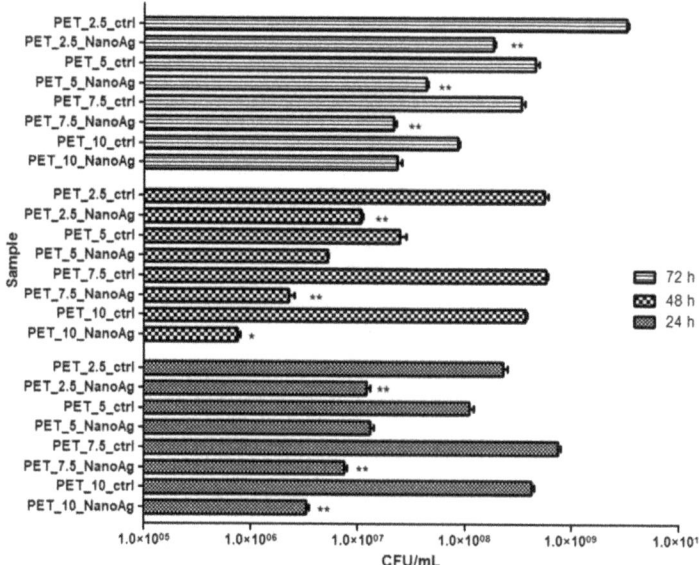

Figure 9. Graphic representation of CFU/mL, representing the number of *P. aeruginosa* viable cells included in the monospecific biofilms developed on the surface of the materials, quantified after 24 h, 48 h, and 72 h at 37 °C. * $p \leq 0.001$, ** $p \leq 0.05$ comparing control PET and NanoAg PET obtained at the same flow rate.

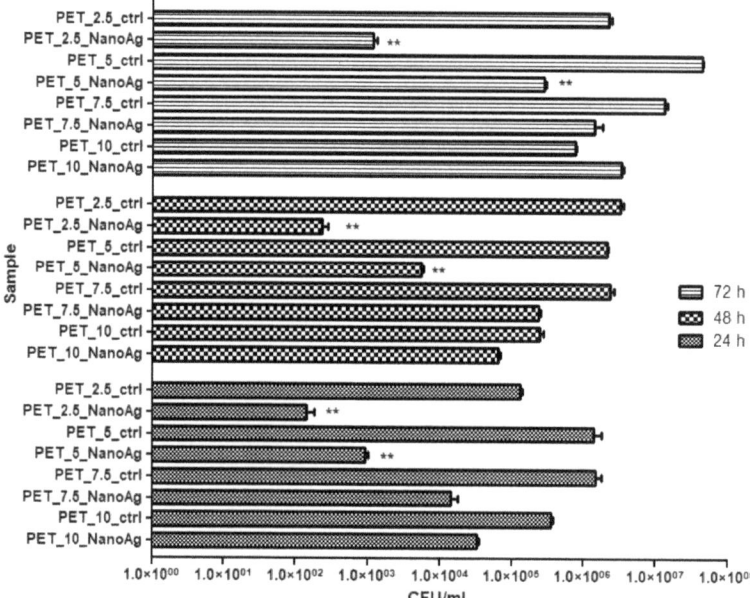

Figure 10. Graphic representation of CFU/mL representing the number of *C. albicans* cells viable cells included in the monospecific biofilms developed on the surface of the materials, quantified after 24 h, 48 h, and 72 h at 37 °C. * $p \leq 0.001$, ** $p \leq 0.05$ comparing control PET and NanoAg PET obtained at the same flow rate.

3.3. In Vitro and In Vivo Biological Response

3.3.1. In Vitro Biocompatibility

The cytotoxicity of recycled PET nanostructured membranes was analyzed using human diploid cells in culture. The results obtained by applying the MTT method showed that the proliferation and activity of diploid cells in the culture underwent changes in the presence of the analyzed materials, depending on the rate of deposition of the fibers by electrospinning; additionally, the majority of cases proved that the addition of NanoAg seemed to slightly reduce the cytotoxicity of the obtained materials, as compared with PET controls. However, these results had no statistical relevance (p-values were higher than 0.05).

The results obtained by applying the MTT assay revealed that a high percentage of the seeded cells remained metabolically active after covering with NanoAg, suggesting a good biocompatibility of the recycled PET containing NanoAg nanoparticles in vitro (Figure 11).

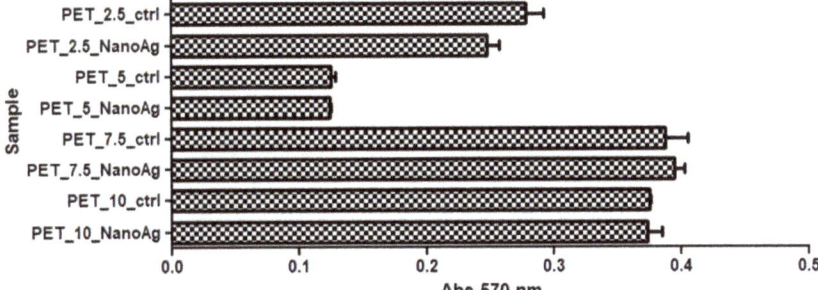

Figure 11. Effects of PET_X_NanoAg on MTT (3-(4,5-dimethylthiazolyl-2)-2,5-diphenyltetrazolium bromide) specific activities in amniotic fluid stem cells (AFSC).

3.3.2. In Vivo Biocompatibility and Inflammatory Response

The subcutaneous implant of the different nanofiber mats showed no adverse local or systemic inflammatory effects. CRP is an inflammation marker, which highlights the activation of a pro-inflammatory cascade. Figure 12 shows the effects of PET_X_NanoAg biomaterials implanted subcutaneously in mice on the CRP serum level. At 24 h post-implantation, the CRP blood level was elevated for all experimental groups, followed by a gradual decrease for up to seven days. Compared to the control ($p < 0.001$), PET_2.5_NanoAg induced significantly lower CRP levels at all time intervals. These results suggest that PET_X_NanoAg biomaterials are well tolerated by the body, and inflammation, together with other potential associated complications, which might lead to implant rejection, is avoided [40,41].

Histopathological analysis of the skin and subcutis of the control animals at days one and seven after implantation showed no significant pathological changes. Inflammatory infiltrate, necrosis, neovascularization, and fibrosis were not observed at either time point. After 24 h post-implantation, PET control samples induced significant edema at the implanting sites, which increased with the rate of fiber deposition. Assessment of inflammatory response revealed the presence of inflammatory cells, such as neutrophils, monocytes, lymphocytes, and macrophages. PET_X_NanoAg samples showed a decreased inflammatory reaction compared with PET-implanted samples at the same rate of electrospinning. In all implants, few eosinophils were noticed (Table 2).

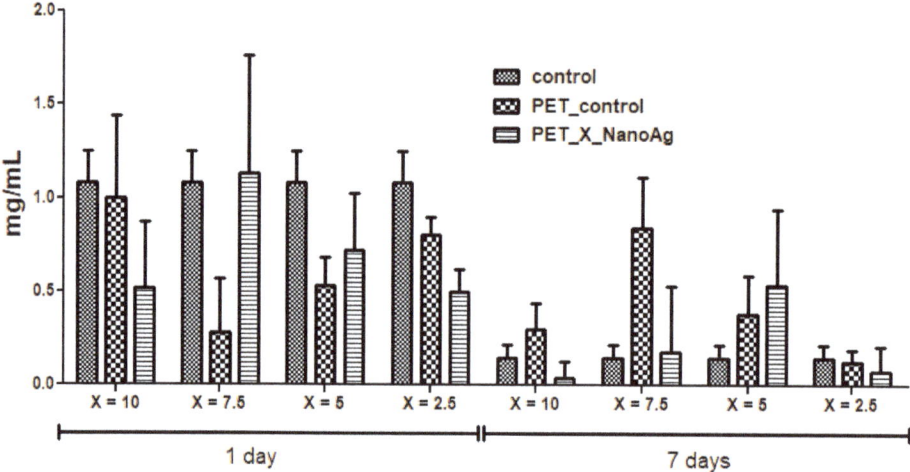

Figure 12. The effects of PET_X_NanoAg subcutaneous implantation in mice on the C-reactive protein (CRP) levels at 24 h and seven days post-surgery.

Table 2. Tissue reactions by histometric scoring used to grade inflammation, fibrosis, necrosis, and neovascularization in the tissue surrounding subcutaneous implants.

Nanofibers	Explan Tation (days)	Edema	PMN	MONO LYM	MO	GC	PC	EOS	FC	NV
Control mice	1	−	+	−	−	−	−	−	−	−
	7	−	−	+	+	−	−	−	−	−
PET_10_ctrl	1	++++	++++	+++	++	+	−	+	+	−
	7	+++	++	++++	++++	++	++	+	++++	−
PET_7.5_ctrl	1	+++	+++	+	+	+	+	+	+	−
	7	++	+	++	+++	++	+	+	+++	−
PET_5_ctrl	1	+	+++	sp	+	sp	−	+	+	−
	7	++	+	++	+++	+	+	+	++	−
PET_2.5_ctrl	1	+	+++	sp	+	sp	−	+	+	−
	7	++	+	++	+++	+	+	+	++	+
PET_10_NanoAg	1	−	+++	++	++	−	−	+	+	−
	7	−	+	+++	+++	−	+	+	+++	+
PET_7.5_NanoAg	1	−	++	sp	sp	−	+	+	+	−
	7	−	+	++	++	−	+	+	+++	+
PET_5_NanoAg	1	−	++	sp	+	−	−	+	+	−
	7	−	+	+	+++	−	+	+	++	+
PET_2.5_NanoAg	1	−	++	sp	+	−	−	+	+	−
	7	−	+	+	+	−	+	sp	+	++

PMN: polymorphonuclear neutrophils; MONO: monocytes; LYM: lymphocytes; EOS: eosinophils; MO: macrophages; PC: plasma cell; GC: giant cell; FC: fibrocytes, NV: neovascularization. Tissue reactions are rated from − (not present), and sp (sporadic) to ++++ (extensive).

On the seventh day post-implantation, the edema reaction persisting in high-purge-speed PET implants and a fibrous capsule of varying thickness were present in all PET-implanted tissue samples (57–76 μm). Consistent with a granulomatous reaction, mainly macrophages, plasma cells, monocytes, lymphocytes, and neutrophils were present at the interface between the mats and this capsule (Figure 13). Some of these macrophages showed marked evidence of phagocytic activity. Giant cells were observed in PET 10 and 7 mL/h samples.

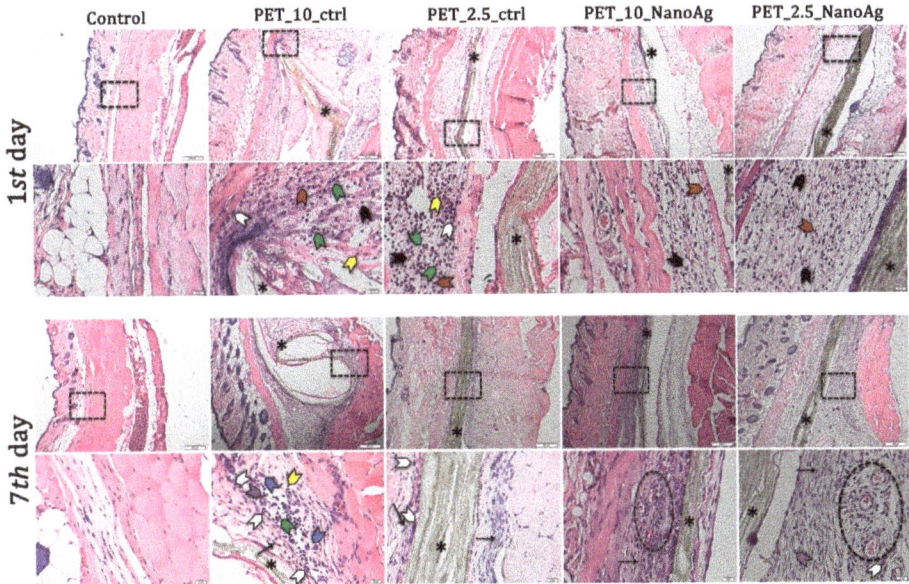

Figure 13. Representative histological images of PET_X_NanoAg mats-implanted sites in mice—days one and seven post-implantation. Neutrophils (black arrowhead); monocytes (green arrowhead); eosinophils (red arrowhead); macrophages (white arrowhead); plasma cells (purple arrowhead); giant cells (blue arrowhead); lymphocytes (yellow arrowhead); * implant (asterisk). Cells were stained with hematoxylin and eosin (H&E) stain. Scale bars = 200 and 20 μm.

The PET_X_NanoAg samples induced the occurrence of fibrotic capsules (35 and 40 μm) with purge speed with lower thickness as compared with PET in the same electrospinning conditions (Figure 14). Attached cells on the PET_X_NanoAg surface and extensive neovascularization of tissue surrounding the nanofiber mat were noticed.

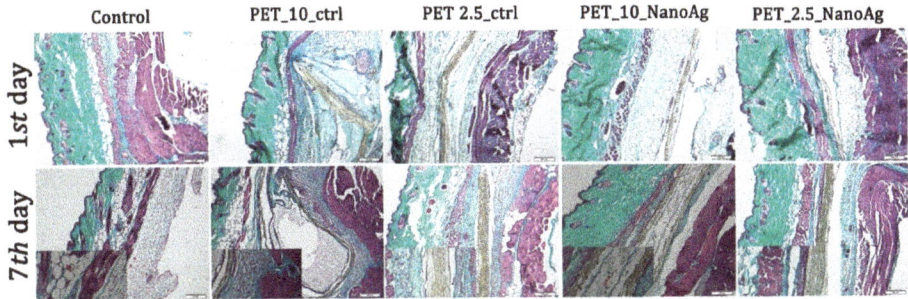

Figure 14. Gomori's trichrome stain of PET control and PET_X_NanoAg-implanted tissues.

Injection or implantation of a biomaterial results in an acute inflammation response, which is most often followed by a chronic inflammatory reaction [42], characterized by the infiltration of polymorphonuclear neutrophils (PMN), macrophages, and eventually lymphocytes [43]. The inflammatory reactions toward the novel in situ PET_X_NanoAg materials were weak, being within the limits of a typical, normal reaction to implanted materials characterized by the accumulation of the inflammatory cells on the materials surface. Similar responses were observed in the immediate post-implant period against other implanted materials with increased biocompatibility [44,45].

Implants with prolonged stay in the host tissue generally alter the tissue wound-healing response in chronic inflammatory conditions, producing fibrous encapsulation of the foreign body, with the presence of hallmark giant cells [46]. The fibrous capsule often isolates the implanted materials from normal host tissue sites, being characterized by poor vascularization and reduced bactericidal capability, predisposing these sites to infection [43]. Results from this study showed no well-defined collagen formation around implants in the case of PET_X_NanoAg after seven days post-implantation, a reaction comparable with that induced by other previously reported biocompatible materials [47,48].

Immunohistochemistry staining was performed for tissue sections to analyze the inflammatory response toward the implanted nanofibers (Figure 15). An increased immunopositivity for TNF-α levels on PET-implanted tissues, as compared to those obtained for the PET_X_NanoAg samples, was observed at both time points.

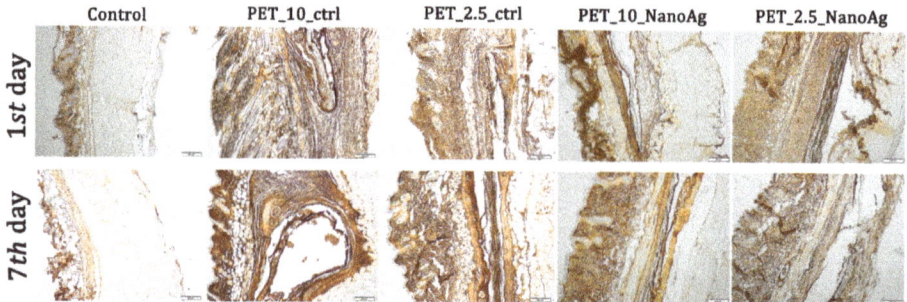

Figure 15. Expression and specific distribution of tumor necrosis factor (TNF)-α at implantation site at 24 h and seven days after implantation; scale bar = 200 μm.

The progression of events in inflammation and the foreign body response require the extravasation and migration of macrophages to the implant site, which produces and releases platelet-derived growth factor (PDGF), tumor necrosis factor (TNF-α), and interleukin-6 (IL-6) [43]. In our study, the NanoAg covering of PET materials reduced TNF-α expression and consequently reduced inflammation and foreign body response at the implantation site [49,50].

4. Discussion

This study focused on the development of antimicrobial fibrous networks consisting of PET materials through the electrospinning technique. With the various applications of electrospun networks, the addition of silver nanoparticles onto the surface of the fibers could potentially be implemented for antimicrobial purposes.

The mechanism of toxicity could be associated with the surface oxidation of the silver nanoparticles and the subsequent release of silver ions, or with the generation of reactive oxygen species and the consequent destabilization of the bacterial membrane [51]. Therefore, an advantage of this study is represented by the formation of the silver nanoparticles on the surface, compared to their direct encapsulation, which could considerably reduce their release. While the material characterization through the GIXRD and FT-IR techniques confirmed the formation of silver nanoparticles on the surface of the PET fibers, a tendency of nanoparticle agglomeration at the nodes was observed in the SEM images. Similar results were previously reported in the literature, either by grafting the nanoparticles on the plasma-treated PET [52] or by using the reduction method [53], and it was stated these clusters could be responsible for a slightly reduced antibacterial property [35,54]. In this regard, there are several solutions reported for enhancing the homogeneous distribution of the silver nanoparticles onto the surface of the fibers, such as sonochemical coating [55], plasma treatment of the silver nitrate-containing polymer solution [56], or chemically reducing the silver nitrate in the polymer matrix prior to the fiber fabrication. Moreover, it was previously reported in the literature that concentrations of silver nanoparticles as low as 0.05% can considerably reduce the incidence of surgery-related infections [57], with demonstrated bacteriostatic effects [58]. Studies reported that the effects of silver nanoparticles are strongly related to the size of the nanoparticles, with 10 nm being related to both the formation of silver ions during dissolution and the penetration of nanoparticles through the bacterial wall [59].

Furthermore, green synthesis methods could also be applied for the production of silver nanoparticles, thus avoiding the use of potentially toxic reducing agents. Examples of such agents can be found in the literature, most commonly involving chitosan [60] and other polysaccharides, plant extracts [61–63], or microbial extracts [64], all exhibiting enhanced antibacterial properties. In the present study, the investigated biomaterials proved to be efficient against the three types of bacteria, both in the planktonic and attached states, thus confirming their potential in anti-infective applications.

Despite their wide use as antimicrobial agents, silver nanoparticles are often associated with cytotoxic effects on the normal cells and have a tendency to accumulate in vital organs, such as the spleen, liver, kidney, and brain. Therefore, they must be considered "double-edged swords" for biomedical applications [65]. In this respect, silver nanoparticles are usually embedded in a composite matrix that has a significant role in controlling the release of the silver ions. In this study, the formation of silver nanoparticles on the surface of the PET biomaterials proved to reduce the cytotoxic effects of the uncoated materials determined by the MTT assay. Similarly, the in vivo biocompatibility tests demonstrated the anti-inflammatory potential of the NanoAg samples as compared to the PET samples, as fewer inflammatory cells were present at the implantation site in the former case. It could be hypothesized that the composite material could delay the release of the silver ions and, subsequently, the release of the pro-inflammatory factors, thus improving the potential for the long-term use of these biomaterials. This is in accordance with previous studies, which demonstrated foreign body reactions of PET materials, including commercial sutures for orthopedic purposes [66]. Additionally, there are studies suggesting the influence of the fiber size, mesh porosity, or contact surface, with one group reporting a minimum foreign body reaction of a PET mesh compared to the highly biocompatible bulk PET material [67].

This study could, therefore, represent a starting point for the development of antimicrobial membranes, which could be used as wound dressings or biomedical coatings, as they exhibit good antimicrobial properties and no inflammatory or cytotoxic effects.

5. Conclusions

The obtained membranes, composed of recycled PET nanofibers obtained by electrospinning at four different flow rates, decorated with silver nanoparticles, were characterized by GIXRD, FT-IR, SEM, TEM, and SAED. Results proved the formation of the silver nanoparticles on the surface of the fibers, with a slight tendency of agglomeration at the nodes. The dimensions of the fibers varied between 30 and 100 nm, while the silver nanoparticles ranged in size between 8 and 20 nm. Furthermore, the antimicrobial properties of the materials showed good antimicrobial and antibiofilm activity against Gram-positive and Gram-negative bacteria, as well as fungal strains. The biocompatibility tests were performed both in vitro, on human AFSC cells, and in vivo, through the subcutaneous implantation of the fibrous networks in CD1 mice. Results showed acceptable levels of toxicity in the in vitro and in vivo assays, with lower cytotoxic and inflammatory effects for the silver nanoparticle-decorated fibers. These results recommend the obtained materials for different antimicrobial applications, both in industry and in the biomedical field, opening promising new perspectives for the PET materials.

Author Contributions: A.M.G., A.H., M.C.C., A.F., B.S.V., and E.A. conceived and designed the experiments; A.E.S., M.-S.D.-B., performed the synthesis of PET fibers; A.F., A.E.S., M.-S.D.-B., A.M.G., and B.S.V. performed the physico-chemical characterization; A.M.H., C.C., and M.C.C. performed the in vitro experiments; S.G., C.B., M.R., H.H., and A.H. performed the in vivo experiments; all authors analyzed the obtained data; E.A., A.F., M.C.C., A.M.H., A.H., and C.C. wrote the paper.

Acknowledgments: This research was supported by the Executive Unit for Financing Higher Education, Research, Development and Innovation (UEFISCDI), by the National research grant no. 61/2018, project code: PN-III-P1-1.1-PD2016-0605, Romania.

Conflicts of Interest: The authors declare no conflicts of interest.

References

1. Lu, P.; Ding, B. Applications of electrospun fibers. *Recent Pat. Nanotechnol.* **2008**, *2*, 169–182. [CrossRef] [PubMed]
2. Naghibzadeh, M.; Firoozi, S.; Nodoushan, F.S.; Adabi, M.; Khoradmehr, A.; Fesahat, F.; Esnaashari, S.S.; Khosravani, M.; Adabi, M.; Tavakol, S.; et al. Application of electrospun gelatin nanofibers in tissue engineering. *Biointerface Res. Appl. Chem.* **2018**, *8*, 3048–3052.
3. Teleanu, R.I.; Gherasim, O.; Gherasim, T.G.; Grumezescu, V.; Grumezescu, A.M.; Teleanu, D.M. Nanomaterial-based approaches for neural regeneration. *Pharmaceutics* **2019**, *11*, 266. [CrossRef] [PubMed]
4. Huang, Z.-M.; Zhang, Y.Z.; Kotaki, M.; Ramakrishna, S. A review on polymer nanofibers by electrospinning and their applications in nanocomposites. *Compos. Sci. Technol.* **2003**, *63*, 2223–2253. [CrossRef]
5. Zhang, M.; Zhao, X.; Zhang, G.; Wei, G.; Su, Z. Electrospinning design of functional nanostructures for biosensor applications. *J. Mater. Chem. B* **2017**, *5*, 1699–1711. [CrossRef]
6. Shi, X.; Zhou, W.; Ma, D.; Ma, Q.; Bridges, D.; Ma, Y.; Hu, A. Electrospinning of nanofibers and their applications for energy devices. *J. Nanomater.* **2015**, *16*, 122. [CrossRef]
7. Ray, S.S.; Chen, S.-S.; Li, C.-W.; Nguyen, N.C.; Nguyen, H.T. A comprehensive review: Electrospinning technique for fabrication and surface modification of membranes for water treatment application. *RSC Adv.* **2016**, *6*, 85495–85514. [CrossRef]
8. Özçam, A.E.; Roskov, K.E.; Spontak, R.J.; Genzer, J. Generation of functional pet microfibers through surface-initiated polymerization. *J. Mater. Chem.* **2012**, *22*, 5855–5864. [CrossRef]
9. Mahendrasingam, A.; Martin, C.; Fuller, W.; Blundell, D.J.; Oldman, R.J.; MacKerron, D.H.; Harvie, J.L.; Riekel, C. Observation of a transient structure prior to strain-induced crystallization in poly(ethylene terephthalate). *Polymer* **2000**, *41*, 1217–1221. [CrossRef]
10. Monier, M.; Abdel-Latif, D. Synthesis and characterization of ion-imprinted chelating fibers based on pet for selective removal of hg^{2+}. *Chem. Eng. J.* **2013**, *122*, 452–460. [CrossRef]
11. Ma, Z.; Kotaki, M.; Yong, T.; He, W.; Ramakrishna, S. Surface engineering of electrospun polyethylene terephthalate (pet) nanofibers towards development of a new material for blood vessel engineering. *Biomaterials* **2005**, *26*, 2527–2536. [CrossRef] [PubMed]
12. Wang, C.; Li, Y.; Ding, G.; Xie, X.; Jiang, M. Preparation and characterization of graphene oxide/poly(vinyl alcohol) composite nanofibers via electrospinning. *J. Appl. Polym. Sci.* **2013**, *127*, 3026–3032. [CrossRef]
13. Huang, J.; Liu, Y.; You, T. Carbon nanofiber based electrochemical biosensors: A review. *Anal. Methods* **2010**, *2*, 202–211. [CrossRef]
14. Klinge, U.; Park, J.-K.; Klosterhalfen, B. The ideal mesh. *Pathobiology* **2013**, *80*, 169–175. [CrossRef] [PubMed]
15. Longo, U.G.; Lamberti, A.; Maffulli, N.; Denaro, V. Tendon augmentation grafts: A systematic review. *Br. Med. Bull.* **2010**, *94*, 165–188. [CrossRef] [PubMed]
16. Kannan, R.Y.; Salacinski, H.J.; Butler, P.E.; Hamilton, G.; Seifalian, A.M. Current status of prosthetic bypass grafts: A review. *J. Biomed. Mater. Res. Part B Appl. Biomater.* **2005**, *74*, 570–581. [CrossRef] [PubMed]
17. Mansour, S.H.; Ikladious, N.E. Depolymerization of poly(ethylene terephthalate) waste using 1,4-butanediol and triethylene glycol. *J. Elastomers Plast.* **2003**, *35*, 133–148. [CrossRef]
18. Abbas, J.A.; Said, I.A.; Mohamed, M.A.; Yasin, S.A.; Ali, Z.A.; Ahmed, I.H. Electrospinning of polyethylene terephthalate (pet) nanofibers: Optimization study using taguchi design of experiment. *IOP Conf. Ser. Mater. Sci. Eng.* **2018**, *454*, 012130. [CrossRef]
19. Esmaeili, E.; Deymeh, F.; Rounaghi, S.A. Synthesis and characterization of the electrospun fibers prepared from waste polymeric materials. *Int. J. Nano Dimens.* **2017**, *8*, 171–181.
20. Zander, N.E.; Gillan, M.; Sweetser, D. Recycled pet nanofibers for water filtration applications. *Materials* **2016**, *9*, 247. [CrossRef]

21. Sereshti, H.; Amini, F.; Najarzadekan, H. Electrospun polyethylene terephthalate (pet) nanofibers as a new adsorbent for micro-solid phase extraction of chromium(vi) in environmental water samples. *RSC Adv.* **2015**, *5*, 89195–89203. [CrossRef]
22. Jhass, P.; Siaw-Sakyi, V.; Wild, T. Wound infection risk evaluation—A new prediction score—Wire. *Wound Med.* **2017**, *16*, 34–39. [CrossRef]
23. Ditaranto, N.; Basoli, F.; Trombetta, M.; Cioffi, N.; Rainer, A. Electrospun nanomaterials implementing antibacterial inorganic nanophases. *Appl. Sci.* **2018**, *8*, 1643. [CrossRef]
24. Armentano, I.; Arciola, C.R.; Fortunati, E.; Ferrari, D.; Mattioli, S.; Amoroso, C.F.; Rizzo, J.; Kenny, J.M.; Imbriani, M.; Visai, L. The interaction of bacteria with engineered nanostructured polymeric materials: A review. *Sci. World J.* **2014**, *2014*, 410423. [CrossRef] [PubMed]
25. Bahrami, M.K.; Movafeghi, A.; Mahdavinia, G.R.; Hassanpouraghdam, M.B.; Gohari, G. Effects of bare and chitosan-coated Fe_3O_4 magnetic nanoparticles on seed germination and seedling growth of capsicum annuum L. *Res. Appl. Chem.* **2018**, *8*, 3552–3559.
26. Narasaiah, B.P.; Mandal, B.K.; Chakravarthula, S.N. Mitigation of textile industries generated pollution by agro-waste cotton peels mediated synthesized silver nanoparticles. *Biointerface Res. Appl. Chem.* **2018**, *8*, 3602–3610.
27. Sabry, N.M.; Tolba, S.; Abdel-Gawad, F.K.; Bassem, S.M.; Nassar, H.F.; El-Taweel, G.E.; Okasha, A.; Ibrahim, M. Interaction between nano silver and bacteria: Modeling approach. *Biointerface Res. Appl. Chem.* **2018**, *8*, 3570–3574.
28. Samoilova, N.A.; Krayukhina, M.A.; Popov, D.A.; Anuchina, N.M.; Piskarev, V.E. 3′-sialyllactose-decorated silver nanoparticles: Lectin binding and bactericidal properties. *Biointerface Res. Appl. Chem.* **2018**, *8*, 3095–3099.
29. Teleanu, D.M.; Chircov, C.; Grumezescu, A.M.; Teleanu, R.I. Neurotoxicity of nanomaterials: An up-to-date overview. *Nanomaterials* **2019**, *9*, 96. [CrossRef]
30. Teleanu, D.M.; Chircov, C.; Grumezescu, A.M.; Volceanov, A.; Teleanu, R.I. Impact of nanoparticles on brain health: An up to date overview. *J. Clin. Med.* **2018**, *7*, 490. [CrossRef]
31. Wan, Y.Z.; Raman, S.; He, F.; Huang, Y. Surface modification of medical metals by ion implantation of silver and copper. *Vacuum* **2007**, *81*, 1114–1118. [CrossRef]
32. You, C.; Han, C.; Wang, X.; Zheng, Y.; Li, Q.; Hu, X.; Sun, H. The progress of silver nanoparticles in the antibacterial mechanism, clinical application and cytotoxicity. *Mol. Biol. Rep.* **2012**, *39*, 9193–9201. [CrossRef]
33. Sharma, N.; Phutela, K.; Goel, A.; Soni, S.; Batra, N. Exploring the bacterial based silver nanoparticle for their possible application as disinfectants. *Biointerface Res. Appl. Chem.* **2018**, *8*, 3100–3104.
34. Choi, O.; Deng, K.K.; Kim, N.J.; Ross, L., Jr.; Surampalli, R.Y.; Hu, Z. The inhibitory effects of silver nanoparticles, silver ions, and silver chloride colloids on microbial growth. *Water Res.* **2008**, *42*, 3066–3074. [CrossRef] [PubMed]
35. Song, K.; Wu, Q.; Qi, Y.; Kärki, T. 20-electrospun nanofibers with antimicrobial properties. In *Electrospun Nanofibers*; Afshari, M., Ed.; Woodhead Publishing: Sawston, UK, 2017; pp. 551–569.
36. Zargham, S.; Bazgir, S.; Tavakoli, A.; Rashidi, A.S.; Damerchely, R. The effect of flow rate on morphology and deposition area of electrospun nylon 6 nanofiber. *J. Eng. Fibers Fabr.* **2012**, *7*. [CrossRef]
37. Bakar, S.S.S.; Fong, K.C.; Eleyas, A.; Nazeri, M.F.M. Effect of voltage and flow rate electrospinning parameters on polyacrylonitrile electrospun fibers. *IOP Conf. Ser. Mater. Sci. Eng.* **2018**, *318*, 012076. [CrossRef]
38. Khelissa, O.; Abdallah, M.; Jama, C.; Faille, C.; Chihib, N.-E. Bacterial contamination and biofilm formation on abiotic surfaces and strategies to overcome their persistence. *J. Mater. Environ. Sci.* **2017**, *8*, 3326–3346.
39. Sadikot, R.T.; Blackwell, T.S.; Christman, J.W.; Prince, A.S. Pathogen-host interactions in pseudomonas aeruginosa pneumonia. *Am. J. Respir. Crit. Care Med.* **2005**, *171*, 1209–1223. [CrossRef]
40. Balta, C.; Herman, H.; Rosu, M.; Cotoraci, C.; Ivan, A.; Folk, A.; Duka, R.; Dinescu, S.; Costache, M.; Alexandru, P.; et al. Homeostasis of blood parameters and inflammatory markers analysis during bone defect healing after scaffolds implantation in mice calvaria defects. *Rom. Biotechnol. Lett.* **2016**, *22*, 12018–12025.
41. Romero-Gavilan, F.; Sanchez-Perez, A.M.; Araujo-Gomes, N.; Azkargorta, M.; Iloro, I.; Elortza, F.; Gurruchaga, M.; Goni, I.; Suay, J. Proteomic analysis of silica hybrid sol-gel coatings: A potential tool for predicting the biocompatibility of implants in vivo. *Biofouling* **2017**, *33*, 676–689. [CrossRef]
42. Ratner, B.D. *The Biocompatibility of Implant Materials*; Elsevier: Amsterdam, The Netherlands, 2015; pp. 37–51.

43. Anderson, J.M.; Rodriguez, A.; Chang, D.T. Foreign body reaction to biomaterials. *Semin. Immunol.* **2008**, *20*, 86–100. [CrossRef] [PubMed]
44. Bos, G.W.; Hennink, W.E.; Brouwer, L.A.; den Otter, W.; Veldhuis, T.F.J.; van Nostrum, C.F.; van Luyn, M.J.A. Tissue reactions of in situ formed dextran hydrogels crosslinked by stereocomplex formation after subcutaneous implantation in rats. *Biomaterials* **2005**, *26*, 3901–3909. [CrossRef] [PubMed]
45. Wilson, J.T.; Cui, W.; Sun, X.-L.; Tucker-Burden, C.; Weber, C.J.; Chaikof, E.L. In vivo biocompatibility and stability of a substrate-supported polymerizable membrane-mimetic film. *Biomaterials* **2007**, *28*, 609–617. [CrossRef] [PubMed]
46. Jay, S.M.; Skokos, E.A.; Zeng, J.; Knox, K.; Kyriakides, T.R. Macrophage fusion leading to foreign body giant cell formation persists under phagocytic stimulation by microspheres in vitro and in vivo in mouse models. *J. Biomed. Mater. Res. Part A* **2010**, *93*, 189–199.
47. Avula, M.N.; Rao, A.N.; McGill, L.D.; Grainger, D.W.; Solzbacher, F. Foreign body response to subcutaneous biomaterial implants in a mast cell-deficient kit(w-sh) murine model. *Acta Biomater.* **2014**, *10*, 1856–1863. [CrossRef] [PubMed]
48. Hermenean, A.; Codreanu, A.; Herman, H.; Balta, C.; Rosu, M.; Mihali, C.-V.; Ivan, A.; Dinescu, S.; Ionita, M.; Costache, M. Chitosan-Graphene oxide 3d scaffolds as promising tools for bone regeneration in critical-size mouse calvarial defects. *Sci. Rep.* **2017**, *7*, 16641. [CrossRef] [PubMed]
49. Chandorkar, Y.; Bhaskar, N.; Madras, G.; Basu, B. Long-term sustained release of salicylic acid from cross-linked biodegradable polyester induces a reduced foreign body response in mice. *Biomacromolecules* **2015**, *16*, 636–649. [CrossRef] [PubMed]
50. Sumayya, A.S.; Muraleedhara Kurup, G. Biocompatibility of subcutaneously implanted marine macromolecules cross-linked bio-composite scaffold for cartilage tissue engineering applications. *J. Biomater. Sci. Polym. Ed.* **2018**, *29*, 257–276. [CrossRef] [PubMed]
51. De Faria, A.F.; Perreault, F.; Shaulsky, E.; Arias Chavez, L.H.; Elimelech, M. Antimicrobial electrospun biopolymer nanofiber mats functionalized with graphene oxide–silver nanocomposites. *ACS Appl. Mater. Interfaces* **2015**, *7*, 12751–12759. [CrossRef]
52. Reznickova, A.; Novotna, Z.; Kolska, Z.; Svorcik, V. Immobilization of silver nanoparticles on polyethylene terephthalate. *Nanoscale Res. Lett.* **2014**, *9*, 305. [CrossRef] [PubMed]
53. Liu, K.-G.; Abbasi, A.R.; Azadbakht, A.; Hu, M.-L.; Morsali, A. Deposition of silver nanoparticles on polyester fiber under ultrasound irradiations. *Ultrason. Sonochemistry* **2017**, *34*, 13–18. [CrossRef] [PubMed]
54. Park, S.-W.; Bae, H.-S.; Xing, Z.; Kwon, O.H.; Huh, M.; Kang, I.-K. Preparation and properties of silver-containing nylon 6 nanofibers formed by electrospinning. *J. Appl. Polym. Sci.* **2009**, *112*, 2320–2326. [CrossRef]
55. Perelshtein, I.; Applerot, G.; Perkas, N.; Guibert, G.; Mikhailov, S.; Gedanken, A. Sonochemical coating of silver nanoparticles on textile fabrics (nylon, polyester and cotton) and their antibacterial activity. *Nanotechnology* **2008**, *19*, 245705. [CrossRef] [PubMed]
56. Shi, Q.; Vitchuli, N.; Nowak, J.; Caldwell, J.M.; Breidt, F.; Bourham, M.; Zhang, X.; McCord, M. Durable antibacterial ag/polyacrylonitrile (ag/pan) hybrid nanofibers prepared by atmospheric plasma treatment and electrospinning. *Eur. Polym. J.* **2011**, *47*, 1402–1409. [CrossRef]
57. Wang, L.; Hu, C.; Shao, L. The antimicrobial activity of nanoparticles: Present situation and prospects for the future. *Int. J. Nanomed.* **2017**, *12*, 1227–1249. [CrossRef]
58. Maiti, S.; Krishnan, D.; Barman, G.; Ghosh, S.K.; Laha, J.K. Antimicrobial activities of silver nanoparticles synthesized from lycopersicon esculentum extract. *J. Anal. Sci. Technol.* **2014**, *5*, 40. [CrossRef]
59. Kubyshkin, A.; Chegodar, D.; Katsev, A.; Petrosyan, A.; Krivorutchenko, Y.; Postnikova, O. Antimicrobial effects of silver nanoparticles stabilized in solution by sodium alginate. *Biochem. Mol. Biol. J.* **2016**, *2*, 13. [CrossRef]
60. Hasan, K.M.F.; Pervez, M.N.; Talukder, M.E.; Sultana, M.Z.; Mahmud, S.; Meraz, M.M.; Bansal, V.; Genyang, C. A novel coloration of polyester fabric through green silver nanoparticles (g-agnps@pet). *Nanomaterials* **2019**, *9*, 569. [CrossRef]
61. Behravan, M.; Hossein Panahi, A.; Naghizadeh, A.; Ziaee, M.; Mahdavi, R.; Mirzapour, A. Facile green synthesis of silver nanoparticles using berberis vulgaris leaf and root aqueous extract and its antibacterial activity. *Int. J. Biol. Macromol.* **2019**, *124*, 148–154. [CrossRef]

62. Yasir, M.; Singh, J.; Tripathi, M.K.; Singh, P.; Shrivastava, R. Green synthesis of silver nanoparticles using leaf extract of common arrowhead houseplant and its anticandidal activity. *Pharm. Mag.* **2017**, *13*, S840–S844.
63. Sanchez-Navarro, M.d.C.; Ruiz-Torres, C.A.; Nino-Martinez, N.; Sanchez-Sanchez, R.; Martinez-Castanon, G.A.; DeAlba-Montero, I.; Ruiz, F. Cytotoxic and bactericidal effect of silver nanoparticles obtained by green synthesis method using annona muricata aqueous extract and functionalized with 5-fluorouracil. *Bioinorg. Chem. Appl.* **2018**, *2018*, 6506381. [CrossRef] [PubMed]
64. Rudakiya, D.M.; Pawar, K. Bactericidal potential of silver nanoparticles synthesized using cell-free extract of comamonas acidovorans: In vitro and in silico approaches. *3 Biotech* **2017**, *7*, 92. [CrossRef] [PubMed]
65. Liao, C.; Li, Y.; Tjong, S.C. Bactericidal and cytotoxic properties of silver nanoparticles. *Int. J. Mol. Sci.* **2019**, *20*, 449. [CrossRef] [PubMed]
66. Lovric, V.; Goldberg, M.J.; Heuberer, P.R.; Oliver, R.A.; Stone, D.; Laky, B.; Page, R.S.; Walsh, W.R. Suture wear particles cause a significant inflammatory response in a murine synovial airpouch model. *J. Orthop. Surg. Res.* **2018**, *13*, 311. [CrossRef] [PubMed]
67. Veleirinho, B.; Coelho, D.S.; Dias, P.F.; Maraschin, M.; Pinto, R.; Cargnin-Ferreira, E.; Peixoto, A.; Souza, J.A.; Ribeiro-do-Valle, R.M.; Lopes-da-Silva, J.A. Foreign body reaction associated with pet and pet/chitosan electrospun nanofibrous abdominal meshes. *PLoS ONE* **2014**, *9*, e95293. [CrossRef] [PubMed]

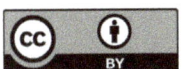

© 2019 by the authors. Licensee MDPI, Basel, Switzerland. This article is an open access article distributed under the terms and conditions of the Creative Commons Attribution (CC BY) license (http://creativecommons.org/licenses/by/4.0/).

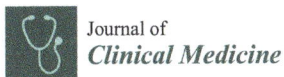

Article

"To Be Microbiocidal and Not to Be Cytotoxic at the Same Time . . . "—Silver Nanoparticles and Their Main Role on the Surface of Titanium Alloy Implants

Aleksandra Radtke [1,2,*], Marlena Grodzicka [1,2], Michalina Ehlert [1,2], Tomasz Jędrzejewski [3], Magdalena Wypij [3] and Patrycja Golińska [3]

1. Faculty of Chemistry, Nicolaus Copernicus University in Toruń, Gagarina 7, 87-100 Toruń, Poland; Marlena.Grodzicka@doktorant.umk.pl (M.G.); m.ehlert@doktorant.umk.pl (M.E.)
2. Nano-implant Ltd., Gagarina 5/102, 87-100 Toruń, Poland
3. Faculty of Biology and Environmental Protection, Nicolaus Copernicus University in Toruń, Lwowska 1, 87-100 Toruń, Poland; tomaszj@umk.pl (T.J.); mwypij@umk.pl (M.W.); golinska@umk.pl (P.G.)
* Correspondence: aradtke@umk.pl; Tel.: +48-600-321-294

Received: 10 February 2019; Accepted: 4 March 2019; Published: 10 March 2019

Abstract: The chemical vapor deposition (CVD) method has been used to produce dispersed silver nanoparticles (AgNPs) on the surface of titanium alloy (Ti6Al4V) and nanotubular modified titanium alloys (Ti6Al4V/TNT5), leading to the formation of Ti6Al4V/AgNPs and Ti6Al4V/TNT5/AgNPs systems with different contents of metallic silver particles. Their surface morphology and silver particles arrangement were characterized by scanning electron microscopy (SEM), energy dispersive X-ray spectrometry (EDS), and atomic force microscopy (AFM). The wettability and surface free energy of these materials were investigated on the basis of contact angle measurements. The degree of silver ion release from the surface of the studied systems immersed in phosphate buffered saline solution (PBS) was estimated using inductively coupled plasma ionization mass spectrometry (ICP-MS). The biocompatibility of the analyzed materials was estimated based on the fibroblasts and osteoblasts adhesion and proliferation, while their microbiocidal properties were determined against Gram-positive and Gram-negative bacteria, and yeasts. The results of our works proved the high antimicrobial activity and biocompatibility of all the studied systems. Among them, Ti6Al4V/TNT5/0.6AgNPs contained the lowest amount of AgNPs, but still revealed optimal biointegration properties and high biocidal properties. This is the biomaterial that possesses the desired biological properties, in which the potential toxicity is minimized by minimizing the number of silver nanoparticles.

Keywords: silver nanoparticles; titanium alloy; titanium dioxide nanotubes; silver ions release; biointegration; antimicrobial activity

1. Introduction

Silver as an antibacterial agent was known and applied in antiquity [1–3], but its wide use in different fields of our contemporary life is a result of more and more detailed studies on the mechanisms of Ag antimicrobial activity [4–6]. Moreover, the development of modern technologies, which allow for the production of silver nanoparticles (AgNPs) of different sizes, shapes, and properties, is of great importance [7–9]. The bactericidal and fungicidal activity of AgNPs has not been fully explained yet, but the three most probable mechanisms are proposed [10–13]. The first of them assumes the capture of free silver ions, which interferes with ATP production and DNA replication. The second one assumes the generation of reactive oxygen species (ROS) by nanoparticles and silver ions. The produced ROS may also have an adverse effect on DNA, the cell membrane and the membrane proteins [14]. The third mechanism takes into consideration the damage of the bacteria cell membrane as a result of its direct contact with AgNPs. In this case, silver nanoparticles joining the proteins of the cell membrane through the connection with sulfur cause a change in its structure [13,15–18]. Extensive use of silver nanoparticles, especially in medicine, forces us to think about the potential toxicity of silver to the human body. In some cases, nanoparticles may be toxic for human organisms and the prolonged use of specimens containing silver may cause argyria [19,20]. The potential risk of AgNPs lies in their ability to bioaccumulation in the body [21]. The harmful effects of nanosilver on human cells act according to similar mechanisms, which was mentioned earlier for bacteria. AgNPs accumulate outside the mitochondria, leading to ROS production, which causes mitochondrial damage and interruption of ATP synthesis. Moreover, the interaction of nanosilver with DNA leads to cell cycle stopping [22–25]. The analysis of previous reports exhibited that the potential toxicity of silver nanoparticles to the human body depends on their size and shape. According to these data, nanoparticles of a diameter smaller than 25 nm and a silver concentration higher than 60 mg/L are considered to be cytotoxic to mammalian cells. Simultaneously, it should be noted that a harmful effect of ionic silver on eukaryotic organisms was noticed at a concentration of 1 mg/L [26,27]. On the other hand, the increase of the AgNPs diameter above 25 nm caused these nanoparticles to be toxic mainly to microorganisms and not harmful to the human body [28,29]. Particles of such sizes are used in different technologies, in which the necessity of a bacteria-free environment exists. One of the interesting directions in the using of AgNPs is combining them with other materials, e.g., polymeric or ceramic ones, in order to form nanocomposites of unique physicochemical properties and bioactivity [30–32]. This approach is developed by us in the design and fabrication of new generation surgical titanium/titanium alloy implants, whose surface is enriched with AgNPs as the anti-inflammatory factor [33,34]. To avoid the inflammation effect after implantation, we enriched the titanium alloy implants' surface with dispersed silver nanoparticles of appropriate diameters using the chemical vapor deposition (CVD) or atomic layer deposition (ALD) techniques. The monitoring of the influence of silver nanoparticles on the adhesion and proliferation of fibroblasts on the implant surface revealed the very diverse biointegration properties of AgNPs-enriched surfaces [35,36]. It should be noted that in our work, two types of Ti6Al4V implants surface were studied, i.e., pure metallic implants and implants with a surface modified by the titania nanotube coating. Analysis of the results of our earlier works revealed that the different surface properties of the tested implants influence the different AgNPs deposition courses and, thereby, their different bioactivities.

Therefore, determining the direct impact of the deposited silver nanoparticles amount, the form in which they act and their size on their biointegration properties and antimicrobial activity is an important issue. Such an analysis is crucial for the production of implants with a surface, which will be microbiocidal enough but at the same time, optimally biointegral. For this purpose, the surfaces of Ti6Al4V and Ti6Al4V/TNT substrates were coated with different amounts of silver using the CVD technique. This technique enables for the deposition of pure silver nanoparticles on the surface of substrates with complex shapes [37]. We set ourselves the goal of enriching the surface of the titanium alloy implant (non-modified and nanotubular modified) with the smallest number of silver nanoparticles, which will have high antimicrobial properties, and which will not interfere with the adhesion and proliferation of fibroblasts and osteoblasts. We wanted, in this way, to create a biomaterial with the desired bioactivity (microbiocidal and biocompatible), minimizing the number of silver precursor used in the CVD process, thereby minimizing the number of silver nanoparticles on the surface of the layer and minimizing the potential silver toxicity. The results of our works are discussed in this paper.

2. Materials and Methods

2.1. Substrates

In all our experiments, the Ti6Al4V foil (grade 5, 99.7% purity, 0.20 mm thick (Strem Chemicals, Inc., Bischheim, France), 7 mm × 7 mm pieces) was used as a substrate. Before the anodization process, the Ti6Al4V foil samples were polished with sandpaper; cleaned by ultrasonication for 15 min in acetone, ethanol, and distilled water; and dried in an argon stream. Then the samples were chemically etched in a 1:4:5 mixture of $HF:HNO_3:H_2O$ for 30 s, rinsed in deionized water and dried in an argon stream. The Ti6Al4V/TNT5 systems were produced using the electrochemical oxidation method in accordance with the previously described procedures [38]. The uniform TNT5 coatings were produced on the surface of Ti6Al4V substrates using a potential of U = 5 V at room temperature (RT) and at an anodization time t = 20 min. After anodization, all the produced Ti6Al4V/TNT5 samples were washed in deionized water (10 min in an ultrasonic bath) and then their surfaces were drying in a stream of argon at RT and additionally dried at 123 °C. The morphology of the produced coatings was studied using a Quanta scanning electron microscope with field emission (SEM, Quanta 3D FEG, Huston, TX, USA).

2.2. Chemical Vapor Deposition of Silver Nanoparticles (AgNPs)

The Ti6Al4V and Ti6Al4V/TNT5 samples were enriched with the AgNPs using the CVD technique, under conditions given in Table 1. $Ag_5(O_2CC_2F_5)_5(H_2O)_3$ has been used as a metallic silver CVD precursor. Its synthesis and physicochemical properties were earlier described [36]. The morphology of created coatings was visualized using a scanning electron microscope (Quanta 3D FEG, Huston, TX, USA). The density of the AgNPs aggregation was illustrated using energy-dispersive X-ray spectroscopy (Quantax 200 XFlash 4010, Bruker AXS, Karlsruhe, Germany)). The surface topography was examined by means of atomic force microscopy (AFM, Veeco Metrology Group (Digital Instruments, Santa Barbara, CA, USA) cooperated with NanoScope IIIa controller and MultiMode microscope) using a contactless module with a force of 20 nN in the 2 × 2 µm area.

Table 1. The silver nanograins CVD parameters.

Precursor	$Ag_5(O_2CC_2F_5)_5(H_2O)_3$
Precursor weight	5, 10, 20, 50
Vaporization temperature (T_V)	230
Carrier gas	Ar
Total reactor pressure (p)	3.0
Flow of the precursor vapors above the substrate	0.2–1.7
Substrate temperature (T_D)	290
Substrates	Ti6Al4V and Ti6Al4V/TNT5
Deposition time	30

CVD: chemical vapor deposition.

2.3. The Wettability and Surface Free Energy of Biomaterials

In order to evaluate how well (or how poorly) the liquid spreads on the surface of the tested biomaterials, the seated drop method was applied. The contact angle was determined using a goniometer with a drop shape analysis software (DSA 10 Krüss GmbH, Hamburg, Germany). Two liquids—distilled water (H_2O) and diiodomethane (CH_2I_2)—were the reagents chosen to measure the contact angle. For distilled water, the volume of the drop in the contact angle measurement was 3 µL, and in the case of diiodomethane, 4 µL. The measurement was carried out immediately after the drops were deposited. In order to determine the surface free energy (SFE), mathematical calculations were made using the Owens–Wendt model [39]. The measurement with both liquids was performed three times for all tested samples.

2.4. Silver Ion Release in the Body Fluid Environment

The studies of silver ions release from the surface of Ti6Al4V/AgNPs and Ti6Al4V/TNT5/AgNPs samples were carried according to the previously used procedure [36]. The pieces of 7 mm × 7 mm samples were immersed in 15 mL of phosphate buffered saline (PBS) in a sealed bottle at a temperature 37 °C for 1, 2, 3, 7, 10, 14, 21, 28 and 34 days. Released concentrations of silver ions in phosphate-buffered saline (PBS) were measured by mass spectrometry with plasma ionization inductively coupled to a quadrupole analyzer using an ICP-MS 7500 CX spectrometer with an Agilent Technologies collision chamber (Agilent Technologies Inc., Tokyo, Japan).

2.5. Biointegration Studies

2.5.1. Cell Culture

Murine fibroblast cell line L929 (American Type Culture Collection, Manassas, VA, USA) was cultured at 37 °C in 5% CO_2 and 95% humidity in a complete RPMI 1640 medium containing 2 mM L-glutamine, heat-inactivated 10% fetal bovine serum (FBS) and antibiotics (100 µg/mL streptomycin and 100 IU/mL penicillin) (all compounds was from Sigma-Aldrich, Darmstadt, Germany). L929 cells were grown in 25 cm^2 cell culture flasks and the culture medium was changed every 2–3 days. The cells were passaged using a cell scraper when reaching 70–80% confluency.

Human osteoblast-like MG 63 cells (European Collection of Cell Cultures, Salisbury, UK) were plated in a 25 cm^2 cell culture flask and cultured with Eagle's Minimum Essential Medium containing 2 mM L-glutamine, 1 mM sodium pyruvate, MEM non-essential amino acid, heat-inactivated 10% FBS and antibiotics (100 µg/mL streptomycin and 100 IU/mL penicillin) (all reagents were purchased from Sigma-Aldrich). The cells were grown at 37 °C in an incubator providing a humidified (95%) atmosphere containing 5% of CO_2. The culture medium was changed every 2–3 days. The cells were passaged using a 0.25% trypsin-EDTA solution (Sigma-Aldrich) when reaching 70–80% of confluency.

2.5.2. Cell Adhesion and Proliferation Detected by the MTT Assay

L929 fibroblasts, as well as MG-63 osteoblasts, in a volume of 1 mL of appropriate complete culture medium were seeded onto the autoclaved tested nanolayers placed in a 24-well culture plate (Corning, NY, USA) at a density of 1×10^4 cells/well for 24, 72 or 120 h, respectively. The cell adhesion (measured after 24 h) and proliferation (evaluated after 72 h and 120 h) was studied by the MTT (3-(4,5-dimethylthiazole-2-yl)-2,5-diphenyl tetrazolium bromide; Sigma Aldrich) assay using the same method as it was reported in Reference [33]. Briefly, after the respective incubation time, the plates were transferred to a new 24-well culture plate. The MTT solution (5 mg/mL; Sigma-Aldrich) in an appropriate culture medium without phenol red (RPMI 1640 medium for L929 fibroblasts or Eagle's Minimum Essential Medium for MG-63 osteoblasts; both from Sigma-Aldrich) was added to each well. After 3 h of incubation, the solution was aspirated and 500 µL of dimethyl sulfoxide (DMSO; 100% v/v; Sigma Aldrich) was added to each well. Finally, the plates were shaken for 10 min and the absorbance was measured at a wavelength of 570 nm with a subtraction of 630 nm (background) using a microplate reader (Synergy HT; BioTek, Winooski, VT, USA). All measurements were done in duplicate in five independent experiments.

2.5.3. Cell Morphology Evaluated by Scanning Electron Microscopy

L929 fibroblasts and MG-63 osteoblasts (1×10^4 cells/well) were incubated on the tested specimens for 24, 72 and 120 h, respectively. Scanning electron microscopy (SEM; Quanta 3D FEG; Carl Zeiss, Göttingen, Germany) analyses were performed to study the morphology changes of the cells grown on the surface of tested plates using the same method as in Reference [33]. Briefly, after the selected incubation time, the samples were fixed in a 2.5% v/v glutaraldehyde (Sigma Aldrich) and dehydrated in a graded series of ethanol (50%, 75%, 90%, and 100%). Finally, the specimens were dried in vacuum-assisted desiccators overnight and stored at room temperature until the SEM analysis was performed.

2.5.4. Statistical Analysis in the MTT Assay

All values are reported as means ± standard error of the means (SEM) and were analyzed using the nonparametric Kruskal–Wallis one-way ANOVA test with the level of significance set at $p < 0.05$. Statistical analyses were performed with GraphPad Prism 7.0 (La Jolla, CA, USA).

2.6. The Evaluation of the Antibacterial Properties of the Ti6Al4V/AgNPs and Ti6Al4V/TNT5/AgNPs Samples

The antimicrobial activity of titanium alloys, Ti6Al4V and Ti6Al4V/TNT5, coated with silver nanograins was studied against Gram-positive (*Staphylococcus aureus* ATCC 6538 and *S. aureus* ATCC 25923=PCM 2054) and Gram-negative (*Escherichia coli* ATCC 8739 and *E. coli* ATCC 25922=PCM 2057) bacteria and yeasts of *Candida albicans* ATCC 10231. Sterile sample plates (7 × 7 mm pieces, 0.2 mm thick) were placed in 1 mL of phosphate buffered saline (PBS) without ions (EURx) for 24 h, and 14 and 28 days to allow for the silver ions to be released. PBS was sterilized with cellulose filters (ø 0.2 μm) prior to use. Ti6Al4V/AgNPs and Ti6Al4V/TNT5/AgNPs plates were then removed and PBS was inoculated with the tested microorganism (final concentration of microorganism in each sample was approximately 5×10^5 c.f.u mL^{-1}). Microbial inoculum density was estimated by colony counts. Briefly, the microbial inoculum (approximately 5×10^5 c.f.u. mL^{-1}) in sterile PBS was diluted (1:1000) and 100 μL was then spread over the surface of Trypticase Soy Agar (TSA, Becton Dickinson, Franklin lake, NJ, USA) or Sabouraud Dextrose Agar (SDA, Becton Dickinson, Franklin lake, NJ, USA). After incubation, the presence of approximately 50 colonies indicated an inoculum density of 5×10^5 c.f.u. mL^{-1}.

Inoculated samples were incubated at 37 °C for 24 h. Subsequently, serial ten-fold dilutions of each sample were prepared. Aliquots (100 μL) of each dilution was spread over the surface of Trypticase Soy Agar (TSA, Becton Dickinson, Franklin lake, NJ, USA) or Sabouraud Dextrose Agar (SDA, Becton Dickinson, Franklin lake, NJ, USA) plates, which had been dried for 15 min prior to inoculation. TSA and SDA media were used for bacterial and fungal growth, respectively. The positive control was Ti6Al4V or Ti6Al4V/TNT5 plates non-coated with AgNPs. Tests were performed in triplicate. Colony forming units were counted on the inoculated plates and compared with the appropriate control plates to estimate the reduction of bacterial or fungal growth.

The antibacterial rate was calculated using the following formula:

$$R = ((B - A)/B) \times 100\%,$$

where R is the antimicrobial rate (%), B is the average number of microorganisms in PBS after the use of uncovered titanium alloys, and A is the average number of microorganisms in PBS after the use of titanium alloys enriched with silver nanoparticles.

3. Results

3.1. The Fabrication of Ti6Al4V/AgNPs and Ti6Al4V/TNT5/AgNPs Systems

Silver nanoparticles were deposited on the surface of Ti6Al4V and Ti6Al4V/TNT5 substrates using the CVD method (*hot wall* reactor, precursor: $Ag_5(O_2CC_2F_5)_5(H_2O)_3$) in the conditions listed in Table 1. The use of the following CVD precursor masses, $m = 5, 10, 20, 50$ mg, made it possible to produce coatings of the AgNPs content: c.a. 0.9, 1.1, 1.3, 2.3 wt% on the surface of Ti6Al4V substrates and 0.6, 1.0, 1.6, 2.3 wt% on the surface of Ti6Al4V/TNT5, respectively (wt% of AgNPs was determined based on the mass sample difference before and after CVD process). Considering the wt% of deposited silver, the studied specimens were marked as Ti6Al4V/0.9–2.3AgNPs and Ti6Al4V/TNT5/0.6–2.3AgNPs.

3.2. Surface Morphology and Topography

SEM images of the Ti6Al4V/0.9–2.3AgNPs and Ti6Al4V/TNT5/0.6–2.3AgNPs samples are presented in Figures 1 and 2. Analysis of these data shows that the precursor mass applied in the CVD experiments and the substrate type are two main factors directly impacting the size and distribution of the deposited nanoparticles (Table 2).

Table 2. The weight % and the diameters of the AgNPs deposited on the surface of the Ti6Al4V and Ti6Al4V/TNT5 substrates using the CVD technique.

Precursor Mass (mg)	Ti6Al4V/AgNPs		Ti6Al4V/TNT5/AgNPs	
	wt%	d (nm)	wt%	d (nm)
5	0.9	18 ± 8	0.6	38 ± 14
10	1.1	45 ± 15	1.0	43 ± 10
20	1.3	68 ± 32	1.6	57 ± 24
50	2.3	53 ± 18	2.3	115 ± 49

The analysis of the SEM images of Ti6Al4V substrates (Figure 1a–d), whose surfaces have been enriched with AgNPs, shows that this surface is evenly covered by dispersed silver grains, whose densities increase with the increase of the nanoparticles weight percent on the substrate surface. The diameter of the nanosilver grains ranges from 18 ± 8 nm up to 53 ± 18 nm. The smallest diameter of nanosilver is observed when 5 mg of the precursor was used. The use of 20 mg of the CVD precursor in the same deposition conditions led to the formation of AgNPs with significant differences in the diameter (from 45 up to 90 nm) and shape (from spherical to rods) of silver grains (Figure 1c). These deposition conditions are probably suitable for the nucleation of spherical grains and their later growth in one direction (formation of rods). The increase of the CVD precursor concentration in vapors (50 mg) caused the deposition of AgNPs of similar diameter and shape, but their arrangement is characterized by a significantly higher density (Figure 1d).

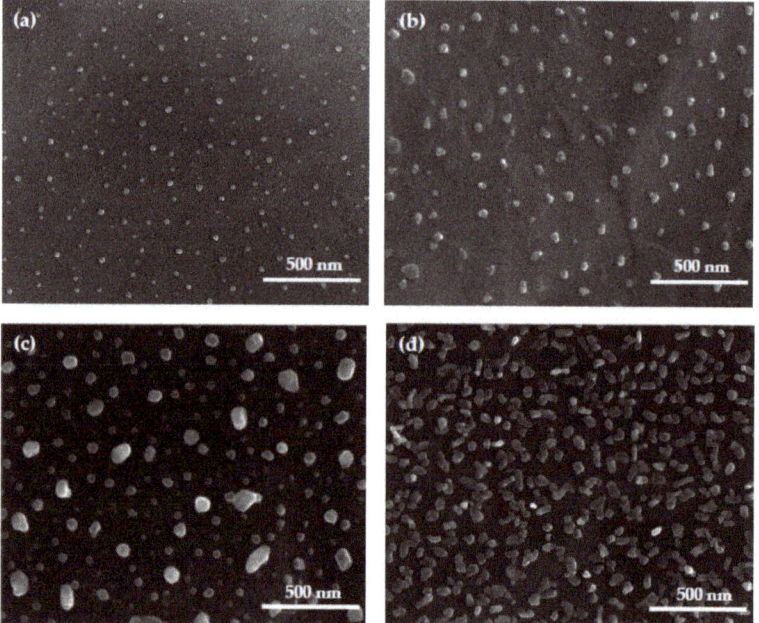

Figure 1. The scanning electron microscopy (SEM) images of Ti6Al4V/0.9AgNPs; $d = 18 \pm 8$ nm (**a**), Ti6Al4V/1.1AgNPs; $d = 45 \pm 15$ nm (**b**), Ti6Al4V/1.3AgNPs; $d = 68 \pm 32$ nm (**c**), Ti6Al4V/2.3AgNPs; $d = 53 \pm 18$ nm (**d**).

SEM images of the Ti6Al4V/TNT5/AgNPs systems are presented in Figure 2a–d. Their analysis shows that on the surface of the TNT5 coating (tubes diameter allow c.a. 28 ± 11 nm), the diameter of the deposited AgNPs changes from 38 ± 14 nm up to 115 ± 49 nm. Both the size of the nanoparticles' diameters and their density on the surface of nanotubes grow along with the increase of the number of silver precursor used in the deposition process. Compared to the growth of the silver nanoparticles on the unmodified surface of the titanium alloy, the silver nanoparticles' growth on the nanotubes is more rational, predictable and does not show any anomalies.

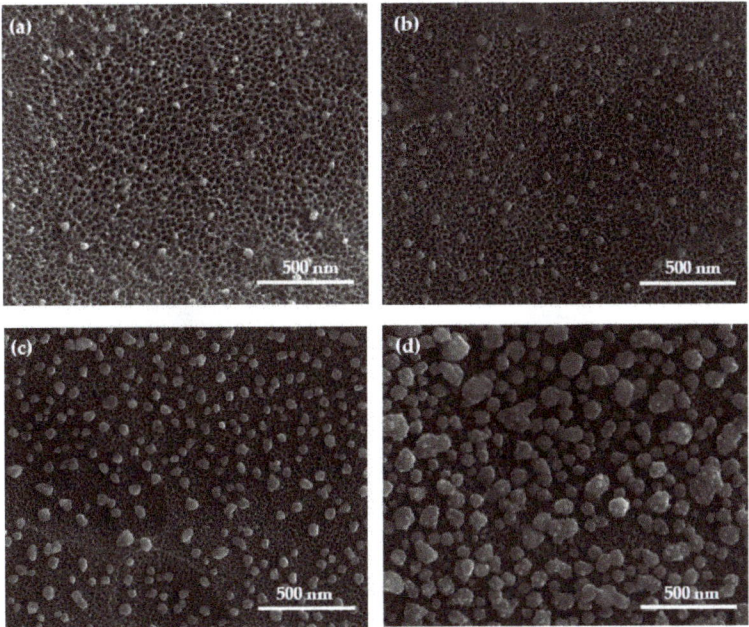

Figure 2. Scanning electron microscopy (SEM) images of Ti6Al4V/TNT5/0.6AgNPs; $d = 38 \pm 14$ nm (**a**), Ti6Al4V/TNT5/1.0AgNPs; $d = 43 \pm 10$ nm (**b**), Ti6Al4V/TNT5/1.6AgNPs; $d = 57 \pm 24$ nm (**c**), Ti6Al4V/TNT5/2.3AgNPs; $d = 115 \pm 49$ nm (**d**).

The surface roughness parameter (R_a) of the studied samples was measured in the 2×2 μm area using software, which is an integral part of the atomic force microscopy (AFM, Veeco (Digital Instruments), Figure 3). The values of the R_a parameters determined for Ti6Al4V and Ti6Al4V/TNT5 samples were used as reference samples. The analysis of these data revealed a significant increase of the roughness parameter value with the increase of the density and size of the AgNPs deposited on the surface of both types of substrates. Moreover, the comparison of the Ti6Al4V/TNT5/AgNPs samples and the Ti6Al4V/AgNPs ones indicate the clear influence of the nanotubular architecture on the increase of the surface roughness, e.g., the value of a R_a parameter of Ti6Al4V/TNT5/1.0AgNPs is about 42% higher than that of Ti6Al4V/1.1AgNPs.

In order to confirm the deposition of silver nanograins on the surface of studied substrates, energy dispersive X-ray spectroscopy (EDS) was applied. The low intense lines, which are found in the EDS spectra of Ti6Al4V/0.9AgNPs and Ti6Al4V/TNT5/0.6AgNPs, show the presence of dispersed silver nanoparticles on the surface of the used substrates (Figure 4). The increase of AgNPs' density on the substrates' surface and their size caused a significant increase of the integral intensity of the Ag lines in the EDS spectra.

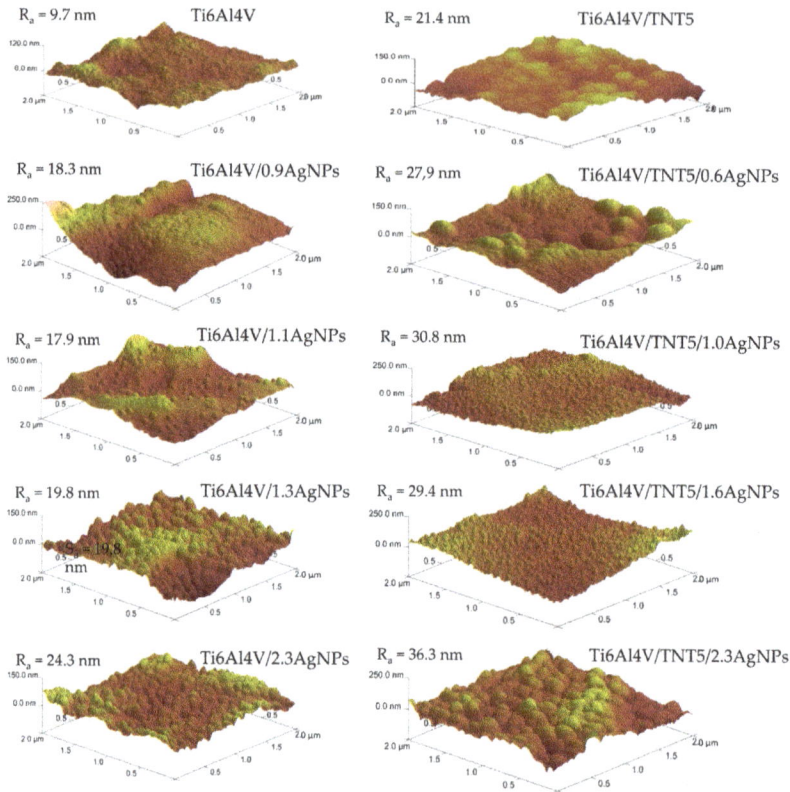

Figure 3. Atomic forces microscopy (AFM) images and R$_a$ parameters determined for the Ti6Al4V, Ti6Al4V/AgNPs, Ti6Al4V/TNT5, and Ti6Al4V/TNT5/AgNPs samples.

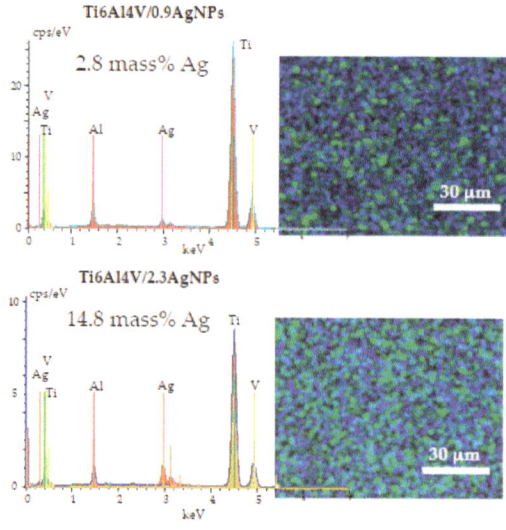

Figure 4. *Cont.*

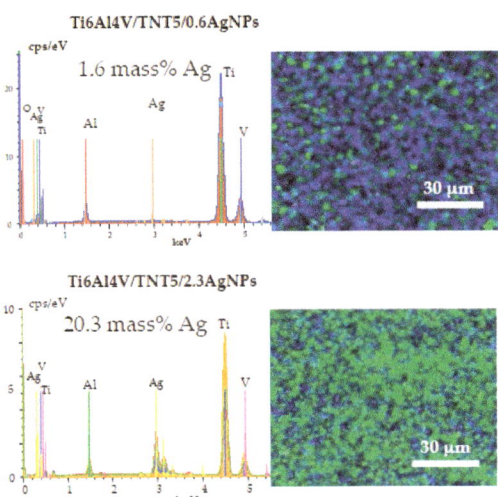

Figure 4. The energy dispersive X-ray spectroscopy (EDS) spectra and maps images of Ti6Al4V/0.9AgNPs, Ti6Al4V/2.3AgNPs, Ti6Al4V/TNT5/0.6AgNPs, and Ti6Al4V/TNT5/2.3AgNPs (AgNPs are marked as the green dots on the presented map images).

3.3. Wettability and Surface Free Energy of Biomaterials

In order to estimate the value of the surface free energy based on mathematical calculations, which were performed using the Owens–Wendt method, the contact angle of two different liquids (one of them, polar, and the other one, dispersional) had to be used in the analyses [39]. Therefore, polar water and dispersional diiodomethane were chosen as measuring liquids. The obtained contact angles measurements results, as well as the calculated SFE values, are presented in Figures 5 and 6 and in Table S1. According to these data, the hydrophobic character of the Ti6Al4V surface slightly decreases after depositing small amounts of AgNPs (0.9 wt%), however, with the increase of their density, the coatings' hydrophobicity increases (Figure 5, Table S1). The fabrication of the titania nanotubes layer on the surface of Ti6Al4V leads to the formation of a hydrophilic surface, which becomes more hydrophobic when it is enriched with silver nanoparticles (Figure 5, Table S1).

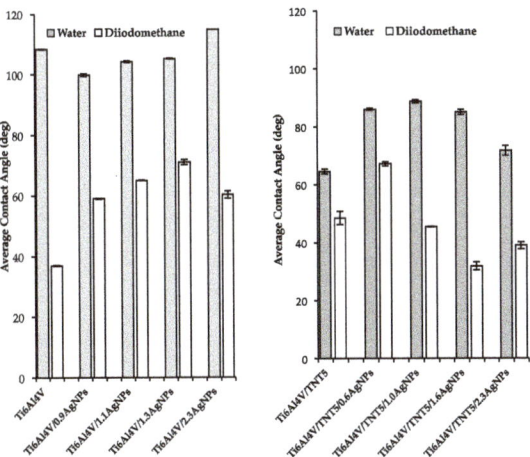

Figure 5. The contact angles values for Ti6Al4V, Ti6Al4V/AgNPs, Ti6Al4V/TNT5, and Ti6Al4V/TNT5/AgNPs.

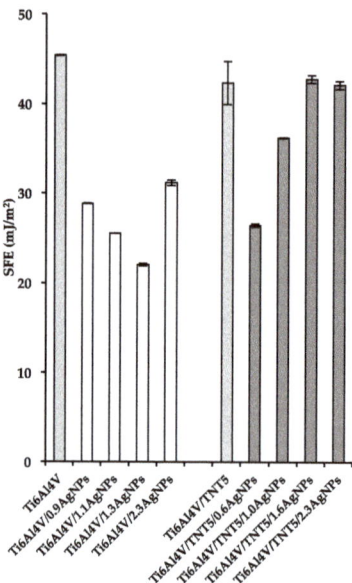

Figure 6. The surface free energy values for Ti6Al4V, Ti6Al4V/AgNPs, Ti6Al4V/TNT5, and Ti6Al4V/TNT5/AgNPs.

The values of the surface free energy (SFE) decreases for all Ti6Al4V/AgNPs samples in comparison to the adequate value for pure Ti6Al4V sample (Figure 6, Table S1). For the sample Ti6Al4V/1.3AgNPs, this is more than two times lower. A different situation is noticed for the Ti6Al4V/TNT and Ti6Al4V/TNT/AgNPs samples. Here, with the exception of the first two silver-enriched systems (Ti6Al4V/TNT/0.6AgNPs and Ti6Al4V/TNT/1.0AgNPs) for which the SFE values are lower than for Ti6Al4V/TNT, two consecutive ones, i.e., Ti6Al4V/TNT/1.6AgNPs and Ti6Al4V/TNT/2.3AgNPs, are characterized by a similar value of free surface energy (Figure 6, Table S1).

3.4. Silver Ion Release in the Body Fluid Environment

The bioactivity of Ti6Al4V and Ti6Al4V/TNT5 samples enriched with silver nanoparticles associated with silver ions releasing from their surface can be estimated on the basis of the Ag^+ ion concentration change studies versus time (5 weeks) for the samples immersed in the phosphate-buffered saline (PBS) solution at human body temperature (37 °C) [36]. Ti6Al4V and Ti6Al4V/TNT5 samples, whose surfaces were enriched with 1.0–1.1 and 2.3 wt% of AgNPs, deposited using 10 and 50 mg of Ag CVD precursor, respectively (Ti6Al4V/1.1AgNPs, Ti6Al4V/2.3AgNPs, Ti6Al4V/TNT5/1.0AgNPs, and Ti6Al4V/TNT5/2.3AgNPs), were used in our studies on the silver ions release effect (Figure 7). The analysis of these data proved the lack of significant differences in the Ag^+ ion release effect for samples containing a high content of AgNPs on their surface, i.e., Ti6Al4V/2.3AgNPs and Ti6Al4V/TNT5/2.3AgNPs. In both cases, the rapid increase of Ag^+ concentration in the PBS solution was noticed in the first 10 days of the experiment, and then the concentration changes remained at the level of 1.7–2 ppm. The deposition of nearly a 2-fold smaller amount of AgNPs on the surface of the studied substrates caused a significant reduction in the concentration of silver ions released. In the case of the Ti6Al4V/1.1AgNPs sample, the maximum Ag^+ release was achieved after 7 days and, in the long-term, it remains at the level of 0.9–1.1 ppm. In the first 10 days, the release of silver ions from the surface of the Ti6Al4V/TNT5/1.0AgNPs sample immersed in the PBS solution was lower than 0.1 ppm. The highest concentration of silver ions was observed after 34 days, i.e., 0.4 ppm. The results of the study showed a significant effect of the number of AgNPs dispersed on the surface of TNT layers on the concentration of silver ions released.

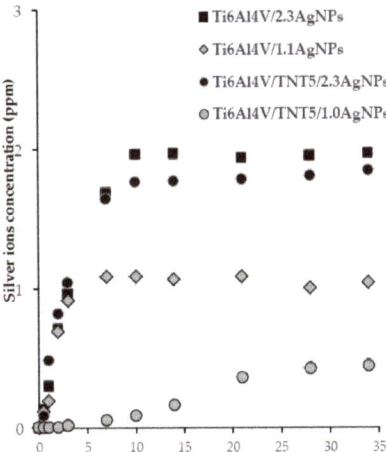

Figure 7. The release amount of Ag$^+$ ions from Ti6Al4V/AgNPs and Ti6Al4V/TNT5/AgNPs samples (containing 2.3 and 1.0–1.1 wt% of AgNPs) immersed in a phosphate buffered saline (PBS) and measured by inductively coupled plasma ionization mass spectrometry (ICP-MS).

3.5. The Evaluation of the Biocompatibility of the Produced Titanium Alloy-Based Materials

The biocompatibility of the studied substrates, whose surfaces were enriched with different amounts of dispersed silver nanoparticles, were evaluated on the basis of the MTT (3-(4,5-dimethylthiazol-2-yl)-2,5-diphenyltetrazolium bromide) assay and Scanning Electron Microscopy (SEM) micrographs. The assays were made for Ti6Al4V, Ti6Al4V/AgNPs and Ti6Al4V/TNT5/AgNPs, using two cell lines: the murine fibroblast cell line L929 and human osteoblast-like MG-63 cells. The level of adhesion (measured after 24 h) and proliferation (assessed after 72 h and 120 h) of the cells growing on the surface of Ti6Al4V/AgNPs and Ti6Al4V/TNT5/AgNPs was compared to that which was observed for the cells cultured on the reference Ti6Al4V alloy foil. As it can be seen, with an increase of the incubation time, more L929 fibroblasts, as well as MG-63 osteoblasts, proliferated on the surface of all the tested biomaterials (Figures 8 and 9). Analysis of the MTT assay data revealed the lack of significant differences in the MG-63 osteoblasts adhesion and proliferation to the surface of the reference Ti6Al4V sample and Ti6Al4V/AgNPs samples, whose surfaces were enriched with various amounts of AgNPs (Figure 8). In contrast, we have noticed that the Ti6Al4V alloy foils covered with nanosilver provoked a slight decrease in the L929 fibroblasts' proliferation after 72 h of incubation ((for Ti6Al4V/1.3AgNPs and Ti6Al4V/2.3AgNPs) Ag nanolayers; $p < 0.05$) and 120 h of incubation for the all tested concentration of nanosilver (relative L929 cells' viability compared to the Ti6Al4V reference sample and expressed as a percentage was presented in the Table below Figure 8A). However, we did not observe any differences in the fibroblasts adhesion measured after 24 h of incubation (Figure 8A).

The results of the MTT assay for Ti6AlV/TNT5/AgNPs are presented in Figure 9. The results were compared to that which was observed for the cells cultured on the reference Ti6Al4V alloy foils. Analysis of these data showed no differences in the cell adhesion (measured after 24 h) for both the tested cells lines. Moreover, L929 fibroblasts cultured on the surface of TNT5 nanotubes' coatings doped by the all tested concentrations of nanosilver showed a higher rate of cell proliferation after 120 h of incubation than the cells that grew on the Ti6Al4V reference layers ($p < 0.001$).

This phenomenon was also observed after 72 h of incubation, but only for the samples enriched with 0.6 wt% of AgNPs ($p < 0.001$, Ti6Al4V/TNT5/0.6AgNPs). On the other hand, MG-63 osteoblasts cultured on the TNT5 nanotubes enriched with silver nanoparticles provoked a decrease in the level proliferation of MG-63 osteoblasts after 120 h of incubation ($p < 0.001$) in comparison to the Ti6Al4V reference alloy ($p < 0.001$) (the relative MG-63 cells viability compared to the Ti6Al4V reference sample and expressed as a percentage was presented in the Table below the Figure 9B). However, it should be clearly emphasized that these samples also showed an increase in the level of proliferation over time.

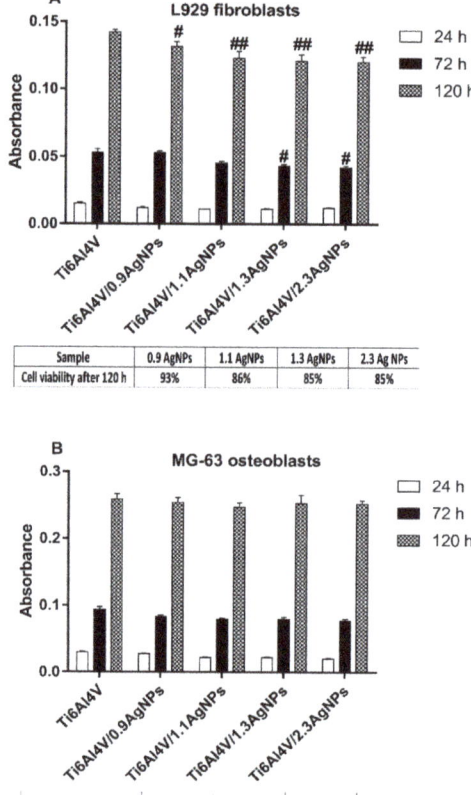

Figure 8. The L929 murine fibroblasts (**A**) and human osteoblasts MG-63 (**B**) adhesion (measured after 24 h) and proliferation (evaluated after 72 h and 120 h) on the surface of Ti6Al4V/AgNPs, detected by the MTT (3-(4,5-dimethylthiazol-2-yl)-2,5-diphenyltetrazolium bromide) assay. The absorbance values are expressed as means ± SEM of five independent experiments. Hash marks indicate significant differences at the appropriate incubation time between the cells incubated on the reference Ti6Al4V alloy foils (Ti6Al4V) compared to the specimen coatings doped by the different concentrations of Ag (# $p < 0.05$, ## $p < 0.01$). Tables below Figure 8A,B presented relative L929 cells or MG-63 cell viability (%) compared to the Ti6Al4V reference sample measured after 120 h of incubation.

Biointegration of titania nanolayers enriched with silver nanoparticles were also assessed by the analysis of SEM micrographs. Comparative SEM images showing the morphology, adhesion and proliferation of the cells growing on the surface of Ti6Al4V alloy and Ti6Al4V/AgNPs, as well as on Ti6Al4V/TNT5/AgNPs, are presented in Figures 10 and 11, respectively. These data clearly demonstrate the high biocompatibility of both types of tested nanolayers, supporting the results from the MTT assay. As it can be seen, L929 fibroblasts cultured on the surface of Ti6Al4V/AgNPs, as well as on the surface of Ti6Al4V/TNT5/AgNPs, showed the increase in cell proliferation over time (compare micrographs in Figure 10d–i). A similar phenomenon was also observed for the MG-63 osteoblasts (compare micrographs in Figure 11d–i). Importantly, the cells, especially MG-63 osteoblasts, start to grow in layers on top of each other (Figure 11k), and moreover, the cells grow with a multilayer structure on most of the surfaces of the nanolayers after 120 h of incubation time (see micrographs in Figure 11f,i,j). Finally, the SEM images also show that L929 fibroblasts, as well as MG-63 osteoblasts, form numerous filopodia which attach the cells to the surface of specimens by penetrating deep into the nanolayers (arrows in Figures 10l and 11l, respectively). These thin, actin-rich plasma-membrane protrusions were also generated between the cells (arrows in Figures 10j–k and 11k, respectively).

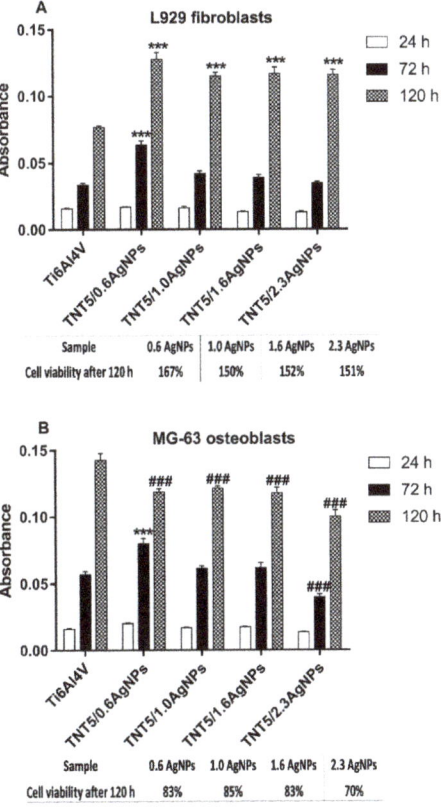

Figure 9. The effect of TNT5/AgNPs coatings on the L929 fibroblasts (A) and MG-63 osteoblasts (B) adhesion (measured after 24 h) and proliferation (evaluated after 72 h and 120 h), detected by the MTT assay. The absorbance values are expressed as means ± SEM of five independent experiments. Asterisks indicate significant differences at the appropriate incubation time when the level of cell proliferation on the surface of specimens coating doped by the different concentrations of Ag was higher compared to the reference Ti6Al4V alloy foils (Ti6Al4V) (*** $p < 0.001$). Hash marks denote significant differences at the appropriate incubation time when the level of cell proliferation on the samples enriched with AgNPs was lower in comparison with the reference Ti6Al4V alloy foils (### $p < 0.001$). Tables below Figure 9A,B presented relative L929 or MG-63 cells viability (%) compared to the Ti6Al4V reference sample measured after 120 h of incubation.

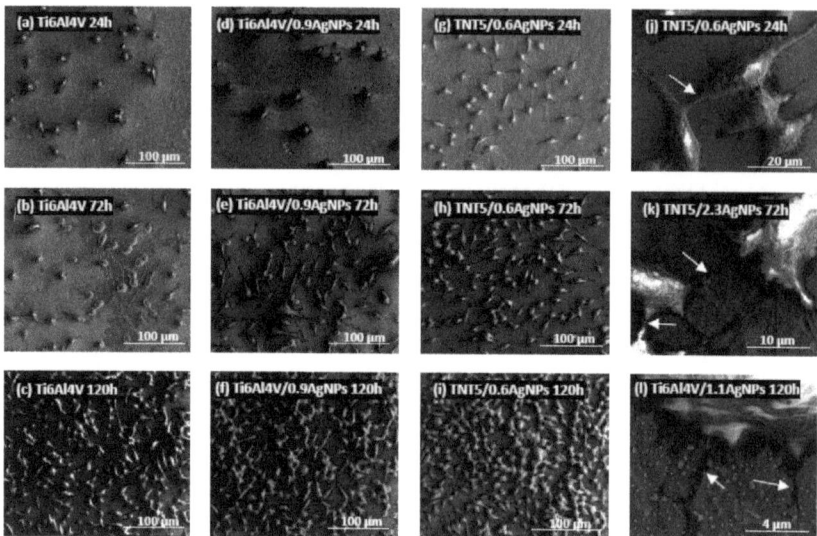

Figure 10. The scanning electron microscopy (SEM) images presenting adhesion (after 24 h) and proliferation (after 72 h and 120 h) of the murine L929 fibroblasts growing on the surface of reference Ti6Al4V alloy foils (**a–c**), (Ti6Al4V/0.9AgNPs) (**d–f**) or Ti6Al4V/TNT5/0.6AgNPs (**g–i**). Arrows in the micrographs indicate numerous filopodia spreading between the fibroblasts (**j–k**) or filopodia, which attached the cells to the surface of nanocoatings (**l**).

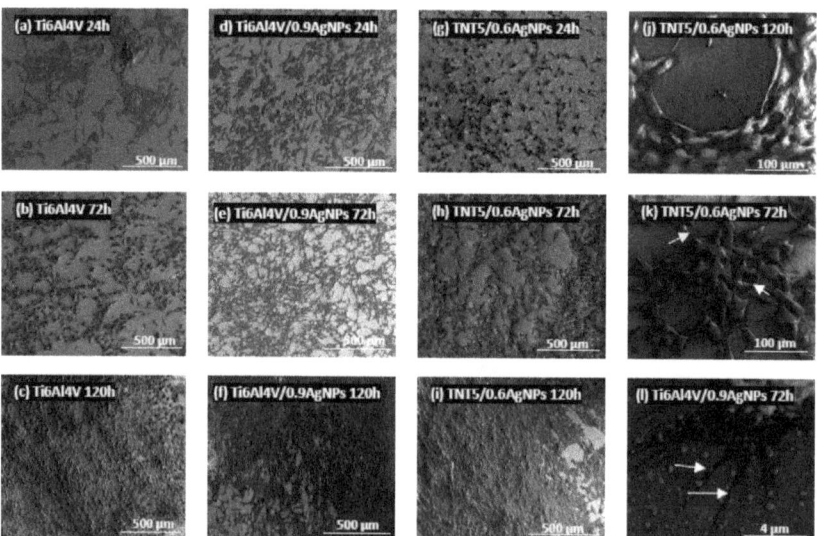

Figure 11. The scanning electron microscopy (SEM) micrographs showing the human osteoblast-like MG-63 cells adhesion (after 24 h) and proliferation (after 72 h and 120 h) growing on the surface of references Ti6Al4V alloy foils (**a–c**), (Ti6Al4V/0.9AgNPs) (**d–f**) or Ti6Al4V/TNT5/0.6AgNPs (**g–i**). The micrograph (**j**) presents the multilayer growth of cells on the surface of Ti6Al4V/TNT5/0.6AgNPs sample. Arrows indicate numerous filopodia, which attached the osteoblasts to the nanocoatings surface (**l**) and filopodia spreading between the cells (**k**).

3.6. Antimicrobial Activity of Silver-Coated Titanium Alloys

The antimicrobial activity of silver nanoparticles is widely known. Titanium alloys (surface non-modified and nanotubular modified), enriched with various amount of nanosilver grains (Ti6Al4V/AgNPs and Ti6Al4V/TNT5/AgNPs) were found to be extremely biocidal against the tested bacteria and fungi when compared to silver non-coated titanium alloy. Biocidal activity was found after 24 h, 14 days and 28 days of silver ion release into PBS. The Ti6Al4V/AgNPs and Ti6Al4V/TNT5/AgNPs composites reduced more than 99% of the growth of all tested microorganisms, independently from the number of silver nanoparticles deposited on their surface (Tables 3–5). The number of bacterial colonies after treatment with Ti6Al4V/AgNPs and Ti6Al4V/TNT5/AgNPs was reduced at least 100-fold when compared to Ti6Al4V, as presented in Figure S1 for *E. coli* ATCC25922 7.0×10^5 c.f.u. mL^{-1} (**a**) and 3.8×10^5 c.f.u. mL^{-1} (**b**), respectively.

Table 3. The reduction of microbial growth (%) in PBS after the use of Ti6Al4V/AgNPs and Ti6Al4V/TNT5/AgNPs alloys for 24 h of ion release.

Ti Alloys	Microorganisms				
	E. coli ATCC8739	*E. coli* ATCC25922	*S. aureus* ATCC6538	*S. aureus* ATCC25923	*C. albicans* ATCC10231
Ti6Al4V	-	-	-	-	-
Ti6Al4V/0.9 AgNPs	99.57	>99.99	>99.99	99.93	99.96
Ti6Al4V/1.1 AgNPs	99.97	99.99	>99.99	99.98	99.97
Ti6Al4V/1.3 AgNPs	99.94	99.80	99.93	99.96	99.67
Ti6Al4V/2.3 AgNPs	99.96	99.83	99.99	99.85	99.93
Ti6Al4V/TNT5	-	-	-	-	-
Ti6Al4V/TNT5/0.6 AgNPs	99.90	99.94	99.94	99.99	>99.99
Ti6Al4V/TNT5/1.0 AgNPs	>99.99	>99.99	99.61	>99.99	>99.99
Ti6Al4V/TNT5/1.6 AgNPs	99.95	99.90	99.46	>99.99	99.99
Ti6Al4V/TNT5/2.3 AgNPs	99.70	99.99	99.95	99.71	>99.99

Key: -; no reduction (control). PBS: phosphate buffered saline solution.

Table 4. The reduction of microbial growth (%) in PBS after the use of Ti6Al4V/AgNPs and Ti6Al4V/TNT5/AgNPs alloys for 14 days of ion release.

Ti Alloys	Microorganisms				
	E. coli ATCC8739	*E. coli* ATCC25922	*S. aureus* ATCC6538	*S. aureus* ATCC25923	*C. albicans* ATCC10231
Ti6Al4V	-	-	-	-	-
Ti6Al4V/0.9 AgNPs	>99.99	>99.99	>99.99	>99.99	>99.99
Ti6Al4V/1.1 AgNPs	>99.99	>99.99	>99.99	>99.99	>99.99
Ti6Al4V/1.3 AgNPs	>99.99	>99.99	>99.99	>99.99	>99.99
Ti6Al4V/2.3 AgNPs	>99.99	>99.99	>99.99	>99.99	>99.99
Ti6Al4V/TNT5	-	-	-	-	-
Ti6Al4V/TNT5/0.6 AgNPs	>99.99	>99.99	>99.99	>99.99	>99.99
Ti6Al4V/TNT5/1.0 AgNPs	>99.99	>99.99	>99.99	>99.99	>99.99
Ti6Al4V/TNT5/1.6 AgNPs	>99.99	>99.99	>99.99	>99.99	>99.99
Ti6Al4V/TNT5/2.3 AgNPs	>99.99	>99.99	>99.99	>99.99	>99.99

Key: -; no reduction (control).

Table 5. The reduction of microbial growth (%) in PBS after the use of Ti6Al4V/AgNPs and Ti6Al4V/TNT5/AgNPs alloys for 28 days of ion release.

Ti Alloys	Microorganisms				
	E. coli ATCC8739	E. coli ATCC25922	S. aureus ATCC6538	S. aureus ATCC25923	C. albicans ATCC10231
Ti6Al4V	-	-	-	-	-
Ti6Al4V/0.9 AgNPs	99.94	>99.99	99.78	99.58	>99.99
Ti6Al4V/1.1 AgNPs	99.84	99.98	99.91	99.49	>99.99
Ti6Al4V/1.3 AgNPs	99.91	99.98	99.84	99.87	>99.67
Ti6Al4V/2.3 AgNPs	99.89	99.83	99.83	99.87	>99.99
Ti6Al4V/TNT5	-	-	-	-	-
Ti6Al4V/TNT5/0.6 AgNPs	>99.99	>99.99	>99.99	>99.99	>99.99
Ti6Al4V/TNT5/1.0 AgNPs	>99.99	99.99	99.99	99.99	>99.99
Ti6Al4V/TNT5/1.6 AgNPs	99.90	99.84	99.99	>99.99	>99.99
Ti6Al4V/TNT5/2.3 AgNPs	99.66	99.88	99.81	99.76	>99.99

Key: -; no reduction (control).

4. Discussion

The studies on the relationship between the number of silver nanoparticles (AgNPs) deposited on the surface of Ti6Al4V and Ti6Al4V/TNT5 substrates, their size and their distribution, and the wettability and bioactivity of the produced systems were the purpose of our investigations. The following two factors determined the choice of the substrate used in our research: (a) the common use of the Ti6Al4V alloy as a material in implantology, and (b) the use of titania nanotube coatings (TNT) to modify the titanium/titanium alloys surfaces and to provide them with biocompatible properties. The electrochemical anodization method, with the use of constant potential (U = 5 V), was applied in the TNT5 coatings production. The results of our earlier works revealed that the TNT5 layer consists of densely packed titania nanotubes of diameters 35–45 nm and length c.a. 150 nm. Simultaneously, this type of coating exhibited optimal biointegration properties [34]. The above-mentioned coating enrichment with AgNPs using the CVD technique lad to the deposition of the dispersed metallic grains mainly on their surface, as in the case of the pure alloys substrates [36]. To achieve better control over the dispersion and growth of deposited AgNPs, low flow values of precursor vapors over the substrate surface were used during the CVD process. Depending on the precursor mass applied in the CVD experiments (i.e., 5, 10, 20, 50 mg) and the defined carrier gas flow, the amounts of the precursor which flow above the substrate surface, were 0.2, 0.3, 0.7, and 1.7 mg·min^{-1}, respectively. The analysis of the SEM images confirmed the clear influence of the experimental conditions on the size and density of the deposited AgNPs (Table 2 and Figures 1 and 2). Moreover, it should be noted that the type of used substrate also affects the increase of the deposited AgNPs' size and density. The diameter of the AgNPs deposited on the surface of Ti6Al4V/TNT5 was bigger than the ones, which were deposited on the surface of the Ti6Al4V substrates (Table 2).

In our work, the biointegration of the studied samples was evaluated using two cell lines: mouse L929 fibroblasts and human osteoblasts-like MG-63 cells. According to earlier reports, the long-term success of an implant placement depends not only on the integrity of osseointegration, but also on the contact with the surrounding soft tissue [40]. In recent years, the MG-63 cell line has become a standard model for bone research in addition to primary human osteoblasts and this cell line is also well-established for studying the effects of surface nanotopography on osteoblast-like cells [41]. In addition, established permanent cell lines of soft tissue, such as L929 fibroblasts, are widely used to test the cytotoxicity of dental materials when employing in vitro methods of experimentation [42]. Moreover, fibroblasts are the most common cells in connective tissue, one of the main components of peri-implant soft tissue, which is key to the formation of the peri-implant mucosal seal and helping to prevent epithelial ingrowth [40]. Therefore, the study of the biointegration of the nanomaterials using two selected cell lines allowed for a comprehensive examination of implant biocompatibility.

It is well-established that cellular behavior, such as cell adhesion and proliferation or morphologic change (including the formation of filopodia) is determined by the surface properties of nanomaterials, thus, the cellular response measured by these parameters are required to assess the biointegration of implants [43]. In our study, the biointegration level of the tested specimens was examined using an MTT assay (for evaluation of cell adhesion and proliferation) and scanning electron microscopy images analysis (for assessment of cell adhesion, proliferation and morphology). The results of the MTT assays related to the cell adhesion (measure after 24 h) and proliferation (measured after 72 h and 120 h) revealed that there were no differences in the MG-63 osteoblasts adhesion and proliferation between the reference Ti6Al4V layers and Ti6Al4V/AgNPs (Figure 8B). On the other hand, the Ti6Al4V/AgNPs induced a significant decrease in the L929 fibroblast proliferation, especially after 120 h of incubation for the all tested concentration of nanosilver (Figure 8A). Surprisingly, the different results were obtained for Ti6Al4V/TNT5/AgNPs samples. L929 fibroblasts cultured on the surface of Ti6Al4V/TNT5 samples enriched with all tested concentration of AgNPs showed a higher rate of cell proliferation after 120 h of incubation than the cells that grow on the Ti6Al4V reference layers (Figure 9A). In contrast, the same nanolayers induced a decrease in the level of proliferation of the MG-63 osteoblasts after 120 h of incubation (Figure 9B). However, it should be clearly emphasized that for the all tested samples, we have noticed an increase in the L929 fibroblast and MG-63 osteoblast proliferation over time, which is confirmed not only by the MTT assay results, but also through the analysis of the comparative SEM micrographs (compare the images in Figures 10 and 11). Importantly, the cells, especially the MG-63 osteoblasts, have almost overgrown the entire surface of the nanolayers enriched with AgNPs (Figure 11f,i,j). The high level of biocompatibility of the tested nanomaterials was also confirmed by the cellular behavior associated with the formation of filopodia by the fibroblasts, as well as the osteoblasts, between the cells (arrows in Figure 10j,k and Figure 11k, respectively). These actin-based cell protrusions also attached the cells to the coating's surface (arrows in Figures 10l and 11l, respectively) by penetration inside the porous nanolayer, functioning as anchorage points enhancing cell proliferation. Filopodia are regarded as one of the most important cellular sensors, collecting information on whether the surface is suitable for cell attachment and proliferation, cell-cell interacting and allowing for cell migration toward the destination [44]. Therefore, filopodia formation is evidence of the biocompatible properties of tested nanomaterials.

Although it is believed that silver has cytotoxicity to some cells at certain concentrations [45], it is well-known that eukaryotic cells exhibit a far bigger target for attacking silver ions than prokaryotic cells and that they show more structural and functional redundancy. Therefore, a higher silver ion concentration is required to achieve comparable toxic effects, relative to bacterial cells [46]. Similar to our results, Reference [47] demonstrated that Ag-decorated TiO_2 nanotubes exhibited monotonically increasing trend in the fibroblasts' cell line proliferation and, at the same time, these specimens may cause a decrease in osteoblast proliferation [48]. Importantly, in our study, the viability of MG-63 osteoblasts cultured on the TNT5 samples enriched with nanosilver was 70% or more after 120 h of incubation in comparison to the Ti6Al4V references alloy (Table below Figure 9B). According to the ISO 10993-1:2018 standards [49] (Biological evaluation of medical devices: Part 1: evaluation and testing within a risk management process), if the cell viability was reduced to <70% of the blank, it would have a cytotoxicity potential. Therefore, our results indicate reasonable biocompatibility of TNT5 enriched with all tested concentration of nanosilver. As we have described above, Ti6Al4V alloy foils enriched with all tested concentrations of silver nanograins induced a slight decrease in L929 fibroblast proliferation without affecting the proliferation of osteoblasts. However, these results also demonstrate reasonable biocompatibility of the tested nanomaterials because the viability of the cells after 120 h of incubation was 85% or more compared to the reference Ti6Al4V specimens (Table below the Figure 8A). Our results corresponding with the findings from the other authors who have shown that silver deposited titanium reduced fibroblasts proliferation by 20% in comparison with titanium control samples [50] or titanium samples coated with the silver alloys, which did not have a cytotoxic effect on osteoblast cells [51].

To summarize, our results from the MTT assay and analysis of comparative SEM micrographs, including an increase in the cell proliferation over time, filopodia formation and viability of cell higher than 70% for the all tested samples, clearly demonstrate the biocompatible properties of the tested nanomaterials that can be used in dentistry or maxillofacial surgery. This conclusion is based on the statement that a favorable cellular interaction with the biomaterial's surface is critical for the long-term success of the implants [52].

Implant-associated infections are one of the critical issues for dental and maxillofacial implantology and can result in serious complications, such as the need for complex revision procedures, as well as poor prognoses, patients suffering, and even death [53,54]. The infections associated with implants are caused mainly by bacterial colonization and biofilm formation on the surface of the implanted specimen, which affects the adjacent tissues [55]. It is known that the most effective way to prevent biofilm buildup on implants is to prohibit the initial bacterial adhesion because the biofilms are quite difficult to remove after formation. One of the approaches is to directly impregnate an implant device with antibiotics to prevent the initial adhesion of bacteria onto the implant surface [53,56]. Although these antibiotic-impregnated surfaces displayed significant therapeutic effects, the potential toxicity and increased microbial drug resistance through the slow-release doses have become increased risks in surgery [53,55]. Therefore, postoperative infection rates could be greatly reduced by improving the antimicrobial properties of the implant surface by its modifications with metal ions such as Ag and Zn [54,55,57]. Silver-containing coatings have attracted increasing attention due to the nontoxicity of the active Ag^+ to human cells and its antimicrobial activity [53,58]. Thus, the surface-modification of titanium alloys with silver coating, which was also performed in the present study, is considered a strategy to prevent the development of peri-implant infections [54]. Based on the results obtained from ICP-MS, which showed a significant release of silver ions from all Ti6Al4V/AgNPs and Ti6Al4V/TNT5/AgNPs immersed into a PBS solution after 14 and 28 days, we presumed that such ions could be responsible for antimicrobial properties. Although superior microbiocidal activity was also observed for all the studied samples after a 24-h ion release time, the ICP-MS did not confirm the presence of silver ions in the case of nanotubular modified titanium alloy surfaces enriched with the smallest amount of silver (Figure 5). This might be due to the low content of released ions, which was not detectable. Thus, the limited sensitivity of ICP-MS is not without meaning. A high biocidal effect of Ti6Al4V/AgNPs and Ti6Al4V/TNT5/AgNPs was observed even at the lowest concentrations of Ag deposited on the surface of the tested alloys. We assert that the required Ag dose in the implants is typically low, which makes it possible to introduce Ag into biocompatible coatings [55]. Therefore, the incorporation of a sufficient amount of Ag to enhance the antibacterial ability of porous coatings could lead to the production of a surface that retains biocompatible and relatively long-term antibacterial activity. On the other hand, the optimization of the fabrication of Ti-Ag specimens by a decrease of the Ag amount on their surface might also improve the adhesion and proliferation of fibroblasts and osteoblasts, thus affecting the better integration of implants with human tissues.

We assert that the inhibitory effect of silver nanoparticles is mainly associated with silver ions present in nanoparticles, but it is not the sole mechanism of antimicrobial activity induced by nanosilver [59]. The major difference between the effectiveness of silver nanoparticles and silver ions against bacteria is that AgNPs act in nanomolar concentrations, while ions act in micromolar ranges [60]. Silver nanoparticles, due to their small size, can easily penetrate and disrupt the membranes of bacteria. Both silver species (nanoparticles and ions) may react with protein thiol groups (key respiratory enzymes) and/or phospholipids of the bacterial membrane [61–63]. This leads to an increase in the membrane permeability and may cause more pronounced effects such as the loss (by leakage) of cellular contents, including ions (mainly K^+), proteins and reducing sugars and a decrease of the ATP level [60,64,65]. Silver species may also interact with nucleic acids, which may probably result in the impairment of DNA replication [59,60,66,67]. All of these effects may culminate in the loss of cell viability [60,68]. It is also suggested that silver ions generate free radicals inside cells, which are involved in the antimicrobial activity of silver nanoparticles and released silver ions [69]. Some authors claimed that the thickness of the peptidoglycan layer of gram-positive bacteria might prevent the action of the silver ions as they found a higher inhibitory activity from the silver ion solution against *E. coli* than against *S. aureus* [70]. However, the microbiocidal activity of silver nanoparticles has been found against both Gram-positive (e.g., *Staphylococcus aureus*) or Gram-negative (e.g., *Escherichia coli*) and even yeasts [69,71,72], which is consistent with our results. The results of our study, where surface modified titanium alloys affected the inhibition of the growth of both Gram-positive and Gram-negative bacteria or fungi, are in good accordance with a previous report [58] where TiO_2 nanotubes enriched with Ag demonstrated superior bactericidal properties against the planktonic bacteria. Similar findings were reported by Reference [54]. The authors showed the strong bactericidal activity that titanium specimens incorporated with silver against *Staphylococcus aureus*. Moreover, the number of bacteria decreased as the dosage of the incorporated Ag increased, suggesting that the antibacterial ability increased with the content of deposited Ag [54].

5. Conclusions

The combination of antibacterial ability and biocompatibility, as well as non-cytotoxicity, studied in vitro, indicates that the optimal AgNPs enriching method could provide a promising strategy for the fabrication of a long-term antibacterial surface and, thus, an attractive biomaterial which successfully solves the growing problem of peri-implant infection. By taking into account the obtained results, it can be stated that all studied samples revealed very high antimicrobial activity, resulting from the release of Ag^- ions from silver nanoparticles, as well as high biocompatibility. Moreover, they are all characterized by a relatively simple synthesis. However, among studied systems, Ti6Al4V/TNT5/0.6AgNPs contained the lowest amount of AgNPs, but revealed to still have optimal biointegration properties and high biocidal properties. Thus, it can be taken into account as a biomaterial possessing the desired biological properties and, at the same time, as a biomaterial in which the potential harm is minimized by minimizing the number of silver nanoparticles.

Supplementary Materials: The following are available online at http://www.mdpi.com/2077-0383/8/3/334/s1, Table S1: The results of the contact angle measurements, which were made three times using distilled water and diiodomethane and the results of the surface free energy (SFE) of biomaterials used in Owens-Wendt method, Figure S1: Reduction of colony number of *Escherichia coli* ATCC25922=PCM2057 after treatment with silver ions released from Ti6Al4V/AgNPs (b–e) and Ti6Al4V/TNT5/AgNPs (g–j) for 24 h. Number of bacterial colonies after treatment with Ti6Al4V/AgNPs and Ti6Al4V/TNT5/AgNPs was reduced at least 100 fold when compared to Ti6Al4V (7.0×10^5 c.f.u. mL^{-1}) (a) and Ti6Al4V/TNT5 (3.8×10^5 c.f.u. mL^{-1}) (b).

Author Contributions: Conceptualization, A.R.; methodology, A.R.; formal analysis, A.R. T.J., P.G.; investigation, A.R., M.G., M.E., T.J., M.W., P.G.; writing—original draft preparation, A.R.; writing—review and editing, A.R.; visualization, A.R.; supervision, A.R.; project administration, A.R.; funding acquisition, A.R.

Funding: This research was funded by the Regional Operational Programme of the Kuyavian-Pomeranian Voivodeship (1.3.1. Support for research and development processes in academic enterprises), within the grant obtained by Nano-implant Ltd. The APC was funded by Nano-implant Ltd.

Conflicts of Interest: The authors declare no conflict of interest.

References

1. Murr, L.E. Nanoparticulate materials in antiquity: The good, the bad and the ugly. *Mater. Charact.* **2009**, *60*, 261–270. [CrossRef]
2. Solomon, S.D.; Bahadory, M.; Jeyarajasingam, A.V.; Rutkowsky, S.A.; Boritz, C. Synthesis and Study of Silver Nanoparticles. *J. Chem. Educ.* **2007**, *84*, 322–325.
3. Aleksander, J.W. History of the medical use of silver. *Surg. Infect.* **2009**, *10*, 289–292. [CrossRef] [PubMed]
4. Dizaj, S.M.; Lotfipour, F.; Barzegar-Jalali, M.; Zarrintan, M.H.; Adibkia, K. Antimicrobial activity of the metals and metal oxide nanoparticles. *Mater. Sci. Eng. C* **2014**, *44*, 278–284. [CrossRef] [PubMed]
5. Prabhu, S.; Poulose, E.K. Silver nanoparticles: Mechanism of antimicrobial action, synthesis, medical applications, and toxicity effects. *Int. Nano Lett.* **2012**, *2*, 1–10. [CrossRef]

6. Lemiere, J.A.; Harrison, J.J.; Turner, R.J. Antimicrobial activity of metals: Mechanisms, molecular targets and applications. *Nat. Rev. Microbiol.* **2013**, *11*, 371–384. [CrossRef] [PubMed]
7. Solanki, J.N.; Murthy, Z.V.P. Controlled Size Silver Nanoparticles Synthesis with Water-in-Oil Microemulsion Method: A Topical Review. *Ind. Eng. Chem. Res.* **2011**, *50*, 12311–12323. [CrossRef]
8. Wang, H.; Qiao, X.; Chen, J.; Ding, S. Preparation of silver nanoparticles by chemical reduction method. *Colloids Surf. A Physicochem. Eng. Asp.* **2005**, *256*, 111–115. [CrossRef]
9. Agnihotri, S.; Mukherji, S.; Mukherji, S. Size-controlled silver nanoparticles synthesized over the range 5–100 nm using the same protocol and their antibacterial efficacy. *RSC Adv.* **2014**, *4*, 3974–3983. [CrossRef]
10. Reidy, B.; Haase, A.; Luch, A.; Dawson, K.A.; Lynch, I. Mechanisms of Silver Nanoparticle Release, Transformation and Toxicity: A Critical Review of Current Knowledge and Recommendations for Future Studies and Applications. *Materials* **2013**, *6*, 2295–2350. [CrossRef] [PubMed]
11. Dakal, T.C.; Kumar, A.; Majumdar, R.S.; Yadav, V. Mechanistic Basis of Antimicrobial Actions of Silver Nanoparticles. *Front. Microbiol.* **2016**, *7*, 1–17. [CrossRef] [PubMed]
12. Durán, N.; Marcato, P.D.; De Conti, R.; Alves, O.L.; Costa, F.T.M.; Brocchi, M. Potential use of silver nanoparticles on pathogenic bacteria, their toxicity and possible mechanisms of action. *J. Braz. Chem. Soc.* **2010**, *21*, 949–959. [CrossRef]
13. de Lima, R.; Seabra, A.B.; Durán, N. Silver nanoparticles: A brief review of cytotoxicity and genotoxicity of chemically and biogenically synthesized nanoparticles. *J. Appl. Toxicol.* **2012**, *32*, 867–879. [CrossRef] [PubMed]
14. Fu, P.P.; Xia, Q.; Hwang, H.M.; Ray, P.C.; Yu, H. Mechanisms of nanotoxicity: Generation of reactive oxygen species. *J. Food Drug Anal.* **2014**, *22*, 64–75. [CrossRef] [PubMed]
15. Chen, X.; Schluesener, H.J. Nanosilver: A nanoproduct in medical application. *Toxicol. Lett.* **2008**, *176*, 1–12. [CrossRef] [PubMed]
16. Young, X.; Yujie, X.; Byung Kwon, L.; Skrabalak, S.E. Shape-Controlled Synthesis of Metal Nanocrystals: Simple Chemistry Meets Complex Physics, Nanostructure. *Angew. Chem. Int. Ed.* **2009**, 60–103.
17. Abdeen, S.; Geo, S.; Sukanya, S.; Praseetha, K.P.; Dhanya, R.P. Biosynthesis of Silver nanoparticles from Actinomycetes for therapeutic applications. *Int. J. Nano Dimens.* **2014**, *5*, 155–162.
18. Leśniak, W.; Bielińska, A.U.; Sun, K.; Janczak, K.W.; Shi, X.; Baker, J.R.; Balogh, L.P. Silver/dendrimer nanocomposites as biomarkers: Fabrication, characterization, in vitro toxicity, and intracellular detection. *Nano Lett.* **2005**, *5*, 2123–2130.
19. Kobayashi, Y.; Katakami, H.; Mine, E.; Nagao, D.; Konno, M.; Liz-Marzan, L.M. Silica coating of silver nanoparticles using a modified Stober method. *J. Colloid Interface Sci.* **2005**, *283*, 392–396. [CrossRef] [PubMed]
20. Sotiriou, G.A.; Pratsinis, S.E. Engineering nanosilver as an antibacterial, biosensor and bioimaging material. *Curr. Opin. Chem. Eng.* **2011**, *1*, 3–10. [CrossRef] [PubMed]
21. Marambio-Jones, C.; Hoek, E.M.V. A review of the antibacterial effects of silver nanomaterials and potential implications for human health and the environment. *J. Nanopart. Res.* **2009**, *12*, 1531–1551. [CrossRef]
22. De Matteis, V.; Malvindi, M.A.; Galeone, A.; Brunetti, V.; De Luca, E.; Kote, S.; Kshirsagar, P.; Sabella, S.; Bardi, G.; Pompa, P.P. Negligible particle-specific toxicity mechanism of silver nanoparticles: The role of Ag+ ion release in the cytosol. *Nanomed. Nanotechnol. Biol. Med.* **2015**, *11*, 731–739. [CrossRef] [PubMed]
23. Zhang, C.; Hu, Z.; Deng, B. Silver nanoparticles in aquatic environments: Physiochemical behavior and antimicrobial mechanisms. *Water Res.* **2016**, *88*, 403–427. [CrossRef] [PubMed]
24. AshaRani, P.V.; Hande, M.P.; Valiyaveettil, S. Anti-proliferative activity of silver nanoparticles. *BMC Cell Biol.* **2009**, *10*, 1–14. [CrossRef] [PubMed]
25. Zheng, J.; Wu, X.; Wang, M.; Ran, D.; Xu, W.; Yang, J. Study on the inter-action between silver nanoparticles and nucleic acids in the presence of cetyltrimethylammonium bromide and its analytical application. *Talanta* **2008**, *74*, 526–532. [CrossRef] [PubMed]
26. Beer, C.; Foldbjerg, R.; Hayashi, Y.; Sutherland, D.S.; Autrup, H. Toxicity of silver nanoparticles—Nanoparticle or silver ion? *Toxicol. Lett.* **2012**, *208*, 286–292. [CrossRef] [PubMed]
27. Kim, S.; Choi, J.E.; Choi, J.; Chung, K.H.; Park, K.; Yi, J.; Ryu, D.Y. Oxidative stress-dependent toxicity of silver nanoparticles in human hepatoma cells. *Toxico. In Vitro* **2009**, *23*, 1076–1084. [CrossRef] [PubMed]

28. Bouwmeester, H.; Poortman, J.; Peters, R.J.; Wijma, E.; Kramer, E.; Makama, S.; Puspitaninganindita, K.; Marvin, H.J.P.; Peijnenburg, A.A.C.M.; Hendriksen, P.J.M. Characterization of Translocation of Silver Nanoparticles and Effects on Whole-Genome Gene Expression Using an In Vitro Intestinal Epithelium Coculture Model. *ACS Nano* **2011**, *5*, 4091–4103. [CrossRef] [PubMed]
29. He, D.; Bligh, M.W.; Waite, T.D. Effects of aggregate structure on the dissolution kinetics of citrate-stabilized silver nanoparticles. *Environ. Sci. Technol.* **2013**, *47*, 1–32. [CrossRef] [PubMed]
30. Bressan, E.; Ferroni, L.; Gardin, C.; Rigo, C.; Stocchero, M.; Vindigni, V.; Cairns, W.; Zavan, B. Silver nanoparticles and mitochondrial interaction. *Int. J. Dent.* **2013**, *2013*, 312747. [CrossRef] [PubMed]
31. Moosa, A.A.; Muhsen, M.F. Ceramic Filters Impregnated with Silver Nanoparticles for Household Drinking Water Treatment. *Am. J. Mater. Sci.* **2017**, *6*, 232–239.
32. Raghavendra, G.M.; Jayaramudu, T.; Varaprasad, K.; Sadiku, R.; Ray, S.S.; Rajua, K.M. Cellulose–polymer–Ag nanocomposite fibers for antibacterial fabrics/skin scaffolds. *Carbohydr. Polym.* **2013**, *93*, 553–560. [CrossRef] [PubMed]
33. Lewandowska, Ż.; Piszczek, P.; Radtke, A.; Jędrzejewski, T.; Kozak, W.; Sadowska, B. The evaluation of the impact of titania nanotube covers morphology and crystal phase on their biological properties. *J. Mater. Sci. Mater. Med.* **2015**, *26*, 163. [CrossRef] [PubMed]
34. Piszczek, P.; Lewandowska, Ż.; Radtke, A.; Jedrzejewski, T.; Kozak, W.; Sadowska, B.; Szubka, M.; Talik, E.; Fiori, F. Biocompatibility of Titania Nanotube Coatings Enriched with Silver Nanograins by Chemical Vapor Deposition. *Nanomaterials* **2017**, *7*, 274. [CrossRef] [PubMed]
35. Radtke, A.; Jędrzejewski, T.; Kozak, W.; Sadowska, B.; Więckowska-Szakiel, M.; Talik, E.; Mäkelä, M.; Leskelä, M.; Piszczek, P. Optimization of the Silver Nanoparticles PEALD Process on the Surface of 1-D Titania Coatings. *Nanomaterials* **2017**, *7*, 193. [CrossRef] [PubMed]
36. Radtke, A.; Grodzicka, M.; Ehlert, M.; Muzioł, T.M.; Szkodo, M.; Bartmanski, M.; Piszczek, P. Studies on Silver Ions Releasing Processes and Mechanical Properties of Surface-Modified Titanium Alloy Implants. *Int. J. Mol. Sci.* **2018**, *19*, 962. [CrossRef] [PubMed]
37. Szłyk, E.; Piszczek, P.; Grodzicki, A.; Chaberski, M.; Goliński, A.; Szatkowski, J.; Błaszczyk, T. CVD of AgI Complexes with Tertiary Phosphines and Perfluorinated Carboxylates—A New Class of Silver Precursors. *Chem. Vap. Depos.* **2001**, *7*, 111–116. [CrossRef]
38. Radtke, A.; Topolski, A.; Jędrzejewski, T.; Kozak, W.; Sadowska, B.; Więckowska-Szakiel, M.; Szubka, M.; Talik, E.; Nielsen, L.P.; Piszczek, P. The Bioactivity and Photocatalytic Properties of Titania Nanotube. *Nanomaterials* **2017**, *7*, 197. [CrossRef] [PubMed]
39. Owens, D.K.; Wendt, R.C. Estimation of the surface free energy of polymers. *J. Appl. Polym. Sci.* **1969**, *13*, 1741–1747. [CrossRef]
40. Furuhashi, A.; Ayukawa, Y.; Atsuta, I.; Okawachi, H.; Koyano, K. The difference of fibroblast behavior on titanium substrata with different surface characteristics. *Odontology* **2012**, *100*, 199–205. [CrossRef] [PubMed]
41. Burmester, A.; Luthringer, B.; Willumeit, R.; Feyerabend, F. Comparison of the reaction of bone-derived cells to enhanced $MgCl_2$-salt concentrations. *Biomatter* **2014**, *4*, e967616. [CrossRef] [PubMed]
42. Thrivikraman, G.; Madras, G.; Basu, B. In vitro/In vivo assessment and mechanisms of toxicity of bioceramic materials and its wear particulates. *RSC Adv.* **2014**, *4*, 12763–12781. [CrossRef]
43. Lord, M.S.; Foss, M.; Besenbacher, F. Influence of nanoscale surface topography on protein adsorption and cellular response. *Nano Today* **2010**, *5*, 66–78. [CrossRef]
44. Ebrahimi, M.; Pripatnanont, P.; Suttapreyasri, S.; Monmaturapoj, N. In vitro biocompatibility analysis of novel nano-biphasic calcium phosphate scaffolds in different composition ratios. *J. Biomed. Mater. Res. B Appl. Biomater.* **2014**, *102*, 52–61. [CrossRef] [PubMed]
45. Braydich-Stolle, L.; Hussain, S.; Schlager, J.; Hofmann, M.C. In vitro cytotoxicity of nanoparticles in mammalian germ line stem cells. *Toxicol. Sci.* **2005**, *88*, 412–419. [CrossRef] [PubMed]
46. Alt, V.; Bechert, T.; Steinrucke, P.; Wagener, M.; Seidel, P. An in vitro assessment of the antibacterial properties and cytotoxicity of nanoparticulate silver bone cement. *Biomaterials* **2004**, *25*, 4383–4391. [CrossRef] [PubMed]
47. Lan, M.Y.; Liu, C.P.; Huang, H.H.; Lee, S.W. Both enhanced biocompatibility and antibacterial activity in Ag-decorated TiO_2 nanotubes. *PLoS ONE* **2013**, *8*, e75364. [CrossRef] [PubMed]
48. Esfandiari, N.; Simchi, A.; Bagheri, R. Size tuning of Ag-decorated TiO_2 nanotube arrays for improved bactericidal capacity of orthopedic implants. *J. Biomed. Mater. Res.* **2014**, *102*, 2625–2635. [CrossRef] [PubMed]

49. ISO 10993-1:2018 Standards. Biological Evaluation of Medical Devices—Part 1: Evaluation and Testing Within a Risk Management Proces. Available online: https://www.iso.org/standard/68936.html (accessed on 10 January 2019).
50. Kheur, S.; Singh, N.; Bodas, D.; Rauch, J.Y.; Jambhekar, S.; Kheur, M.; Rajwade, J. Nanoscale silver depositions inhibit microbial colonization and improve biocompatibility of titanium abutments. *Colloids Surf. B Biointerfaces* **2017**, *159*, 151–158. [CrossRef] [PubMed]
51. Ewald, A.; Glückermann, S.K.; Thull, R.; Gbureck, U. Antimicrobial titanium/silver PVD coatings on titanium. *Biomed. Eng. Online* **2006**, *5*, 22. [CrossRef] [PubMed]
52. Cevc, G.; Vierl, U. Nanotechnology and the transdermal route: A state of the art review and critical appraisal. *J. Controll. Release* **2010**, *141*, 277–299. [CrossRef] [PubMed]
53. Zhao, L.; Chu, P.K.; Zhang, Y.; Wu, Z. Antibacterial coatings on titanium implants. *J. Biomed. Mater. Res. B Appl. Biomater.* **2009**, *91*, 470–480. [CrossRef] [PubMed]
54. He, X.; Zhang, X.; Wang, X.; Qin, L. Review of antibacterial activity of titanium-based implants surfaces fabricated by micro-arc oxidation. *Coatings* **2017**, *7*, 45. [CrossRef]
55. Zhang, P.; Zhang, Z.; Li, W. Antibacterial TiO_2 coating incorporating silver nanoparticles by microarc oxidation and ion implantation. *J. Nanomater.* **2013**, *2013*, 8.
56. De Giglio, E.; Cometa, S.; Ricci, M.A.; Cafagna, D.; Savino, A.M.; Sabbatini, L.; Orciani, M.; Ceci, E.; Novello, L.; Tantillo, G.M.; et al. Ciprofloxacin modified electrosynthesized hydrogel coatings to prevent titanium-implant-associated infections. *Acta Biomater.* **2011**, *7*, 882–891. [CrossRef] [PubMed]
57. Rodriguez, O.; Stone, W.; Schemitsch, E.H.; Zalzal, P.; Waldman, S.; Papini, M.; Towler, M.R. Titanium addition influences antibacterial activity of bioactive glass coatings on metallic implants. *Heliyon* **2017**, *3*, e00420. [CrossRef] [PubMed]
58. Zhao, L.; Wang, H.; Huo, K.; Cui, L.; Zhang, W.; Ni, H.; Zhang, Y.; Wu, Z.; Chu, P.K. Antibacterial nano-structured titania coating incorporated with silver nanoparticles. *Biomaterials* **2011**, *32*, 5706–5716. [CrossRef] [PubMed]
59. Morones, J.R.; Elechiguerra, L.J.; Camacho, A.; Holt, K.; Kouri, B.J. The bactericidal effect of silver nanoparticles. *Nanotechnology* **2005**, *16*, 2346–2353. [CrossRef] [PubMed]
60. Lok, C.N.; Ho, C.M.; Chen, R.; He, Q.Y.; Yu, W.Y.; Sun, H. Proteomic analysis of the mode of antibacterial action of silver nanoparticles. *J. Proteome. Res.* **2006**, *5*, 916–924. [CrossRef] [PubMed]
61. Panáček, A.; Kvitek, L.; Prucek, R.; Kolar, M.; Vecerova, R. Silver colloid nanoparticles: Synthesis, characterization, and their antibacterial activity. *J. Phys. Chem. B* **2006**, *110*, 16248–16253. [CrossRef] [PubMed]
62. Ghosh, S.; Patil, S.; Ahire, M.; Kitture, R.; Kale, S.; Pardesi, K. Synthesis of silver nanoparticles using *Dioscorea bulbifera* tuber extract and evolution of its synergistic potential in combination with antimicrobial agents. *Int. J. Nanomed.* **2012**, *7*, 483–496.
63. Chauhan, R.; Kumar, A.; Abraham, J. A Biological approach to the synthesis of silver nanoparticles with *Streptomyces* sp. JAR1 and its antimicrobial activity. *Sci. Pharm.* **2013**, *81*, 607–621. [CrossRef] [PubMed]
64. Kim, S.H.; Lee, H.S.; Ryu, D.S.; Choi, S.J.; Lee, D.S. Antibacterial activity of silver–nanoparticles against *Staphylococcus aureus* and *Escherichia coli*. *Korean J. Microbiol. Biotechnol.* **2011**, *39*, 77–85.
65. Li, J.; Rong, K.; Zhao, H.; Li, F.; Lu, Z.; Chen, R. Highly selective antibacterial activities of silver nanoparticles against *Bacillus subtilis*. *J. Nanosci. Nanotechnol.* **2013**, *13*, 6806–6813. [CrossRef] [PubMed]
66. Feng, Q.L.; Wu, J.; Chen, G.O.; Cui, F.Z.; Kim, T.N.; Kim, J.O. A mechanistic study of the antibacterial effect of silver ions on *Escherichia coli* and *Staphylococcus aureus*. *J. Biomed. Mater. Res. Part A* **2000**, *52*, 662–668. [CrossRef]
67. Manivasagan, P.; Venkatesan, J.; Senthilkumar, K.; Sivakumar, K.; Kim, S.K. Biosynthesis, antimicrobial and cytotoxic effect of silver nanoparticles using a novel *Nocardiopsis* sp. MBRC-1. *Biol. Med. Res. Int.* **2013**, 1–9.
68. Rai, M.K.; Deshmukh, S.D.; Ingle, A.P.; Gade, A.K. Silver nanoparticles: The powerful nanoweapon against multidrug-resistant bacteria. *J. Appl. Microbiol.* **2012**, *112*, 841–852. [CrossRef] [PubMed]
69. Kim, J.S.; Kuk, E.; Yu, K.N.; Kim, J.H.; Park, S.J.; Lee, H.J.; Kim, S.H.; Park, Y.K.; Park, Y.H.; Hwang, C.Y.; et al. Antimicrobial effects of silver nanoparticles. *Nanomedicine* **2007**, *3*, 95–101. [CrossRef] [PubMed]
70. Jung, W.K.; Koo, H.C.; Kim, K.W.; Shin, S.; Kim, S.H.; Park, Y.H. Antibacterial activity and mechanism of action of the silver ion in *Staphylococcus aureus* and *Escherichia coli*. *Appl. Environ. Microbiol.* **2008**, *74*, 2171–2178. [CrossRef] [PubMed]

71. Mohan, Y.M.; Lee, K.; Premkumar, T.; Geckeler, K.E. Hydrogel networks as nanoreactors: A novel approach to silver nanoparticles for antibacterial applications. *Polymer* **2007**, *48*, 158–164. [CrossRef]
72. Wypij, M.; Czarnecka, J.; Swiecimska, M.; Dahm, H.; Rai, M.; Golinska, P. Synthesis, characterization and evaluation of antimicrobial and cytotoxic activities of biogenic silver nanoparticles synthesized from Streptomyces xinghaiensis OF1 strain. *World J. Microbiol. Biotechnol.* **2018**, *34*, 2. [CrossRef] [PubMed]

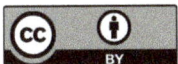

© 2019 by the authors. Licensee MDPI, Basel, Switzerland. This article is an open access article distributed under the terms and conditions of the Creative Commons Attribution (CC BY) license (http://creativecommons.org/licenses/by/4.0/).

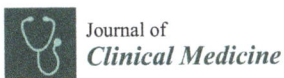

Article

The Morphology, Structure, Mechanical Properties and Biocompatibility of Nanotubular Titania Coatings before and after Autoclaving Process

Aleksandra Radtke [1,2,*], Michalina Ehlert [1,2], Tomasz Jędrzejewski [3] and Michał Bartmański [4]

1. Faculty of Chemistry, Nicolaus Copernicus University in Toruń, Gagarina 7, 87-100 Toruń, Poland; m.ehlert@doktorant.umk.pl
2. Nano-implant Ltd., Gagarina 5/102, 87-100 Toruń, Poland
3. Faculty of Biology and Environmental Protection, Nicolaus Copernicus University in Toruń, Lwowska 1, 87-100 Toruń, Poland; tomaszj@umk.pl
4. Faculty of Mechanical Engineering, Gdańsk University of Technology, Gabriela Narutowicza 11/12, 80-233 Gdańsk, Poland; michal.bartmanski@pg.edu.pl
* Correspondence: aradtke@umk.pl; Tel.: +48-600-321-294

Received: 29 January 2019; Accepted: 20 February 2019; Published: 23 February 2019

Abstract: The autoclaving process is one of the sterilization procedures of implantable devices. Therefore, it is important to assess the impact of hot steam at high pressure on the morphology, structure, and properties of implants modified by nanocomposite coatings. In our works, we focused on studies on amorphous titania nanotubes produced by titanium alloy (Ti6Al4V) electrochemical oxidation in the potential range 5–60 V. Half of the samples were drying in argon stream at room temperature, and the second ones were drying additionally with the use of immersion in acetone and drying at 396 K. Samples were subjected to autoclaving and after sterilization they were structurally and morphologically characterized using Raman spectroscopy, diffuse reflectance infrared Fourier transform spectroscopy (DRIFT) and scanning electron microscopy (SEM). They were characterized in terms of wettability, mechanical properties, and biocompatibility. Obtained results proved that the autoclaving of amorphous titania nanotube coatings produced at lower potentials (5–15 V) does not affect their morphology and structure regardless of the drying method before autoclaving. Nanotubular coatings produced using higher potentials (20–60 V) require removal of adsorbed water particles from their surface. Otherwise, autoclaving leads to the destruction of the architecture of nanotubular coatings, which is associated with the changing of their mechanical and biointegration properties.

Keywords: titanium dioxide; nanotubes; autoclaving; titanium alloy; biocompatibility; wettability; mechanical properties

---

1. Introduction

Titanium and its alloys (Ti6Al4V, Ti5Al25Fe, and Ti6Al7Nb) are commonly used as biomaterials for orthopedic, dental, or neurosurgery applications [1–3]. This choice is determined by the beneficial properties of titanium, which is characterized by the excellent corrosion resistance, light weight, high strength, chemical stability, and modulus of elasticity much closer to that one of bone, compared to other metals. Unfortunately, its surface does not form a direct connection with the living bone [3–5]. And the most significant factor influencing the efficiency of implantology is the interaction between the body cells and the implanted artificial biomaterial [4–6]. In a wide range of clinical applications, implant rejections still occur mainly due to osseointegration defects and infection [7,8]. Many techniques are used to modify the surface topography of implants in order to improve cell adhesion and osteogenic differentiation on them. It has been concluded that the surface roughness is conducive to the osseointegration process, influences the adhesion of osteoblasts, increases their enzymatic activity and determines the amount and type of proteins they synthesize [6,7,9–11]. The appropriate porosity of the implant is ensured, by scaffolds manufactured on its surface, which are characterized by the specific structure, morphology, and wettability [12,13]. According to previous reports, the fabrication of the titanium dioxide nanotubes coating (TNT) on the surface of titanium or titanium alloys implants, improves the adhesion and proliferation of osteoblast cells, and promotes the faster growth of bone and vascular tissue [14,15]. TNT coatings on the surfaces of medical devices, fabricated of titanium or titanium alloys, are commonly produced by their electrochemical anodization [5,7,16–20]. The main advantages of this technique are: the mild processing conditions, low costs, possibilities of large-scale production, and, which is the most important, very good control of structural and morphological properties [16,21]. By changing the type and composition of the electrolyte solution, the anodizing voltage, the temperature and duration of anodizing, it is possible to control the diameter and length of the nanotubes [17,21]. For medical applications, it is particularly important to control the diameters of the produced tubes, as their size influences on the coating biocompatibility degree. Considering earlier reports it should be noted that TNT coatings, which consist of nanotubes with different tube sizes (30–100 nm) could enhance osteoblast cell functions [22,23]. Park et al. suggest something opposite - that nanotubes of smaller sizes than 15 nm strongly enhance cell activities and cell functions deteriorate with increasing tube sizes [24]. Results of our works confirm this suggestion. However, this applies to TNT coatings consisted of nanotubes with 25–35 diameters [25]. Zaho et al. noted that the observed divergences might be caused by the used sterilization method and its possible influence on morphology, structure and the biocompatibility of titania nanotubes [26]. Among the sterilization procedures, which are commonly applied in the clinical practice, i.e., gamma radiation, plasma sterilization, ethylene oxide (EO) sterilization, autoclaving, ultraviolent (UV) irradiation, and ethanol immersion [26–30]—autoclaving is the one, we have used in our research. In this method, the medical device's surface is treated by the hot steam under increased pressure. In the case of implants coated with bioactive TNT layer, such treatment may lead to changes in their surface morphology, structure, mechanical properties, and biocompatibility.

In our works, we have focused on studies on autoclaving procedure influence on the surface architecture rearrangement, mechanical properties and biointegration of nanotubular systems produced via anodic oxidation of titanium alloy at different potentials (5–60 V). Despite intense works on the application of TNT coatings in clinical practice as well as the wide use of autoclaving as the main sterilization procedure, above-mentioned issues have not been sufficiently investigated. Therefore, the results discussed in this paper can be important both for the design and fabrication of Ti6Al4V implants coated with bioactive coating and also for their practical use for clinicians.

2. Experimental Section

2.1. Synthesis and Characterization of Studied Coatings

Scheme 1 presents the experimental procedure applied in our studies. The electrochemical anodization of Ti6Al4V foil samples (Ti6Al4V, grade 5, 99.7% purity, 0.20 mm thick (Strem Chemicals, Inc., Bischheim, France), 5 mm × 50 mm strips) was carried out in accordance with the previously described methodology [25]. The uniform TNT coatings were produced using the following potentials: 5, 10, 15, and 20–60 V (every 10V) at room temperature (anodization time t = 30 min). After the anodization, all produced nanotubular systems (Ti6Al4V/TNT/F samples; F-freshly obtained) were washed 10 minutes in an ultrasonic bath in deionized water (Ti6Al4V/TNT/W samples; W-washed) and then their surfaces were drying in a stream of argon at room temperature (Ti6Al4V/TNT/Ar samples; Ar-dried in stream of argon).

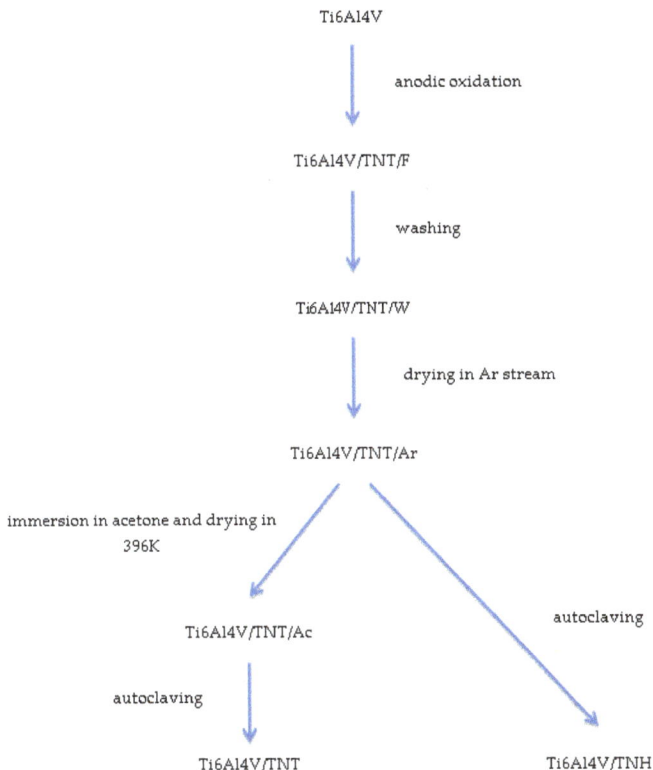

Scheme 1. The scheme of experimental procedure applied in the preparation of the samples.

Due to the fact that the fabricated TiO$_2$ nanotubes could still contain water molecules, adsorbed inside of tubes, which were not removed by the use of the Ar stream, half of the samples were subjected to an additional drying process. These samples were immersed in acetone for 10 min in ultrasonic bath and then were drying at 396 K for 1 h. All produced samples were then autoclaved using IS YESON YS-18L autoclave (Ningbo Haishu Yeson Medical Device Co. Ltd, Zhejiang, China) at 396 K, using $p = 120$ kPa, $t = 30$ min. The surface morphology of studies samples, at every stage of the experimental procedure, was studied, using Quanta scanning electron microscope with field emission (SEM, Quanta 3D FEG, FEI Company, Huston, TX, USA). The structure of the produced coatings was studied using Raman spectroscopy (RamanMicro 200 PerkinElmer (PerkinElmer Inc., Waltham, MA, USA) ($\lambda = 785$ nm)) and diffuse reflectance infrared Fourier transform spectroscopy (DRIFT, Spectrum2000, PerkinElmer Inc., Waltham, MA, USA). The wettability and surface free energy of the produced titania nanocoatings were determined using earlier described methods [25,31]. The contact angle was measured using a goniometer (DSA 10 Krüss GmbH, Hamburg, Germany) with drop shape analysis software (ADVANCE). Each measurement was carried out three times.

2.2. Topography and Mechanical Properties of Studied Coatings

Surface topographies were examined by means of atomic force microscopy (AFM, NaniteAFM, Nanosurf AG, Liestal, Switzerland) using a contactless module with a force of 20 nN in the 50 × 50 µm area. Hardness tests and Young modulus measurements were carried out using a nanoindenter (NanoTest Vantage, Micro Materials Ltd., Wrexham, UK) with a pyramidal, diamond, three-sided Berkovich indenter, at an apical angle of 124.4°. Hardness tests were performed for loads of 10 mN.

The time of load increase from the zero value to the maximum load 10 mN was 15 s. Indentation were performed at one cycle with 5 s dwell at maximum load. Hardness (H), reduced Young's modulus (E_r), and Young's modulus values were determined using the Oliver-Pharr method based on the NanoTest results analysis program. In order to convert the reduced Young's modulus into Young's modulus, a Poisson coefficient of 0.25 was assumed for the coatings.

Tests of coatings adhesion were made using nanoindenter (NanoTest Vantage, Micro Materials Ltd., Wrexham, UK) and the Berkovich indenter, as in the case of the nanoindentation tests.

The parameters of scratch tests were as follows: scratch load 0 to 500 mN, loading rate 3.3 mN/s, scan velocity 3 µm/s, and scan length 500 µm. Based on the dependence of the friction force (F_t) on the normal force (F_n) in the program for the analysis of NanoTest results, the values of critical friction force (L_f) and critical force (L_c), which caused the separation of the layer from the substrate, were determined.

2.3. Analysis of Studied Coatings Biointegration Properties

2.3.1. Cell Culture

Human osteoblast-like MG-63 cells (European Collection of Cell Cultures, Salisbury, UK) were plated in a 25 cm^2 cell culture flask (Corning, Corning, NY, USA) and culture with Eagle's Minimum Essential Medium containing 2 mM L-glutamine, 1 mM sodium pyruvate, Minimum Essential Medium (MEM) non-essential amino acid, heat-inactivated 10% fetal bovine serum (FBS), 100 µg/mL streptomycin and 100 IU/mL penicillin (all compounds from Sigma-Aldrich, Darmstadt, Germany). Cultures were maintained at 37 °C in a 95% humidified atmosphere of 5% CO_2. The culture medium was changed every 2–3 days. The cells were passaged using 0.25% trypsin- ethylenediaminetetraacetic acid (EDTA) solution (Sigma-Aldrich, Darmstadt, Germany) when reaching 70–80% of confluence.

Murine fibroblast cell line L929 (American Type Culture Collection, Manassas, VA, USA) were cultured at 37 °C in 5% CO_2 and 95% humidity in a complete Roswell Park Memorial Institute (RPMI) 1640 medium containing 2 mM L-glutamine, heat-inactivated 10% FBS, 100 µg/mL streptomycin and 100 IU/mL penicillin. L929 cells culture conditions were the same as we have described previously [32].

The cells belong to both cell lines, in a volume of 1 mL of appropriate culture medium, were seeded onto the autoclaved tested specimens placed in a 24-well culture plate (Corning, Corning, NY, USA) at a density of 1×10^4 cells/well for 24 h, 72 h or 120 h, respectively. The cells incubated with the tested plates in the above incubation time were also analyzed for the observation of cell morphology. Cell morphology and proliferation was investigated for the Ti6Al4V/TNH samples as well as for Ti6Al4V/TNT specimens.

2.3.2. Proliferation of L929 Fibroblasts and MG-63 Osteoblasts Detected by MTT Assay

The effect of the tested specimens on the cell proliferation (after 24-, 72- and 120 h, respectively) was studied by the MTT (3-(4,5-dimethylthiazole-2-yl)-2,5-diphenyl tetrazolium bromide; Sigma Aldrich, Darmstadt, Germany) assay using the same method as it was reported in Lewandowska et al. [28]. Briefly, after the respective incubation time, the plates were washed with phosphate buffered saline (PBS) and transferred to a new 24-well culture plate. The MTT (5 mg/mL; Sigma-Aldrich, Darmstadt, Germany) solution in a culture medium without phenol red (RPMI 1640 medium for L929 fibroblasts or Eagle's Minimum Essential Medium for MG-63 osteoblasts; both from Sigma-Aldrich, Darmstadt, Germany) was added to each well. After 3 h of incubation at 37 °C in a humidified atmosphere of 5% CO_2, the solution was aspirated, 500 µL of dimethyl sulfoxide (DMSO; 100% v/v; Sigma Aldrich, Darmstadt, Germany) was added to each well and the plates were shaken for 10 min. The absorbance was measured at the wavelength of 570 nm with the subtraction of the 630 nm background, using a microplate reader (Synergy HT; BioTek, Winooski, VT, USA). The blank groups (the plates incubated without cells) were treated with the same procedures as the experimental groups. All measurements were done in duplicate in five independent experiments.

2.3.3. Cell Morphology

Scanning electron microscopy (SEM; Quanta 3D FEG; Carl Zeiss, Göttingen, Germany) analyses were performed to study the morphology changes of L929 fibroblasts and MG-63 osteoblasts grown on the surface of the tested specimens using the same method as in Lewandowska et al. [32]. Briefly, after the selected incubation time, the samples were washed with PBS to remove the non-adherent cells and were fixed in 2.5% v/v glutaraldehyde (Sigma Aldrich, Darmstadt, Germany) for a minimum of 4 h. Then, the plates were rinsed again with PBS and dehydrated in a graded series of ethanol (50%, 75%, 90%, and 100%). Finally, the specimens were dried in vacuum-assisted desiccators overnight and stored at room temperature until the SEM analysis was performed.

2.3.4. Statistical Analysis in the MTT Assay

All values are reported as means ± standard error of the means (SEM) and were analyzed using analysis of variance (ANOVA) followed by Bonferroni multiple comparisons test with the level of significance set at $p < 0.05$. Statistical analyses were performed with GraphPad Prism 7.0 (GraphPad Software, La Jolla, CA, USA).

3. Results

3.1. Synthesis of Nanotubular Coatings and Analysis of Their Surface Morphology on Different Steps of Experimental Procedure

Titania nanotube (TNT) layers on the surface of Ti6Al4V foil samples were produced according to the earlier described electrochemical oxidation methodology (anodization process) [25] in potentials range U = 5–60 V at room temperature (RT). After washing them in deionized water and drying them in the stream of argon their surface morphology has been checked. SEM images presented Ti6Al4V/TNT/Ar surface nanoarchitecture are visible in Figures 1 and 2. In Table S1 diameters of formed nanotubes and their wall thickness are presented.

In the next stage, the produced Ti6Al4V/TNT5-TNT60/Ar systems were divided into two groups. The first one was autoclaved directly, leading to the production of Ti6Al4V/TNH5-TNH60, and the second one, before autoclaving was subjected to the additional drying process, using immersion in acetone and drying at 396 K for 1 h. This second procedure led to the production of Ti6Al4V/TNT5-TNT60. Figures 1 and 2 present the differences in surface morphology of Ti6Al4V/TNH5-TNH60 and Ti6Al4V/TNT5-TNT60 and their comparison with the initial nanotubes samples, after drying in Ar stream, before the autoclaving process - Ti6Al4V/TNT5-TNT60/Ar. The comparison of SEM images of TNT5/Ar, TNT10/Ar coatings with TNH5, TNH10, TNT5, and TNT10 ones proves that regardless of the method used to dry the samples before autoclaving, the surface morphology after autoclaving remains unchanged, even identical (Figure 1). In the case of TNT15/Ar, TNH15, and TNT15 coatings, the slight surface changes were noticed for the TNH15 sample, which consisted in the partial, incidentally appeared destruction of nanotubes. Analysis of SEM images of TNT20-TNT60 coatings and TNH20-TNH60 ones revealed significant differences in their morphology. The tubular surface architecture of Ti6Al4V/TNT20-60 is identical with the initial samples Ti6Al4V/TNT20-60/Ar. But the surface architecture of Ti6Al4V/TNH20-60 samples is nothing like the starting nanotubes—nanotubular architecture of Ti6Al4V/TNT20-60/Ar was completely destroyed (Figure 2).

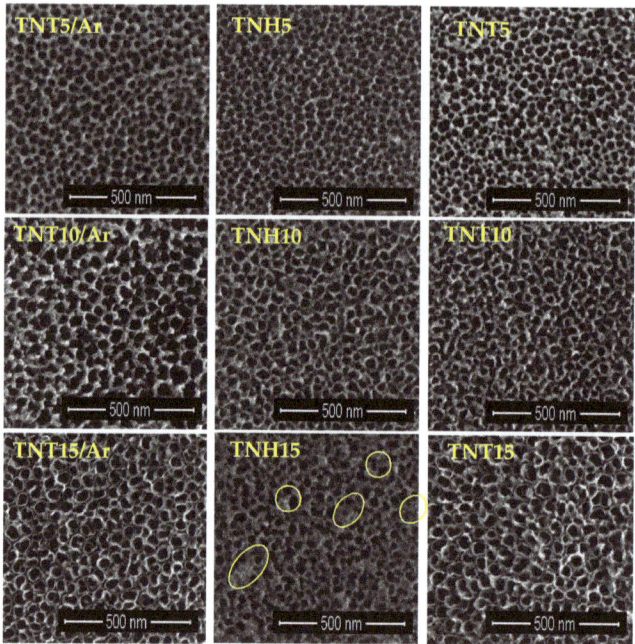

Figure 1. Scanning Electron Microscopy (SEM) images of Ti6Al4V/TNT5-15/Ar, Ti6Al4V/TNH5-TNH15, and Ti6Al4V/TNT5-15 samples surface (selected destruction sites of TiO_2 nanotubes were marked with circles).

A significant influence of preparing procedure of nanotubular coatings for autoclaving and the autoclaving process itself, on surface morphology changes, for nanotubes with higher potential (20–60 V), highlighted a focus for future works in terms of structure, wettability, mechanical properties, and biocompability of two groups of samples obtained at potential 20–60 V: (1) nanotubes coatings, dried after their production in ordinary way, only with Ar stream at RT—which nanotubular morphology during the autoclaving is completely destroyed (we will describe them as Ti6Al4V/TNH20-60 systems, or just TNH20-60 coatings, H—indicates that they are hydrothermally modified) and (2) nanotubes coatings dried additionally using immersion in acetone and slow drying in 396K, which nanotubular morphology during the autoclaving is not changed (we will describe them as Ti6Al4V/TNT20-60 systems or just TNT20-60 coatings).

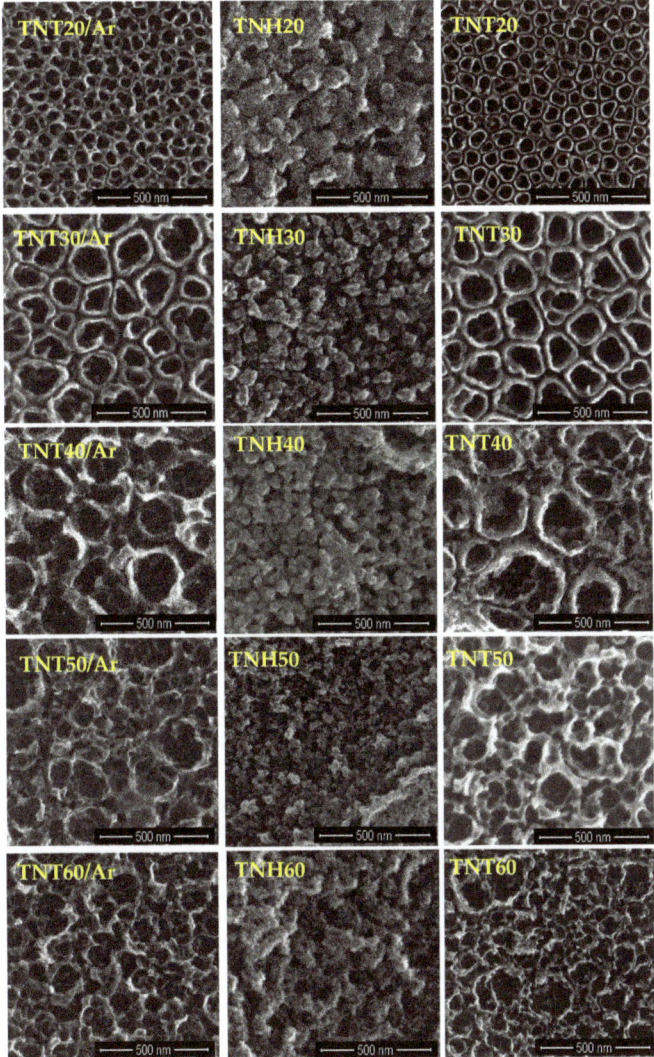

Figure 2. SEM images of Ti6Al4V/TNT20-60/Ar, Ti6Al4V/TNH20-TNH60, and Ti6Al4V/TNT20-60 samples surface.

3.2. Structural Studies on TNH20-60 and TNT20-60 Coatings and Their Wettability Analysis

The Raman and diffuse reflectance infrared Fourier transform spectroscopy (IR DRIFT) methods have been used to study the eventual structural differences between Ti6Al4V/TNH20-TNT60 and Ti6Al4V/TNT20-60 systems, as we suspected that structural changes could follow the already described morphological changes (Figure 3). Analysis of Raman spectra between 300 and 700 cm^{-1} of TNT20-TNT60 coatings confirms the amorphousness of these samples (Figure 3a). Raman spectra of TNH20-TNH60 samples indicate also on the formation of amorphous layers. However, very weak bands, which were found at 450 and 611 cm^{-1} and also at 399, 516, and 639 cm^{-1} indicate on the possible phase transitions and the formation of TiO$_2$ rutile/anatase (TNH20, TNH30, TNH60) nanocrystals (Figure 3b). The strong bands detected between 600 and 950 cm^{-1} in all DRIFT spectra of TNH20-TNH60 samples confirm the formation of TiO$_2$ layers (Figure S1).

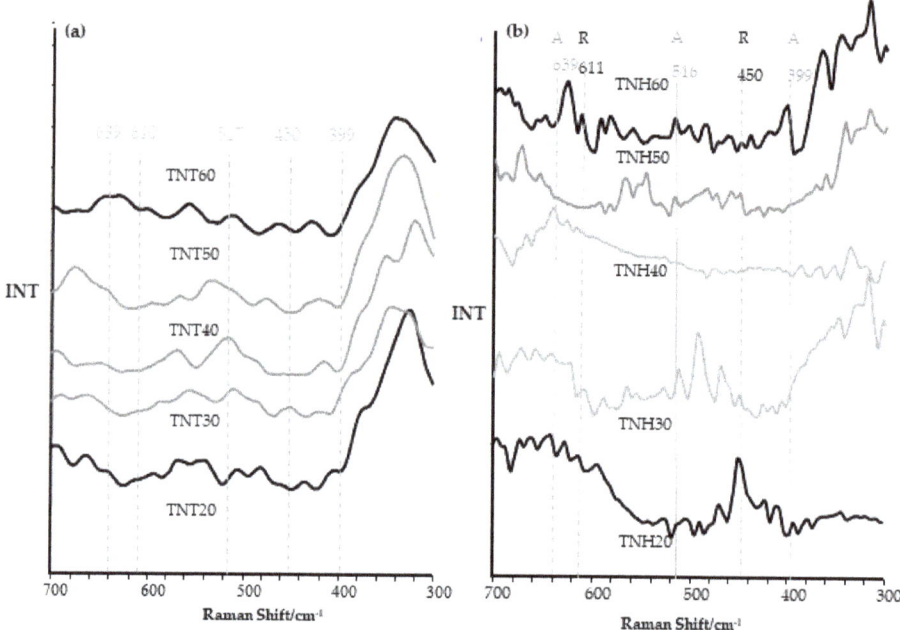

Figure 3. Raman spectra of Ti6Al4V/TNT20-60 (**a**) and Ti6Al4V/TNH20-TNT60 (**b**) samples (A—TiO$_2$ anatase form, R—TiO$_2$ rutile form).

In order to answer the question, what is responsible for the differences in the surface morphology of Ti6Al4V/TNT20-60 and Ti6Al4V/TNH20-TNT60, and at the same time taking into account our suspicion that the reason for the differences may be the water, which is not completely dried during the traditional drying process using a stream of argon, we made detailed Raman and IR DRIFT spectra analyses of Ti6Al4V/TNT20-60/Ar and Ti6Al4V/TNT20-60/Ac systems. Analysis of DRIFT spectra of Ti6Al4V/TNT20-60/Ar samples revealed the presence of weak and very weak bands at 3320–3390 cm^{-1} and 1620–1660 cm^{-1}, which were attributed to ν(OH) (stretching) and δ(HOH) (bending) modes of water molecules, respectively (Figures 4 and 5). Moreover, the very strong band, which was found between 450 and 1000 cm^{-1} was assigned to ν(Ti-O) modes of TiO$_2$, which confirms the formation of titania nanotube layers. In IR spectra of Ti6Al4V/TNT20-60/Ac samples (which after anodization were immersed in acetone and dried at 396 K), the intensity of bands attributed to vibrations of water molecules significantly decreased (Figure 5). According to these data, we can assume that the use of additional drying procedure allows for the removing of water molecules from the nanotubular surface of Ti6Al4V/TNT20-60/Ar, in particular from inside the nanotubes.

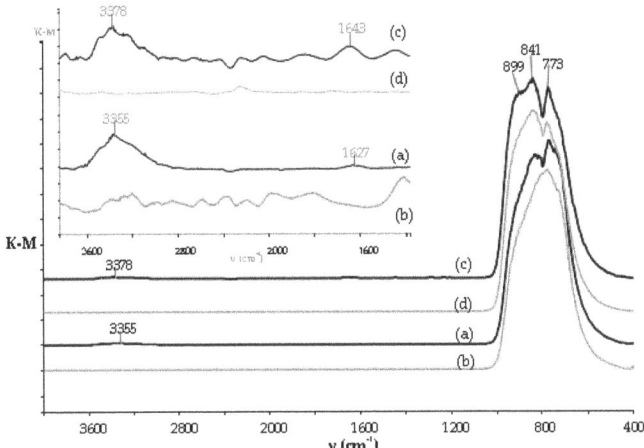

Figure 4. Infrared (IR) spectra (DRIFT) of (**a**) Ti6Al4V/TNT20/Ar and (**c**) Ti6Al4V/TNT50/Ar samples (the samples after drying in the Ar stream) and Ti6Al4V/TNT20/Ac (**b**) and Ti6Al4V/TNT50/Ac (**d**) the samples immersed in acetone and dried at 396 K by 1 h.

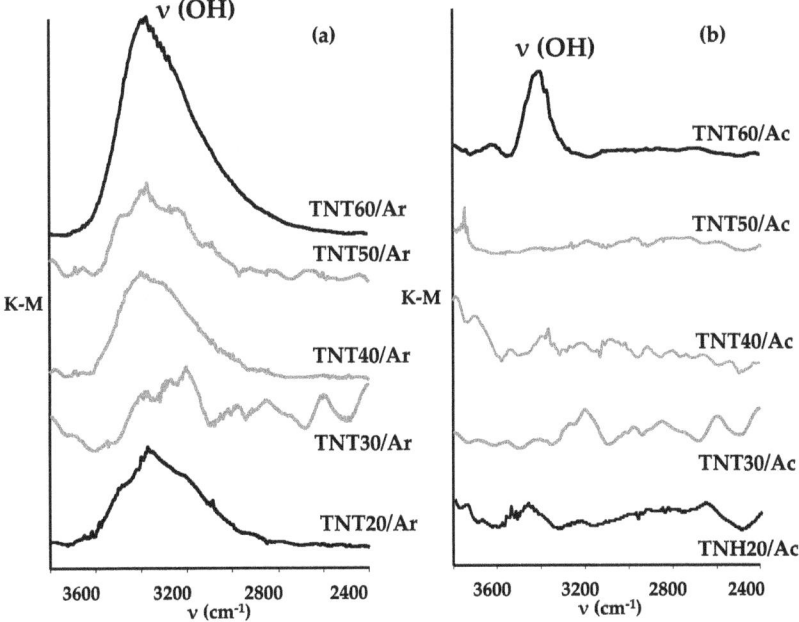

Figure 5. IR DRIFT spectra of (**a**) Ti6Al4V/TNT20-60/Ar and (**b**) Ti6Al4V/TNT20-60/Ac systems.

The results of contact angles measurements for water and diiodomethane, and also changes of surface free energy value (SFE) of Ti6Al4V/TNH20-60 and Ti6Al4V/TNT20-60 are presented in Figure S2 and in Table S2. According to these data, it can be stated that the wettability of Ti6Al4V/TNH20-60 layers is significantly different then adequate values for Ti6Al4V/TNT20-60. However, these differences in the case of TNT60 and TNH60 are not so huge. Analysis of data presented in Figure S2(a) indicate the clear hydrophobic character of Ti6Al4V/TNH20-60 layers, whose tubular architecture was destroyed and much more hydrophilic character of Ti6Al4V/TNT20-60. In the case of Ti6Al4V/TNT20-60 their hydrophilicity decreases from TNT20 to TNT60. The free surface energy (SFE) of the produced coatings was appointed by the Owens-Wendt method [33]. This method required the contact angles measured for two liquids, i.e., water as a polar liquid (Figure S2(a)) and dispersive one such as diiodomethane (Figure S2(b)). The SFE calculations for Ti6Al4V/TNT20-60 samples showed that their values change in the narrow range, i.e. from SFE = 47.6 (mJ/cm^2) up to SFE = 53.7 (mJ/cm^2). In the case of Ti6Al4V/TNH20-60 samples, the SFE value increases from 28.4 to 63.8 (mJ/cm^2) for TNH20-TNH40 and again decreases to 61.0 and 49.2 (mJ/cm^2) for TNH50-TNH60 respectively (Figure S2(c)).

3.3. Topography and Mechanical Properties of Ti6Al4V/TNH20-60 and Ti6Al4V/TNT20-60 Samples

The studies of surface topography and mechanical properties (such us hardness, Young's modulus) were carried out on the reference Ti6Al4V specimens, Ti6Al4V/TNH20-60 and Ti6Al4V/TNT20-60 systems. The studies of adhesion were performed for the same composites without reference Ti6Al4V specimens. The purpose of the research was to determine the relations between roughness parameters S_a, of studied systems.

3.3.1. Surface Topography

Analysis of atomic force microscopy (AFM) images allowed the estimation of differences in surface topography of Ti6Al4V/TNH20-60 and Ti6Al4V/TNT20-60 samples versus pure Ti6Al4V foil as a reference sample. Surface roughness parameter S_a, was determined using software, being an integral part of the device. The AFM topography and S_a parameters value are presented in Figure 6 and in Table S3. As demonstrated by the performed research, the electrochemical anodization of titanium alloy surface and their further autoclaving increases the roughness parameter S_a for all specimens in comparison to the reference titanium alloy. For the layers from TNT20 to TNT50 and TNH20 to TNH50, the increase of roughness with increasing voltage applied during the anodization process was observed. For the TNT60 and TNH60 layers, the decrease of the roughness was noticed compared to earlier TNT50 and TNH50 coatings. Also, the additional drying of Ti6Al4V/TNT/Ar changed surface roughness parameter S_a of Ti6Al4V/TNH20-60—all of them posses the higher S_a values than adequate Ti6Al4V/TNT20-60 systems. The correlation between the S_a parameter and the architecture of the nanotubular layers can be observed (Table 1, Table S1, Figure 2, Figure 6). With increasing the wall thickness of nanotubes, the roughness parameter S_a increased.

Table 1. Mechanical and nanoindentation properties (hardness, Young's modulus and maximum depth of indentation) of reference Ti6Al4V, Ti6Al4V/TNH20-60 and Ti6Al4V/TNT20-60 systems.

Biomaterial Sample	Hardness (GPa)	Young's Modulus (GPa)	Maximum Depth of Indentation (nm)
Ti6Al4V	16.17 ± 3.61	269.74 ± 40.10	162.14 ± 14.95
TNH20	10.24 ± 2.59	293.01 ± 59.43	194.40 ± 24.46
TNH30	9.15 ± 3.19	258.82 ± 57.44	212.80 ± 46.42
TNH40	4.95 ± 2.78	213.74 ± 87.35	323.33 ± 141.30
TNH50	4.43 ± 2.00	192.45 ± 56.42	312.17 ± 78.23
TNH60	6.51 ± 2.80	214.97 ± 52.72	258.13 ± 68.94
TNT20	19.38 ± 6.13	462.76 ± 245.91	143.99 ± 22.26
TNT30	16.81 ± 5.80	370.23 ± 109.44	160.08 ± 38.65
TNT40	9.42 ± 4.12	269.16 ± 79.77	212.39 ± 42.11
TNT50	9.56 ± 5.12	269.14 ± 91.83	217.36 ± 51.49
TNT60	14.32 ± 4.29	320.72 ± 77.26	169.28 ± 26.80

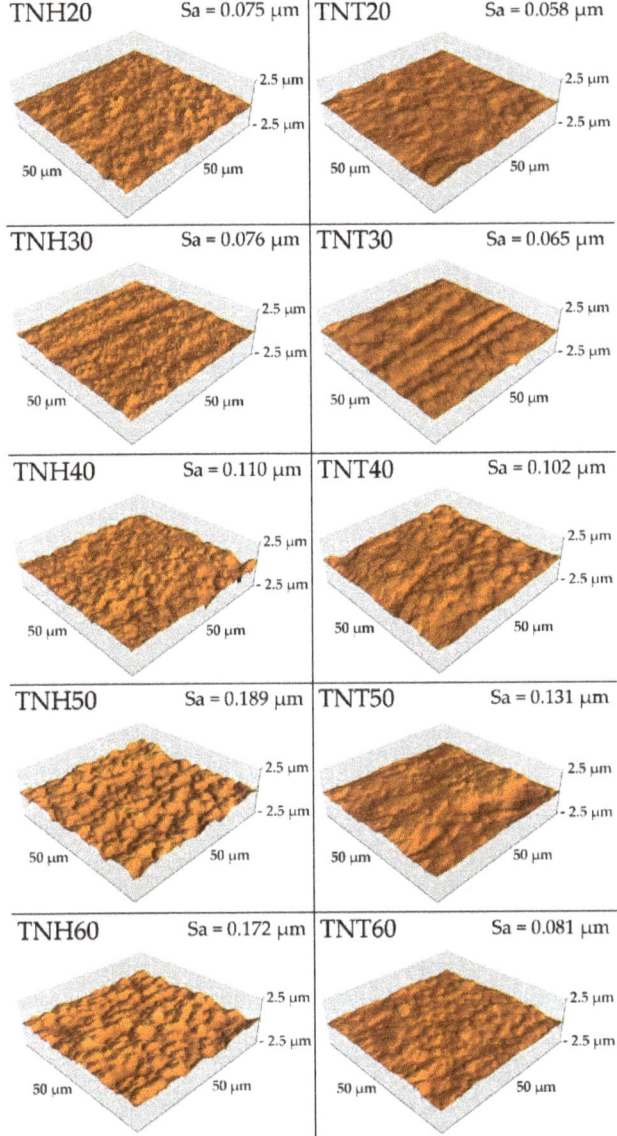

Figure 6. Atomic force microscopy (AFM) topography of Ti6Al4V/TNH20-60 and Ti6Al4V/TNT20-60 systems.

3.3.2. Mechanical Properties (Hardness and Young's Modulus) of Ti6Al4V/TNH20-60 and Ti6Al4V/TNT20-60 Systems

The nanomechanical properties of reference Ti6Al4V specimen, Ti6Al4V/TNH20-60 and Ti6Al4V/TNT20-60 systems, such as hardness and Young's modulus are presented in Table 1. Nanoindentation technique, which is dedicated to mechanical studies of nanometric structures, was used to obtain the results. The anodization of Ti6Al4V samples with the potential 20–60 V and their further treatment (drying in Ar and autoclaving or drying in Ar, immersion in acetone, additional drying and autoclaving) completely changed mechanical properties all of the tested specimens but in a different way for different samples. Only for Ti6Al4V/TNT20 and Ti6Al4V/TNT30 the increase of mechanical properties as compared to the reference material was observed. For TNT40 and TNT50, which among Ti6Al4V/TNT20-60 systems was characterised by the greatest diameter of nanotubes, the deepest decrease in hardness and Young's modulus were demonstrated. In the case of Ti6Al4V/TNH20-TNH60 samples, all tested specimens revealed lower mechanical properties than the reference titanium alloy and about 50% lower hardness than the same specimen additionally dried before hydrothermal treatment—Ti6Al4V/TNT20-60. The remarkable standard deviations for mechanical properties are characteristic for the nanoindentation technique and confirm the accuracy of measurements.

3.3.3. Adhesion Properties

In Table 2 the results of adhesion tests of the Ti6Al4V/TNT20-60 and Ti6Al4V/TNH20-60 systems are presented.

Table 2. Results of nano scratch-tests of Ti6Al4V/TNH20-60 and Ti6Al4V/TNT20-60 systems.

Coating	Nanoscratch-Test Properties	
	Critical Load (mN)	Critical Friction (mN)
TNH20	234.86 ± 53.53	266.87 ± 59.73
TNH30	254.14 ± 53.89	284.31 ± 73.77
TNH40	293.23 ± 54.71	355.05 ± 73.27
TNH50	268.78 ± 83.19	316.54 ± 98.03
TNH60	241.61 ± 68.00	246.25 ± 84.18
TNT20	286.51 ± 77.35	307.92 ± 90.38
TNT30	336.65 ± 41.21	397.86 ± 79.63
TNT40	379.08 ± 46.38	417.66 ± 68.00
TNT50	353.01 ± 12.82	388.39 ± 17.87
TNT60	271.52 ± 46.79	311.04 ± 66.94

The critical load was assumed as the maximum force at which the nanotubular or nanostructural layers were delaminated from titanium alloy substrate, and critical friction as the maximum friction force during layers' delamination. Scratch-tests showed lower values of critical load and critical friction for Ti6Al4V/TNH20-60 systems comparing to Ti6Al4V/TNT20-60 ones. It means that the adhesion of non-tubular coatings is lower than adequate tubular ones. And that additional drying of nanotubular samples before autoclaving increases the adhesion to titanium alloy substrate. The biggest difference in the critical force (delamination force) between Ti6Al4V/TNT20-60 and Ti6Al4V/TNH20-60 systems is visible for samples TNT30 and TNH30 and is equal 25%, while the smallest difference is visible for TNT60 and TNH60 (12%).

3.4. Cell Proliferation Detected by MTT Assay

Biointegration of Ti6Al4V/TNH20-60 and Ti6Al4V/TNT20-60 systems were evaluated based on the results of the MTT (3-(4,5-dimethylthiazol-2-yl)-2,5- diphenyltetrazolium bromide) assays made for the two different cell lines: murine L929 fibroblasts and human osteoblast-like MG 63 cells. The level of proliferation (assessed after 24-, 72- and 120 h) of the cells growing on the Ti6Al4V/TNH20-60 surface was compared to that observed for the cells cultured on the Ti6Al4V/TNT20-60 e.g., TNH20 vs. TNT20. As it can be seen in Figure 7, with an increase of incubation time more L929 fibroblasts (Figure 7A), as well as MG-63 osteoblasts (Figure 7B), proliferated on the surface of the all tested biomaterials ($p < 0.001$).

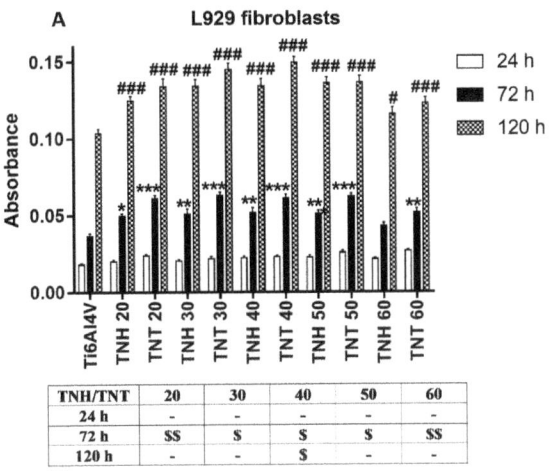

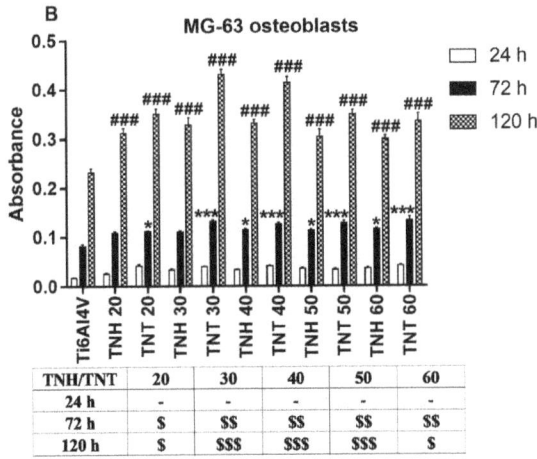

Figure 7. L929 murine fibroblasts (**A**) and human osteoblasts MG-63 (**B**) proliferation (after 24-, 72- and 120 h) on the surface of Ti6Al4V/TNH20-TNH60 and Ti6Al4V/TNT20-TNT60 samples, detected by MTT assay. The absorbance values are expressed as means ± SEM of five independent experiments. Asterisk and hash mark indicate significant differences between the cells incubated with the alloy references samples (Ti6Al4V) compared to the TNH and TNT specimens after 72 h (* $p < 0.05$, ** $p < 0.01$, *** $p < 0.001$) or 120 h (# $p < 0.05$, ## $p < 0.01$, ### $p < 0.001$) of incubation time, respectively. Tables below the graphs A and B present the statistical differences in the proliferation of the cells, between TNH and TNT coatings produced by the electrochemical anodization of the Ti6Al4V foil at the same selected potential ($ $p < 0.05$, $$ $p < 0.01$, $$$ $p < 0.001$).

Analysis of these data revealed also that there were no differences in the cells proliferation after 24 h between the all tested samples and titanium alloy references sample (Ti6Al4V). In contrast, Ti6Al4V/TNH coatings, as well as Ti6Al4V/TNT nanolayers, provoked a significant increase in cells proliferation compared to the Ti6Al4V reference alloy. This phenomenon was the most noticeable after 120 h of incubation both in the culture of fibroblasts (with the exception of TNH60 sample) and osteoblasts ($p < 0.001$). In the tables below the graphs in Figure 7, the statistical differences in the cells biointegration between TNH and TNT coatings produced by the electrochemical anodization of the Ti6Al4V foil at the same selected potential were presented. Analysis of these tables shows that there were no differences in cells proliferation measured after 24 h for both tested cells lines. In contrast, TNT nanolayers caused a greater increase in MG-63 osteoblasts proliferation than TNH coatings, which was noticed after 72 h as well as 120 h of incubation time (Table in Figure 7B). On the other hand, L929 fibroblasts cultured on the surface of TNT samples showed a higher rate of proliferation than the cells that grew on the TNH specimens only after 72 h of incubation time, except for the comparison of TNH40 and TNT40 layers, when the differences were also observed after 120 h (Table in Figure 7A). However, it should be clearly emphasized that all the tested TNH coatings showed a much higher level of biocompatibility than titanium alloy references sample (Ti6Al4V) and TNT coatings even higher than TNH ones.

3.5. Cell Morphology Observed by Scanning Electron Microscopy

SEM images micrographs present L929 murine fibroblasts (Figure 8) and MG-63 human osteoblasts (Figure 9) morphology, and proliferation. The cells showed of both figures were cultured on the surface of Ti6Al4V references sample, Ti6Al4V/TNH40, and Ti6Al4V/TNT40 nanocomposites. These data support the MTT results and clearly demonstrate the high biocompatibility properties of both types of tested nanomaterials, which are mainly related to the increase in cells proliferation level over time (compare micrographs (a–c), (d–f) and (g–i) in Figures 8 and 9, respectively).

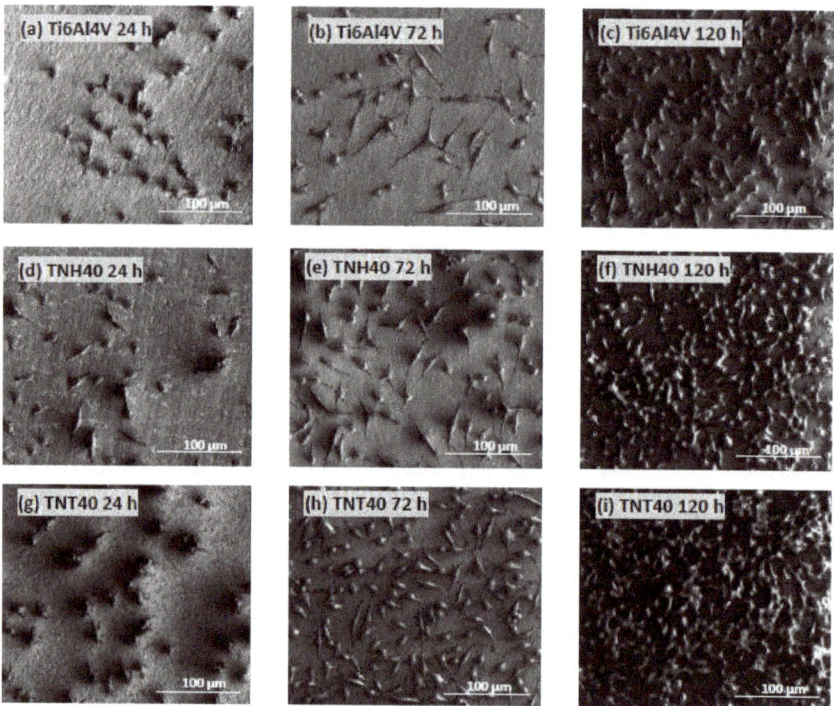

Figure 8. *Cont.*

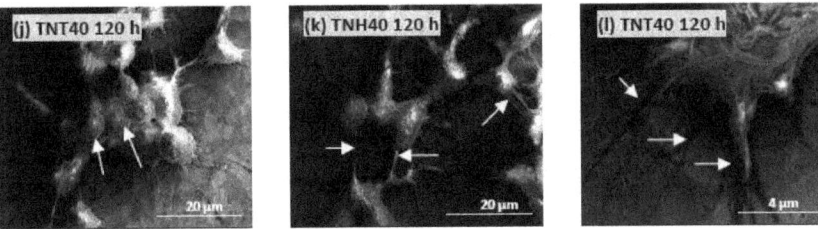

Figure 8. Scanning electron microscopy (SEM) images presenting proliferation of the murine L929 fibroblasts growing on the surface of the titanium alloy references sample (Ti6Al4V; (**a–c**) in comparison with Ti6Al4V/TNH40 sample; (**d–f**) and Ti6Al4V/TNT40 sample; (**g–i**). Arrows in the image (**j**) show the cells growing in layers on top of each other. Arrows in micrographs (**k**) and (**l**) indicate filopodia spread between cells or penetrating deep into the TNT40 nanolayers, respectively

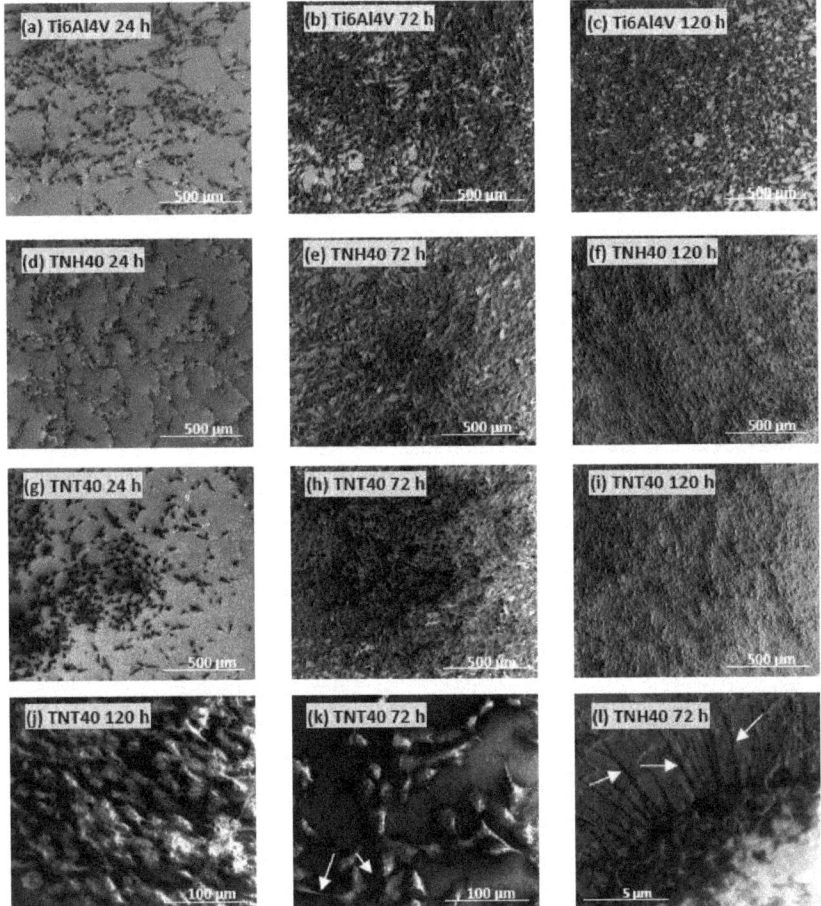

Figure 9. Scanning electron microscopy (SEM) micrographs showing the human osteoblast-like MG-63 cell proliferation on the surface of the references sample (Ti6Al4V; (**a–c**) compared to Ti6Al4V/TNH40 sample; (**d–f**) and the Ti6Al4V/TNT40 sample; (**g–i**). Micrograph (**j**) presents the multilayer growth of cells. Arrows indicate numerous filopodia spreading between cells (**k**) or filopodia, which attached osteoblasts to the nanocoatings surface (**l**).

Importantly, as it can be seen in Figure 8j, L929 fibroblasts also start to grow in layers on top of each other and this phenomenon is much more noticeable during the MG-63 osteoblasts incubation (see, e.g., Figure 9j), when the entire surface of TNH40 as well as TNT40 coatings is overgrown with multilayer structure of growing cells after 120 h of incubation time (Figure 9f,i, respectively). Finally, SEM images show that L929 fibroblasts as well as MG-63 osteoblasts form numerous filopodia, which strongly attach the cells to the nanocoatings surface by penetrating deep into nanolayers (arrows in Figures 8l and 9l, respectively) or the cells generate filopodia between themselves (arrows in Figures 8k and 9k, respectively).

4. Discussion

During designing and manufacturing titanium alloy implants, we focused mainly on ensuring their surface the appropriate physicochemical and mechanical properties, which directly influence on implants biointegration and anti-inflammation activity [34,35]. Providing the basic aseptic and sterile properties to implants is another important issue requiring a solution at the design level. This is particularly important when their surface is modified by a nanocomposite coating. The understanding of how the sterilization process influences on the implant surface properties may be important for the future clinical outcome. The most common method of sterilization is the steam sterilization (autoclaving), during which irreversible damage of microorganisms takes place due to the hydrothermal processes taking place. In our works, we have focused on autoclaving influence on surface layer morphology, structure, wettability, mechanical properties, and bioactivity of Ti6Al4V/TNTU systems produced by anodic oxidation using potentials U = 20–60 V. Spectral studies (DRIFT) of TNT coatings after anodization (dried only Ar stream at room temperature) proved the presence of traces of water on their surface (Figure 4). It can be a result of the adsorption of water molecules on the titania layer surface coming from washing of samples in deionized water after anodization. In other cases, the use of additional drying procedures to remove adsorbed water from the TNT layers surface is necessary. The good results were obtained by the immersion of samples in acetone (10 min., ultrasonic bath) and then their drying at 396 K for 1h. DRIFT spectra presented in Figures 3 and 4 confirmed the decrease of intensity of bands assigned to water molecules.

Analysis of SEM images of TNT5-15 and TNH5-15 coatings exhibited the lack of significant differences between surface morphology of samples produced at the same conditions but subjected to different drying procedure. It suggests that the surface morphology of TNT layers composed of densely packed nanotubes of diameter 25–70 nm, does not change as a result their interaction with hot water vapor (396 K) under high pressure (120 kPa) (Figure 1). The results of our earlier studies of Ti6Al4V/TNTU composites (TNTU layers were produced using electrochemical oxidation at potentials U = 3–20 V) revealed that coatings, which consisted of densely packed tubes of diameter c.a. 20 nm (TNT4-TNT8) exhibited the hydrophobic character, which decreased with the increase of their diameter and separation (TNT10-TNT20) [25]. Analysis of these data suggests that the hydrophobic character of TNT coatings produced at lower potentials (U = 5–10 V), causes that the use of Ar stream to remove of adsorbed water traces should be sufficient. Although, on the surface of TNH15 sample the slight changes, which were the result of the destruction of small tubular architecture fragments, have been found (Figure 1). The autoclaving of Ti6Al4V/TNT/Ar systems led to the complete destruction of their tubular architecture, while the surface morphology of Ti6Al4V/TNT/Ar samples remained unchanged (Figure 2). The affecting of the TNT layers drying on the stabilization of their tubular architecture was also proved by the results of our previous works on the use of TNT coatings, as the substrates in chemical vapor deposition (CVD) of silver nanoparticles [36,37]. According to these reports, the amorphous TNT coatings kept their tubular architecture during their heating up to 693 K in the stream of dry argon (carrier gas). Simultaneously, the autoclaving of all produced materials after CVD experiments did not change their surface morphology and amorphousness. The coatings consisted of anatase or anatase/rutile nanocrystals were formed during heating of the TNT coatings above 693 K [32]. The results of Liu et al investigations revealed that the annealing of amorphous

TNT layers at 723 K for 1h led to the phase transitions up to TiO$_2$ anatase form (thermally annealed and "water annealed" samples) or the anatase/rutile mixture (hydrothermally treated sample) [38]. According to this report, the hydrothermal treatment led to faceting or granularization of the tube walls, while the use of both other methods mentioned above, led to destroying their tubular architecture. The destruction effect of autoclaving carried out on amorphous TNT layers (tubes of diameters 15 and 50 nm), was also noticed by Junkar et al. [39]. In this case, the observed surface morphology changes have been explained as a combined result of the effect of moisture and temperature c.a. 365 K, which caused the crystallization of amorphous TNT layers. The results of Lamberti et al. studies also revealed that amorphous titania nanotubes crystallized into TiO$_2$ anatase form after exposure to water vapor in ambient conditions [40]. The transformation of TNT layers to anatase or anatase/brukite phase, treated by the hot deionized water (365 K) for 35h, were noticed by Liao et al [41]. Studies of Liu J. et al. showed that the nanotubular architecture of the amorphous titania nanotubes remained almost unchanged during the hydrothermal reaction at 403–453K for 1h [42]. The prolongation of the hydrothermal reaction time to 4, 6h caused that TiO$_2$ nanotubes were converted into nanoparticulate aggregations, which narrow the tubes' diameters up to their closure. Considering previous reports, it should be noted that that phase transitions of amorphous titania nanotubes to polycrystalline TiO$_2$ forms and surface morphology changes TNT layers can result in the water molecules interactions with the nanotube walls, which probable catalyzes the rearrangement of TiO$_6^{2-}$ octahedra and initiate crystallization processes [39,40,42].

Discussing the observed changes of TNH20-TNH60 coatings morphology after their autoclaving, it should be pointed out the possible influence of water molecules adsorbed on/inside the TNT coating surface. The adsorbed water molecules on the TNT surface in contact with the hot steam under the higher pressure accelerates the tubular architecture destroying and simultaneously favors the phase transition of the amorphous nanotubes to TiO$_2$ polycrystalline forms. Analysis of Raman spectra of TNH20-TNH60 layers revealed the appearance of very weak bands at 450 and 611 cm^{-1} and at 399, 516, and 639 cm^{-1}, which would indicate on the formation of rutile or rutile/anatase nanocrystals (Figure 5).

The comparison of TNH20-TNH60 and TNT20-TNT60 wettability data revealed a significant hydrophobic character of TNH20-TNH50 coatings, although the trend of changes is not strictly defined. The contact angle increases in the row: TNH20<TNH30<TNH40 and decreases in the row: TNH40>TNH50>TNH60, pointing out the sample TNH40 as the most hydrophobic. SEM analysis of this sample surface showed that coating is characterized by very dense packing, which does not allow the penetration of water molecules when measuring the contact angle. In comparison, TNT coatings are more hydrophilic, however their hydrophilicity decreases with the increase of diameter of tubes, and the lowest contact angle value is assigned to TNT20. What should be underlined the contact angle of TNH60 and TNT60 is almost identical, but this similarity should not come as a surprise—if you look at SEM images of both systems, you can also see some similarity in the morphology of the surface (Figure 2 and Figure S2).

The use of AFM technique permitted to characterize the topography and, dedicated for studied coatings and layers, S$_a$ roughness parameters. It was proven than roughness of the implant's surface would indeed be an important factor determining the proper osseointegration process between implants and bone. The high value of the surface roughness brought out better osteoblast adhesion after implementation in primary stabilization phase [43]. In this study, the positive effect of anodization of titanium alloy resulting in higher surface roughness was proved as compared with reference Ti6Al4V and additionally confirmed by biological tests. The same effect was reported previously [44,45]. Analysis of AFM images of TNH20-60 and TNT20-60 proved the influence of the presence of trace of water on/inside nanotubes and further autoclaving on the surface topography. The S$_a$ parameters are higher for TNH20-60 coatings than for TNT20-60 ones, pointing out that disappearance of nanotubular architecture and the creation of granular nanoarchitecture leads to more porous surface and gives higher values of S$_a$ (Figures 2 and 6).

The mechanical properties of all studied specimens were measured by nanoindentation technique. Noticeable standard deviations were obtained, which can be mostly attributed to the morphology of TiO_2 layers (such as presence of pores and nanotubular architecture). For Ti6Al4V specimen hardness was equal to 16.17 ± 3.61 GPa, and only TNT20 and TNT30 specimens demonstrated higher values of hardness. The mechanical properties, such as hardness and Young's modulus, and adhesion strength of layers for long-term and load-bearing implants determine their applicability for the living organisms. It has been proven that high difference between mechanical properties of bone and implants can increase a danger of a so-called "shielding effect" and in consequence of destabilization and loosening of the implants [46,47]]. Mechanical properties of nanotubular layers obtained by nanoindentation technique were dependent on the morphology of TiO_2. It was observed that increasing hardness followed indenter penetration depth increase. The influence of microstructural features such as columns' type, crystalline or amorphous character of the layer and porosity on mechanical properties of TiO_2 has been proven [48]. The tubular' architecture of the layers on titanium alloy determine mechanical properties. The nanotube walls are characterized by very high mechanical properties, such as hardness. The decrease of measured properties of the layers TNH20-60, compared with TNT20-60, can be explained by homogenization of the surface and the disappearance of nanotubular architecture on all of the specimens TNH20-60. The increase in packing density and porosity of TiO_2 were already reported to cause an increase of hardness and Young's modulus value [49]. According to SEM images (Figure 2) of specimens with visible nanotubular architecture (TNT20-60), the porosity and packing density are the highest for TNT20 and TNT30 specimens, which possess the highest mechanical properties. The highest value of hardness of TNH20 among all TNH specimens may be due to confirmed presence of rutile in the structure of TNH20 tubular layer, the highest among all TNH20-60 specimens [50]. The ratio of H (hardness) to E (Young's modulus) H^2/E^3 describes the resistance of the material to plastic deformation [51]. The highest value of H^2/E^3 was noticed for Ti6Al4V specimens (0.058 GPa), which suggests better tribological properties of reference specimen than TNT and TNH layers [52]. Nanoscratch-test was used in the past to study adhesion of thin oxide layer on titanium alloys [53,54]. Adhesion between the layer and the implant surface is one of the most important factors deciding on the possibility of using this modification technique for the biomaterials. Loosening of layer crystals to the tissue surrounding the implant can cause inflammatory states. In this study, TNT20-60 layers, which have higher mechanical properties, were characterized by better adhesion to the titanium substrate. TNH20-60 samples are characterized by decreased the critical force (delamination force) due to decreased hardness of the layers. Furthermore, decrease of adhesion of the layers was caused by change in the roughness of the surface. For all tested TNH specimens, the roughness was higher than for adequate TNT coatings. Cedillo-Gonzalez et al. [55] proved that higher roughness of the layers reduced adhesion.

In the present study, the biointegration of tested nanomaterials was investigated using two cell lines: mouse L929 fibroblasts and human osteoblast-like MG-63 cells. Since it is well known that the long-term success of an implant depends not only on the integrity of osseointegration but also on the contact with surrounding soft tissue [56], the use of both osteoblasts and fibroblasts cell lines in *in vitro* studies allowed for a comprehensive examination of implant biocompatibility. Moreover, it is well established that cellular behavior, such as adhesion, morphologic change, including formation of filopodia, and proliferation is determined by surface properties of nanomaterials, thus cellular response measured by these parameters are required to assess the biointegration of implants [57]. In our study, this response was estimated using MTT assay and scanning electron microscopy images analysis. The results of MTT assays related to the cell proliferation (measured after 24- 72- and 120 h) revealed the promising biocompatible properties both of TNT20-TNT60 as well as TNH20-TNH60 samples, which were observed both during fibroblast as well as osteoblasts culture (Figure 7A,B, respectively). Moreover, the analysis of these data revealed a slight deterioration of proliferation properties of TNH20-TNH60 samples in comparison to TNT20-TNT60 ones, both for fibroblast as well as osteoblasts culture. These findings were confirmed by SEM micrographs analysis that unambiguously indicate the increase in the number of cells over time that was greater for TNT40 and TNH40 surface compared to the Ti6Al4V references sample (Figures 8 and 9, respectively). Importantly, the cells, especially MG-63 osteoblasts, have overgrown entire surface of TNT40 and TNH40 nanocoatings forming multilayer structure of growing cells (Figure 9j). Since it is believed that the stimulation of post-confluent osteoblasts proliferation result in the formation multilayered nodules that later become mineralize [58], we presume that the tested specimens can stimulate bone regeneration *in vivo* due to the high osseointegration level. Finally, the biocompatibility of tested nanomaterials was also confirmed by the filopodia's formation between the cells (arrows in Figures 8k and 9k, respectively) growing on the tested nanomaterials, which attached also the cells to the coating's surface (arrows in Figures 8l and 9l, respectively) by penetration inside the porous nanolayer. Consequently, the porous surface caused a stronger cell adhesion by functioning as anchorage points for fibroblasts as well as osteoblasts. Filopodia are actin-based cell protrusions, which are regarded as one of the most important cellular sensors. They are used to collect space information and for sensing the substrate to determine areas suitable for cell attachment and proliferation, cell-cell interaction and allow cell migration toward the destination [59]. Therefore, formation of multiple filopodia, together with other presented results, clearly demonstrate the biocompatible properties of the tested nanomaterials.

5. Conclusions

The results of our works proved that amorphous titania nanotube coatings, used to modify the surface of medical devices made of titanium alloys, requires the removing of water remains on/inside nanotubular surface before autoclaving procedure—if we want, of course, the nanotube architecture remains on the surface. Additional drying affects the TiO_2 tubes surface stabilization, making them resistant to the effects of hot water vapors under higher pressure, which are present during the sterilization process made by autoclaving. Otherwise, nanotubular coatings containing traces of water on the surface or inside the nanotubes during autoclaving can be subjected to the destruction of their tubular architecture and to promoting of amorphous TiO_2 tubes phase transformation into polymorphic nanocrystals or crystalline powders. Such coatings revealed different mechanical and biointegration properties compared to nanotubular ones.

Supplementary Materials: The following are available online at http://www.mdpi.com/2077-0383/8/2/272/s1, Figure S1: IR DRIFT spectra of TNH20-TNH60; Figure S2: The values of contact angles for water (a) and diiodomethane (b), and surface free energy (c) of Ti6Al4V/TNT20-60 and Ti6Al4V/TNH20-60 samples; Table S1: Diameters and wall thickness of titania nanotubes produced on the surface of Ti6Al4V substrates in the potential range of 5–60V; Table S2: Contact angles values for Ti6Al4V/TNT20-60 and Ti6Al4V/TNH20-60, measured for water and diiodomethane, and surface free energy values obtained according to Owens-Wendt method; Table S3: Surface roughness parameters (S_a) of Ti6Al4V, Ti6Al4V/TNT20-60 and Ti6Al4V/TNH20-60 systems, as determined based on the AFM image analysis.

Author Contributions: Conceptualization, A.R.; methodology, A.R.; formal analysis, A.R., T.J., M.B; investigation, A.R., M.E., T.J., M.B.; writing—original draft preparation, A.R.; writing—review and editing, A.R.; visualization, A.R.; supervision, A.R.

Funding: This research was funded by the Regional Operational Programme of the Kuyavian-Pomeranian Voivodeship (1.3.1. Support for research and development processes in academic enterprises), within the grant obtained by Nano-implant Ltd. The APC was funded by Nano-implant Ltd.

Acknowledgments: A.R. and M.B. would like to thank Piotr Piszczek and Andrzej Zieliński for valuable conversations enriching the discussion presented in the manuscript.

Conflicts of Interest: The authors declare no conflict of interest.

References

1. Tsimbouri, P.M.; Fisher, L.; Holloway, N.; Sjostrom, T.; Nobbs, A.H.; Meek, R.M.; Su, B.; Dalby, M.J. Osteogenic and bactericidal surfaces from hydrothermal titania nanowires on titanium substrates. *Sci. Rep.* **2016**, *18*, 1–12. [CrossRef] [PubMed]
2. Orapiriyakul, W.; Young, P.S.; Damiati, L.; Tsimbouri, P.M. Antibacterial surface modification of titanium implants in orthopaedics. *J. Tissue Eng.* **2018**, *9*, 1–16. [CrossRef] [PubMed]
3. Wyatt, M.; Hooper, G.; Frampton, C.; Rothwell, A. Survival outcomes of cemented compared to uncemented stems in primary total hip replacement. *World J. Orthop.* **2014**, *5*, 591–596. [CrossRef] [PubMed]
4. Ning, C.; Wang, S.; Zhu, Y.; Zhong, M.; Lin, X.; Zhang, Y.; Tan, G.; Li, M.; Yin, Z.; Yu, P.; et al. Ti nanorod arrays with a medium density significantly promote osteogenesis and osteointegration. *Sci. Rep.* **2016**, *6*, 1–7. [CrossRef] [PubMed]
5. Parcharoen, Y.; Kajitvichyanukul, P.; Sirivisoot, S.; Termsuksawa, P. Hydroxyapatite electrodeposition on anodized titanium nanotubes for orthopedic applications. *Appl. Surf. Sci.* **2014**, *311*, 54–61. [CrossRef]
6. Li, Z.; Qiu, J.; Du, L.Q.; Jia, L.; Liu, H.; Ge, S. TiO_2 nanorod arrays modified Ti substrates promote the adhesion, proliferation and osteogenic differentiation of human periodontal ligament stem cells. *Mater. Sci. Eng. C* **2017**, *76*, 684–691. [CrossRef] [PubMed]
7. Huo, K.; Zhang, X.; Wang, H.; Zhao, L.; Liu, X.; Chu, P.K. Osteogenic activity and antibacterial effects on titanium surfaces modified with Zn-incorporated nanotube arrays. *Biomaterials* **2013**, *34*, 3467–3478. [CrossRef] [PubMed]
8. Neoh, K.G.; Hu, X.; Zheng, D.; Kang, E.T. Balancing osteoblast functions and bacterial adhesion on functionalized titanium surfaces. *Biomaterials* **2012**, *33*, 2813–2822. [CrossRef] [PubMed]
9. Yao, X.; Peng, R.; Ding, J. Cell-material interactions revealed via material techniques of surface patterning. *Adv. Mater.* **2013**, *25*, 5257–5286. [CrossRef] [PubMed]
10. Klokkevold, P.; Nishimura, R.D.; Adachi, M.; Caputo, A. Osseointegration enhanced by chemical etching of the titanium surface. A torque removal study in the rabbit. *Clin. Oral Implant. Res.* **1997**, *8*, 442–447. [CrossRef]
11. Bächle, M.; Kohal, R.J. A systematic review of the influence of different titanium surfaces on proliferation, differentiation and protein synthesis of osteoblast-like MG63 cells. *Clin. Oral Implant. Res.* **2004**, *15*, 683–692. [CrossRef] [PubMed]
12. Radtke, A.; Topolski, A.; Jędrzejewski, T.; Kozak, W.; Sadowska, B.; Więckowska-Szakiel, M.; Piszczek, P. Bioactivity Studies on Titania Coatings and the Estimation of Their Usefulness in the Modification of Implant Surfaces. *Nanomaterials* **2017**, *7*, 90. [CrossRef] [PubMed]
13. Gao, A.; Hang, R.; Bai, L.; Tang, B.; Chu, P.K. Electrochemical surface engineering of titanium-based alloys for biomedical application. *Electrochim. Acta* **2018**, *271*, 699–718. [CrossRef]
14. Qin, J.; Yang, D.; Maher, S.; Lima-Marques, L.; Zhou, Y.; Chen, Y.; Atkins, G.J.; Losic, D. Micro- and Nano-structured 3D Printed Titanium Implants with Hydroxyapatite Coating for Improved Osseointegration. *J. Mater. Chem. B* **2018**, *6*, 3136–3144. [CrossRef]
15. Le Guéhennec, L.; Soueidan, A.; Layrolle, P.; Amouriq, Y. Surface treatments of titanium dental implants for rapid osseointegration. *Dent. Mater.* **2007**, *23*, 844–854. [CrossRef] [PubMed]
16. Gong, D.; Grimes, C.A.; Varghese, O.K.; Hu, W.; Singh, R.S.; Chen, Z.; Dickey, E.C. Titanium oxide nanotube arrays prepared by anodic oxidation. *J. Mater. Res.* **2001**, *16*, 3331–3334. [CrossRef]
17. Radtke, A.; Bal, M.; Jędrzejewski, T. Novel Titania Nanocoatings Produced by Anodic Oxidation with the Use of Cyclically Changing Potential: Their Photocatalytic Activity and Biocompatibility. *Nanomaterials* **2018**, *8*, 712. [CrossRef] [PubMed]
18. Wang, D.; Liu, Y.; Yu, B.; Zhou, F.; Liu, W. TiO_2 Nanotubes with Tunable Morphology, Diameter and Length: Synthesis and Photo-Elecrtical/Catalytic Performance. *Chem. Mater.* **2009**, *21*, 1198–1206. [CrossRef]
19. Nyein, N.; Tanc, W.K.; Kawamura, G.; Matsuda, A.; Lockman, Z. TiO_2 nanotube arrays formation in fluoride/ethylene glycol electrolyte containing LiOH or KOH as photoanode for dye-sensitized solar cell. *J. Photochem. Photobiol. A Chem.* **2017**, *343*, 33–39. [CrossRef]
20. Tai, M.A.; Razak, K.A.; Jaafar, M.; Lockma, Z. Initial growth study of TiO_2 nanotube arrays anodised in KOH/fluoride/ethylene glycol electrolyte. *Mater. Des.* **2017**, *128*, 195–205. [CrossRef]

21. Mansoorianfar, M.; Tavoosi, M.; Mozafarinia, R.; Ghasemi, A.; Doostmohammadi, A. Preparation and characterization of TiO$_2$ nanotube arrays on Ti6Al4V surface for enhancement of cell treatment. *Surf. Coat. Technol.* **2017**, *321*, 409–415. [CrossRef]
22. Brammer, K.S.; Oh, S.; Cobb, C.J.; Bjursten, L.M.; Heyde, H.V.; Jin, S. Improved bone forming functionality on diameter-controlled TiO$_2$ nanotube surface. *Acta Biomater.* **2009**, *5*, 3215–3223. [CrossRef] [PubMed]
23. Das, K.; Bose, S.; Bandyopadhyay, A. TiO$_2$ nanotubes on Ti: Influence of nanoscale morphology on bone cell–materials interaction. *J. Biomed. Mater. Res. A* **2009**, *90*, 225–237. [CrossRef] [PubMed]
24. Park, J.; Bauer, S.; Schlegel, K.A.; Neukam, F.W.; von der Mark, K.; Schmuki, P. TiO$_2$ nanotube surfaces: 15 nm—An optimal length scale of surface topography for cell adhesion and differentiation. *Small* **2009**, *5*, 666–671. [CrossRef] [PubMed]
25. Radtke, A.; Topolski, A.; Jędrzejewski, T.; Sadowska, B.; Więckowska-Szakiel, M.; Szubka, M.; Talik, E.; Nielsen, L.P.; Piszczek, P. The bioactivity and photocatalytic properties of titania nanotube coatings produced with the use of the low-potential anodization of Ti6Al4V alloy surface. *Nanomaterials* **2017**, *7*, 197. [CrossRef] [PubMed]
26. Zhao, L.; Meia, S.; Wanga, W.; Chub, P.K.; Wua, Z.; Zhanga, Y. The role of sterilization in the cytocompatibility of titania nanotubes. *Biomaterials* **2010**, *31*, 2055–2063. [CrossRef] [PubMed]
27. Harrell, C.R.; Djonov, V.; Fellabaum, C.; Volarevic, V. Risks of Using Sterilization by Gamma Radiation: The Other Side of the Coin. *Int. J. Med. Sci.* **2018**, *15*, 274–279. [CrossRef] [PubMed]
28. Shintani, H.; Sakudo, A.; Burke, P.; McDonnell, G. Gas plasma sterilization of microorganisms and mechanisms of action. *Exp. Ther. Med.* **2010**, *1*, 731–738. [CrossRef] [PubMed]
29. Ravikumar, M.; Hageman, D.J.; Tomaszewski, W.H.; Chandra, G.M.; Skousen, J.L.; Capadona, J.R. The effect of residual endotoxin contamination on the neuroinflammatory response to sterilized intracortical microelectrodes. *J. Mater. Chem. B* **2014**, *2*, 2517–2529. [CrossRef] [PubMed]
30. Ecker, M.; Danda, V.; Shoffstall, A.J.; Mahmood, S.F.; Joshi-Imre, A.; Frewin, C.L.; Voit, W.E. Sterilization of Thiol-ene/Acrylate Based Shape Memory Polymers for Biomedical Applications. *Macromol. Mater. Eng.* **2017**, *302*, 1600331. [CrossRef]
31. Yuan, Y.; Lee, T.R. Chapter 1 Contact Angle and Wetting Properties. In *Surface Science Techniques, Springer Series in Surface Sciences*; Bracco, G., Holst, B., Eds.; Springer: Berlin/Heidelberg, Germany, 2013; pp. 3–34.
32. Lewandowska, Ż.; Piszczek, P.; Radtke, A.; Jędrzejewski, T.; Kozak, W.; Sadowska, B. The Evaluation of the Impact of Titania Nanotube Covers Morphology and Crystal Phase on Their Biological Properties. *J. Mater. Sci. Mater. Med.* **2015**, *26*, 163. [CrossRef] [PubMed]
33. Owens, D.K.; Wendt, R.C. Estimation of the surface free energy of polymers. *J. Appl. Polym. Sci.* **1969**, *13*, 1741–1747. [CrossRef]
34. Zhao, G.; Schwartz, Z.; Wieland, M.; Rupp, F.; Geis-Gerstorfer, J.; Cochran, D.L.; Boyan, B.D. High surface energy enhances cell response to titanium substrate microstructure. *J. Biomed. Mater. Res. A* **2005**, *74*, 49–58. [CrossRef] [PubMed]
35. Mavrogenis, A.F.; Dimitriou, R.; Parvizi, J.; Babis, G.C. Biology of implant osseointegration. *J. Musculoskelet. Neuronal. Interact.* **2009**, *9*, 61–71. [PubMed]
36. Radtke, A.T.; Jędrzejewski, W.; Kozak, B.; Sadowska, M.; Więckowska-Szakiel, E.; Talik, M.; Mäkelä, M.; Leskelä, P. Optimization of the silver clusters PEALD process on the surface of 1-D titania coatings. *Nanomaterials* **2017**, *7*, 193. [CrossRef] [PubMed]
37. Piszczek, P.; Lewandowska, Ż.; Radtke, A.; Jędrzejewski, T.; Kozak, W.; Sadowska, B.; Szubka, M.; Talik, E.; Fiori, F. Biocompatibility of Titania Nanotube Coatings Enriched with Silver Nanograins by Chemical Vapor Depositiom. *Nanomaterials* **2017**, *7*, 274. [CrossRef] [PubMed]
38. Liu, N.; Albu, S.P.; Lee, K.; So, S.; Schmuki, P. Water annealing and other low temperature treatments of anodic TiO$_2$ nanotubes: A comparison of properties and efficiencies in dye sensitized solar cells and for water splitting. *Electrochim. Acta* **2012**, *82*, 98–102. [CrossRef]
39. Junkar, I.; Kulkarni, M.; Drašer, B.; Rugelj, N.; Mazare, A.; Flašker, A.; Drobne, D.; Humpoliček, P.; Resnik, M.; Schmuki, P.; et al. Influence of various sterilization procedures on TiO$_2$ nanotubes used for bimedical devices. *Bioelectrochemistry* **2016**, *109*, 79–86. [CrossRef] [PubMed]
40. Lamberti, A.; Chidoni, A.; Shahzad, N.; Bianco, S.; Quaglio, M.; Pirri, C.F. Ultrafast room-temperature crystallization of TiO$_2$ Nanotubes exploiting water-vapor treatment. *Sci. Rep.* **2015**, *5*, 7808. [CrossRef] [PubMed]

41. Liao, Y.; Que, W.; Zhong, P.; Zhang, J.; He, Y. A facile method to crystallize amorphous anodized TiO_2 nanotubes at low temperature. *Acs Appl. Mater. Interfaces* **2011**, *3*, 2800–2804. [CrossRef] [PubMed]
42. Liu, J.; Liu, Z.; Zahang, T.; Zhai, J.; Jiang, L. Low-temperature crystallization of anodized TiO_2 nanotubes at the solid-gas interface and their photoelectrochemical properties. *Nanoscale* **2013**, *5*, 6139–6144. [CrossRef] [PubMed]
43. Feng, B.; Weng, J.; Yang, B.C.; Qu, S.X.; Zhang, X.D. Characterization of surface oxide films on titanium and adhesion of osteoblast. *Biomaterials* **2003**, *24*, 4663–4670. [CrossRef]
44. Goodarzi, S.; Moztarzadeh, F.; Nezafati, N.; Omidvar, H. Titanium dioxide nanotube arrays: A novel approach into periodontal tissue regeneration on the surface of titanium implants. *Adv. Mater. Lett.* **2016**, *7*, 209–215. [CrossRef]
45. Bezerra, H.; Inês, M.; Bernardi, B.; Maria, T.; Carlos, A.; Nara, A.; Rastelli, D.S. Titanium dioxide and modified titanium dioxide by silver nanoparticles as an anti-biofilm filler content for composite resins. *Dent. Mater.* **2018**, *35*, 36–46. [CrossRef]
46. Niinomi, M.; Nakai, M.; Hieda, J. Development of new metallic alloys for biomedical applications. *Acta Biomater.* **2012**, *8*, 3888–3903. [CrossRef] [PubMed]
47. Abdel-Hady Gepreel, M.; Niinomi, M. Biocompatibility of Ti-alloys for long-term implantation. *J. Mech. Behav. Biomed. Mater.* **2013**, *20*, 407–415. [CrossRef] [PubMed]
48. Dikici, T.; Toparli, M. Microstructure and mechanical properties of nanostructured and microstructured TiO_2 films. *Mater. Sci. Eng. A* **2016**, *661*, 19–24. [CrossRef]
49. Munirathinam, B.; Neelakantan, L. Role of crystallinity on the nanomechanical and electrochemical properties of TiO_2 nanotubes. *J. Electroanal. Chem.* **2016**, *770*, 73–83. [CrossRef]
50. Rayón, E.; Bonache, V.; Salvador, M.D.; Bannier, E.; Sánchez, E.; Denoirjean, A.; Ageorges, H. Nanoindentation study of the mechanical and damage behaviour of suspension plasma sprayed TiO_2 coatings. *Surf. Coat. Technol.* **2012**, *206*, 2655–2660. [CrossRef]
51. Chernozem, R.V.; Surmeneva, M.A.; Krause, B.; Baumbach, T.; Ignatov, V.P.; Tyurin, A.I.; Loza, K.; Epple, M.; Surmenev, R.A. Hybrid biocomposites based on titania nanotubes and a hydroxyapatite coating deposited by RF-magnetron sputtering: Surface topography, structure, and mechanical properties. *Appl. Surf. Sci.* **2017**, *426*, 229–237. [CrossRef]
52. Dearnaley, G.; Arps, J. Biomedical applications of diamond-like carbon (DLC) coatings: A review. *Surf. Coat. Technol.* **2005**, *200*, 2518–2524. [CrossRef]
53. Ossowska, A.; Beutner, R.; Scharnweber, D.; Zielinski, A. Properties of composite oxide layers on the Ti13Nb13Zr alloy. *Surf. Eng.* **2017**, *33*, 841–848. [CrossRef]
54. Catauro, M.; Bollino, F.; Giovanardi, R.; Veronesi, P. Modification of Ti6Al4V implant surfaces by biocompatible TiO_2/PCL hybrid layers prepared via sol-gel dip coating: Structural characterization, mechanical and corrosion behavior. *Mater. Sci. Eng. C* **2017**, *74*, 501–507. [CrossRef] [PubMed]
55. Iventh Cedillo-Gonzalez, E.; Montorosi, M.; Mugoni, C.; Montorosi, M.; Siligardi, C. Improvement of the adhesion between TiO_2 nanofilm and glass substrate by roughness modifications. *Phys. Procedia* **2013**, *40*, 19–29. [CrossRef]
56. Furuhashi, A.; Ayukawa, Y.; Atsuta, I.; Okawachi, H.; Koyano, K. The difference of fibroblast behavior on titanium substrata with different surface characteristics. *Odontology* **2012**, *100*, 199–205. [CrossRef] [PubMed]
57. Lord, M.S.; Foss, M.; Besenbacher, F. Influence of nanoscale surface topography on protein adsorption and cellular response. *Nano Today* **2010**, *5*, 66–78. [CrossRef]
58. Lengner, C.J.; Steinman, H.A.; Gagnon, J.; Smith, T.W.; Henderson, J.E.; Kream, B.E.; Stein, G.S.; Lian, J.B.; Jones, S.N. Osteoblast differentiation and skeletal development are regulated by Mdm2-p53 signaling. *J. Cell. Biol.* **2006**, *172*, 909–921. [CrossRef] [PubMed]
59. Ebrahimi, M.; Pripatnanont, P.; Suttapreyasri, S.; Monmaturapoj, N. In vitro biocompatibility analysis of novel nano-biphasic calcium phosphate scaffolds in different composition ratios. *J. Biomed. Mater. Res. B Appl. Biomater.* **2014**, *102*, 52–61. [CrossRef] [PubMed]

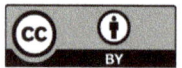

© 2019 by the authors. Licensee MDPI, Basel, Switzerland. This article is an open access article distributed under the terms and conditions of the Creative Commons Attribution (CC BY) license (http://creativecommons.org/licenses/by/4.0/).

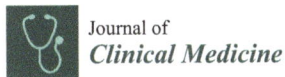

Article

Inflammatory Cell Recruitment in *Candida glabrata* Biofilm Cell-Infected Mice Receiving Antifungal Chemotherapy

Célia F. Rodrigues [1,2,*], Alexandra Correia [3,4], Manuel Vilanova [3,4,5] and Mariana Henriques [1]

1. LIBRO – 'Laboratório de Investigação em Biofilmes Rosário Oliveira', Centre of Biological Engineering, University of Minho, 4710-057 Braga, Portugal; mcrh@deb.uminho.pt
2. Laboratory for Process Engineering Environment Biotechnology and Energy-Department of Chemical Engineering, Faculty of Engineering, University of Porto, 4200-465 Porto, Portugal
3. Instituto de Investigação e Inovação em Saúde, Universidade do Porto, 4200-135 Porto, Portugal; alexandra.correia@ibmc.up.pt (A.C.); vilanova@icbas.up.pt (M.V.)
4. Instituto de Biologia Molecular e Celular, Universidade de Porto, 4200-135 Porto, Portugal
5. Departamento de Imuno-Fisiologia e Farmacologia, Instituto de Ciências Biomédicas de Abel Salazar, Universidade do Porto, 4050-313 Porto, Portugal
* Correspondence: c.fortunae@gmail.com

Received: 26 December 2018; Accepted: 20 January 2019; Published: 26 January 2019

Abstract: (1) Background: Due to a high rate of antifungal resistance, *Candida glabrata* is one of the most prevalent *Candida* spp. linked to systemic candidiasis, which is particularly critical in catheterized patients. The goal of this work was to simulate a systemic infection exclusively derived from *C. glabrata* biofilm cells and to evaluate the effectiveness of the treatment of two echinocandins—caspofungin (Csf) and micafungin (Mcf). (2) Methods: CD1 mice were infected with 48 h-biofilm cells of *C. glabrata* and then treated with Csf or Mcf. After 72 h, the efficacy of each drug was evaluated to assess the organ fungal burden through colony forming units (CFU) counting. The immune cell recruitment into target organs was evaluated by flow cytometry or histopathology analysis. (3) Results: Fungal burden was found to be higher in the liver than in the kidneys. However, none of the drugs was effective in completely eradicating *C. glabrata* biofilm cells. At the evaluated time point, flow cytometry analysis showed a predominant mononuclear response in the spleen, which was also evident in the liver and kidneys of the infected mice, as observed by histopathology analysis. (4) Conclusions: Echinocandins do not have a significant impact on liver and kidney fungal burden, or recruited inflammatory infiltrate, when mice are intravenously (i.v.) infected with *C. glabrata* biofilm-grown cells.

Keywords: *Candida glabrata*; candidemia; echinocandins; resistance; biofilms; infection; micafungin; caspofungin; *in vivo*

---

1. Introduction

Candida glabrata is one of the most common causes of systemic fungal infection (candidemia), surpassed only by *Candida albicans* [1–3]. It is the second most common isolated yeast in the United States of America and the third in Europe, after *Candida parapsilosis*, accounting for 20% of candidemia [2,4]. As a commensal yeast, *C. glabrata* colonizes and adapts to many different niches in the human body and can be isolated from the mucosae of healthy individuals [2,5]. Yet, as an opportunistic pathogen, this fungus can also be the point of origin for mucosal infections and severe candidemia. Its biofilm-forming ability and the ability to rapidly acquire resistance to antifungals (especially to azoles) [2,5,6], which in many cases can be further increased by genetic and genomic mutations (e.g., polymorphisms, the formation of new chromosomes, karyotype variations) [7–9], may contribute to increased virulence.

Risk factors for the development of invasive *C. glabrata* infections in human patients comprise immunosuppression (e.g., cancer chemotherapy, human immunodeficiency virus (HIV) infection, diabetes mellitus, neutropenia), mucosal colonization by *Candida* spp., the use of indwelling medical devices (e.g., vascular catheters), and gastrointestinal surgery [10–12].

During infection, *C. glabrata* virtually colonizes all sites and organs, which reveals a high capacity to adapt to the many different niches inside the human host [1]. Oral and systemic *C. glabrata* infections have high associated morbidity and mortality [13–15] and the rise in incidence infections caused by this yeast is to some extent attributable to its ability to tolerate or resist many antifungals commonly used in clinical practice [2,16,17]. The occurrence of oral candidiasis related to *C. glabrata* is increasing [15,18]. Although *C. glabrata* colonization does not always lead to infection, it is a foreword to infection when the risk of systemic infection is elevated, or the host immunity is compromised. *C. glabrata* infections are a major challenge [15,19,20]. The good biofilm-forming ability and raised enzymatic activity of *C. glabrata* are two of the most important features favoring oral and systemic candidiasis. In fact, biofilms can be formed on both biotic (e.g., gastrointestinal or mouth mucosae) and abiotic surfaces (e.g., indwelling medical devices) [21,22] and biofilm cells are recognized to be more resistant to antifungal treatment than planktonic cells, as well as responsible for more severe infections [2,23–25]. Systemic candidiases are the most prevalent invasive mycoses worldwide with mortality rates close to 40% and *C. glabrata* is frequently recognized as a causative agent [26]. In nearly all these cases, the infections are related to the use of a medical device and biofilm formation on its surface [20]. The contamination of medical devices (mostly catheters) or infusion fluids can occur from the skin of the patient, the hands of health professionals [27], or by migration into medical devices from a previous lesion. Less commonly, *Candida* spp. that commensally colonize the gastrointestinal tract switch to having a pathogenic behavior, being able to infiltrate the intestinal mucosa, disseminate through the bloodstream, and colonize medical devices endogenously (this is more common in cancer patients, since chemotherapy harms the mucosa) [28]. Depending on the clinical situation, the removal of medical devices can be recommended in patients with disseminated *Candida* spp. infection to enable pathogen eradication and to improve the prognosis [29,30]. In contrast, experimental intravenous infection of laboratory animals with *C. glabrata* does not usually cause mortality, since it appears that this species has successfully developed immune evasion strategies enabling it to survive, disseminate, and persist within mammalian hosts [1,31].

Because of the high probability of innate resistance to azoles, echinocandins are recommended as first-line therapy against *C. glabrata* candidemia [32]. Nonetheless, and worryingly, *C. glabrata* is the first *Candida* spp. for which resistance to echinocandins has been identified and described [33,34]. Recently, case reports of echinocandin-resistant *C. glabrata* subsequent to different echinocandin therapies are becoming more common [35–41]. Indeed, one third of those isolates may be multidrug resistant [42] and have specific mutations in one of two "hot spot" regions of the *FKS1* or *FKS2* (1,3-β-glucan synthase) genes, which encode a subunit of the β-1,3-D glucan synthase protein, a target of echinocandins [35,43–45].

Therefore, in this work, a simulation of a hematogenously disseminated *C. glabrata* infection derived exclusively from biofilm cells (as occurs in catheter infections) was performed. CD1 mice were infected with 48 h-biofilm cells of the wild type *C. glabrata* strain ATCC2001, and then treated with the echinocandins caspofungin (Csf) and micafungin (Mcf) in order to evaluate organ fungal burdens after 72 h, the efficacy of each drug after two administrations, and the associated inflammatory response.

2. Experimental Section

2.1. Ethics Statement

This study was performed in strict accordance with the recommendations of the European Convention for the Protection of Vertebrate Animals used for Experimental and Other Scientific

Purposes (ETS 123), the 86/609/EEC directive, and Portuguese rules (DL 129/92). All experimental protocols were approved by the competent national authority (Direcção-Geral de Veterinária), document 0420/000/000/2010. Female CD1 mice, 8–12 weeks old, were purchased from Charles River (Barcelona, Spain) and kept under specific pathogen-free conditions at the Animal Facility of the Instituto de Ciências Biomédicas Abel Salazar, Porto, Portugal. Mice were maintained in individually ventilated cages (five animals per cage) with corncob bedding, and under controlled conditions of temperature (21 ± 1 °C), relative humidity (between 45 and 65%), and light (12 h light/dark cycle). Mice had ad libitum access to food and water. Hiding and nesting materials were provided for enrichment. All procedures such as cage changing, water and food supply, as well as intravenous and intraperitoneal injections were always performed during the day cycle (between 7 a.m. and 7 p.m.).

2.2. Organisms and Growth Conditions

One strain of the American Type Culture Collection (ATCC), *C. glabrata* ATCC2001, was subcultured on Sabouraud dextrose agar (SDA) (Merck, Darmstadt, Germany) for 24 h at 37 °C. Cells were then inoculated in Sabouraud dextrose broth (SDB) (Merck, Darmstadt, Germany) and incubated for 18 h at 37 °C under agitation at 120 rpm. Biofilms were formed in 24-well polystyrene microtiter plates (Orange Scientific, Braine-l'Alleud, Belgium) [46]. For this, 1000 µL of the yeast cell suspension (1×10^5 cells/mL) was added to each well and incubated for 24 h. After 24 h, 500 µL of RPMI 1640 was removed and an equal volume of fresh medium was carefully added. Biofilms allowed to grow, under the same temperature and agitation conditions, for an additional 24 h. After this time (total 48 h), all media were removed and the biofilms carefully washed to remove non-adhered cells. Biofilms were scraped from the 24-well plates, resuspended in ultra-pure water, sonicated (Ultrasonic Processor, Cole-Parmer, IL, USA) for 30 s at 30 W, and then suspension vortexed for 2 min. The suspension was centrifuged at 5000 g for 5 min at 4 °C, as previously optimized [46,47]. The pellets of the biofilm cells were then suspended in RPMI 1640 and the cellular density was adjusted to 5×10^8 cells/mL using a Neubauer counting chamber.

2.3. Antifungal Drugs

Csf and Mcf were kindly provided by MSD® and Astellas®, respectively. Aliquots of 5000 mg/L were prepared using dimethyl-sulfoxide (DMSO). The final concentrations used were prepared with pyrogen-free phosphate buffer saline (PBS) for both drugs.

2.4. Murine Model of Hematogenously Disseminated Infection

Candida glabrata inoculum was prepared following previously described procedures [47,48]. The number of cultivable cells was assessed by colony forming units (CFU) counting and were injected intravenously in the lateral tail vein, with the support of a restrainer. Sample size was determined based on the results of preliminary experiments. On day 0, adult CD1 mice, randomly allocated to each experimental group, received 200 µL of *C. glabrata* biofilm cell suspensions containing 5×10^8 CFU i.v. via the tail vein. Control mice were injected intravenously with 200 µL of pyrogen-free PBS. Treatment with the echinocandins started 24 h post-inoculation and was administered intraperitoneally (i.p.) with a volume of 0.5 mL at 24 and 48 h post-inoculation. Doses were as follows: caspofungin 6 mg/kg and micafungin 12 mg/kg. This experimental scheme (days and dosages) were chosen on the basis of previous pharmacodynamic studies of echinocandins against *C. glabrata* and a need to reach drug exposures in mice that were comparable to those in humans receiving currently licensed echinocandin regimens [32,49,50]. Liver and kidneys were aseptically removed, weighed, homogenized, and quantitatively cultured on Sabouraud dextrose agar (Difco) at 37 °C. Values are expressed as log CFU per gram of liver. Two independent experiments were performed, with at least five animals per infected group.

2.5. Flow Cytometry

For flow cytometry analysis, spleens from infected mice and controls were aseptically removed 72 h post-infection, homogenized in Hanks' Balanced Salt Solution (Sigma Aldrich, Roswell-Park, St. Louis, MO, USA) and, when necessary, red blood cells were lysed. The following monoclonal antibodies (mAb) were used (at previously determined optimal dilutions) for surface antigen staining after pre-incubation with anti-mouse CD16/CD32 for FcγR blocking. For dead cell exclusion, all samples except single-stained controls were first incubated with allophycocyanin (APC) eFluor 780 Fixable Viability Dye (eBioscience, San Diego, CA, USA) diluted 1:1000 in PBS for 30 min at 4 °C. For surface staining, cells were incubated with the following monoclonal antibodies: anti-mouse GR1 Fluorescein isothiocyanate (FITC)-conjugate, anti-mouse CD80 Phycoerythrin (PE)-conjugate, anti-mouse F4/80 Peridinin-chlorophyll protein Cyanin 5.5 (PerCp Cy5.5)-conjugate, anti-mouse CD86 PE-cychrome 7 (PE-Cy7)-conjugate, anti-mouse CD11c BV421-conjugate (all from BD Biosciences, San Jose, CA, USA), anti-mouse CD11b BV510-conjugate, and anti-mouse major histocompatibility complex (MHC) class II APC conjugate (eBiosciences, San Diego, CA, USA). Data acquisition was performed in a FACSCanto™ II system (BD Biosciences, San Jose, CA, USA) using the FACSDIVA™ software (BD) and compensated and analyzed in FLOWJO version 9.7.5. (Tree Star Inc., Ashland, OR, USA). A biexponential transformation was applied to improve data visualization; 10^6 cells were stained per sample.

2.6. Histopathologic Examination and Immunohistochemistry

Livers were fixed in buffered formalin and embedded in paraffin for hematoxylin-eosin (HE) and periodic acid–Schiff (PAS) histopathologic analysis, as previously described [51,52].

2.7. Statistical Analysis

Statistical analysis was carried out with Prism™ 7 (GraphPad™, San Diego, CA, USA). The normality of the data obtained was evaluated using the Kolmogorov–Smirnov test. Accordingly, Kruskal–Wallis and Sidak's multiple comparison tests were applied and data were depicted as means of all independent experiments. Differences among groups were considered significant when $P < 0.05$.

3. Results and Discussion

Candidemia has been increasing in the last decades, especially among individuals under chemotherapy programs, as well as in those who are HIV-positive, hospitalized, or catheterized [2,53]. *C. albicans* is still the most frequent isolated yeast, but *C. glabrata* has become one of the most threatening non-*Candida albicans Candida* (NCAC) spp., mostly due to its high antifungal resistance [2,54]. Though human clinical data demonstrate that immunosuppression is a risk factor for *C. glabrata* infections, it is not an absolute prerequisite for *C. glabrata* candidiasis [55]. Hence, increasing the data on the host immune response to *C. glabrata* and revising the efficacy of chemotherapeutic approaches to treat infections caused by this fungus are of major value. The murine model is a suitable one to address both issues, alone or combined [56].

3.1. Fungal Burden Progression Differs Substantially between Liver and Kidneys

The fungal burden of CD1 mice infected intravenously with *C. glabrata* biofilm cell suspensions and subsequently treated with echinocandins was assessed in the liver and kidneys 72 h post-infection. No differences were observed among the different infected groups.

In contrast to *C. albicans*, which can heavily infect the kidneys [57], a tropism of *C. glabrata* to the liver was clearly noticed. High CFU counts were detected on this organ (Figure 1), in contrast to the low or non-detected CFU counts in the kidneys ($\leq 3 \times 10^4$ CFU/g kidney). The low colonization of this organ, as compared to the liver or brain in immunocompetent mice systemically infected with *C. glabrata*, was also reported by other authors [1,31,58–60]. Nevertheless, Kaur et al. [59],

Srikantha et al. [60], and Brieland et al. [58] stated that *C. glabrata* could be recovered after several days in the kidneys, liver, spleen, hearts, lungs, brains, and lungs. Moreover, Atkinson et al. [61] described that fungal burdens were 10^4 to 10^8 in immunocompromised mice in the spleen and kidneys. Nonetheless, it is important to stress that the differences in mouse strains and immunocompetence status, *C. glabrata* strains, animal age and gender, or even the concentration of the inoculum used do not allow a direct comparison of published data [31]. In addition, past *in vitro* reports have shown that susceptible *C. glabrata* strains can become resistant in less than four days of continuous culture with low doses of drugs, such as fluconazole [1,16] and echinocandins [62–65]. Thus, it is plausible that a fast increase of resistance could have been observed in vivo. Moreover, the inoculum exclusively contained biofilm cells, known to be more resistant than their planktonic counterparts [66–72].

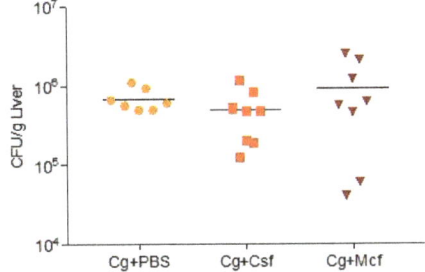

Figure 1. Liver fungal burden of CD1 mice 72 h after intravenously challenged with 1×10^8 biofilm cells plus two cycles of treatment with PBS, caspofungin (Csf), or micafungin (Mcf). Data are representative of two independent experiments. Each symbol represents an individual mouse, and horizontal bars are means of colony forming unit (CFU) numbers for each group. The obtained results are displayed as CFU/liver. Controls (naïve; PBS + Csf; PBS + Mcf), $n = 2$; Cg + Csf, $n = 8$; Cg + Mcf, $n = 8$. No statistical differences were observed among infected groups (evaluated by Kruskal–Wallis (Overall ANOVA $P < 0.05$) and post hoc Sidak's multiple comparison tests). Cg—*Candida glabrata* ATCC2001.

3.2. Host Immune Response to Hematogenously Disseminated Candidiasis

In contrast to the considerable work that has been described on the host immune response to *C. albicans*, the immune mechanisms elicited in the course of *C. glabrata* infections are far less explored.

Neutrophils and macrophages are in the first line of host immune defence against *Candida* spp. cells infecting the bloodstream or the endothelia [73–75]. Clinical observations and experimental studies have demonstrated the main role of polymorphonuclear leukocytes in mediating host protection against systemic *C. albicans* infections [76–78]. In mice, neutrophils have a Gr-1^{high} surface phenotype and macrophages typically express the F4/80 cell surface marker. Previous reports have shown that, in *C. albicans* infections, Gr-1$^+$ splenocytes may have immunosuppressive function and F4/80$^+$ cells may play a pro-inflammatory role [79,80]. The expression of these two surface markers was analyzed using flow cytometry in the spleen of CD1 mice 72 h after i.v. infection with 1×10^8 *C. glabrata* biofilm cells. Myeloid cells (CD11b$^+$) displaying the phenotypes F4/80^{high} Gr-1^{neg}, F4/80^{high} Gr-1^{high}, and F4/80$^{neg/low}$ Gr-1^{high} were respectively considered macrophages, inflammatory monocytes, and neutrophils [81]. The gating strategies employed in this study are shown in Figure 2. As shown in Figure 3A, a significant increase in the numbers of inflammatory monocytes was observed in the spleen of infected mice, while those of neutrophils and macrophages remained within control values. No significant differences, however, were observed among treated groups. These results are in accordance with previous reports [31,82,83]. Unlike *C. albicans* infections, for which high neutrophil infiltration is a commonly observed feature, *C. glabrata* infections are not associated with massive neutrophil infiltration. Indeed, *C. glabrata* infection has mainly been associated with mononuclear cell infiltration and is far less inflammatory. One of the reasons given to explain this disparate outcome is that C. albicans hyphae cause significant host cell damage, which results in the extensive recruitment of myeloid cells and the production of pro-inflammatory cytokines [31,82,83].

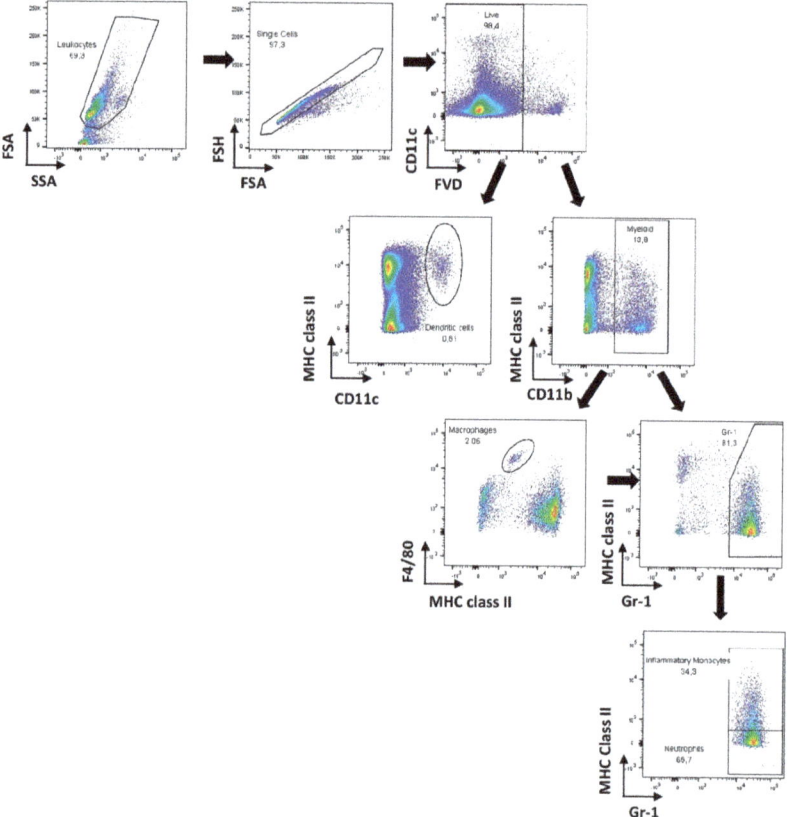

Figure 2. Gating strategy applied for the flow cytometry data analysis. Following leukocyte selection based on Forward Scatter Area (FSA) and Side Scatter Area (SSA), doublets were excluded based on FSA and Forward Scatter Height (FSH) parameters, and dead cells were further excluded by fixable viability dye (FVD) incorporation. Dendritic cells were gated as CD11c^{high} MHC class II$^+$ cells. Myeloid cells were defined as CD11b$^+$ cells that were further divided into macrophages (CD11b$^+$ F4/80^{high} MHC class II^{low}) and Gr-1$^+$ cells. Within the latter, neutrophils were defined as CD11b$^+$ Gr-1$^+$MHC class II$^-$ and inflammatory monocytes were gated as CD11b$^+$ Gr-1$^+$MHC class II$^+$ cells.

Additionally, other reports have shown that C. glabrata is recognized and phagocytized by macrophages at a much higher rate than C. albicans [84]. After recognizing pathogens, macrophages release cytokines that help coordinate the immune response. However, when C. glabrata is internalized by macrophages, it interferes with the phagosome maturation process [85], surviving through autophagy and replicating inside the phagosome until the eventual bursting of the phagocyte [59,85,86]. Here, no elevated numbers of macrophages were detected in the spleen of infected mice as compared to noninfected controls (Figure 3C), which indicates that the recruitment or local proliferation of these cells does not occur in response to C. glabrata.

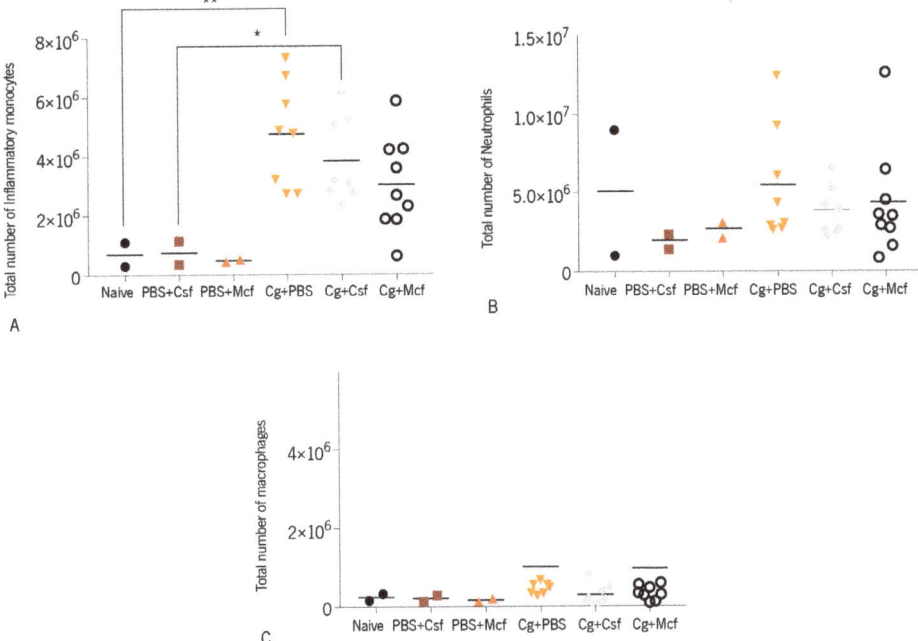

Figure 3. CD1 mice were challenged intravenously with 1×10^8 biofilm cells and then treated with PBS, caspofungin (Csf), or micafungin (Mcf). The obtained results are displayed as the total number of cells of indicated populations: (**A**) inflammatory monocytes, (**B**) neutrophils, and (**C**) macrophages. The numbers of animals used were as follows: controls (naïve; PBS + Csf; PBS + Mcf), $n = 2$; Cg + Csf, $n = 8$; Cg + Mcf, $n = 8$. Statistical differences were evaluated using Kruskal–Wallis and post hoc Sidak's multiple comparison tests (Overall ANOVA $P < 0.05$). Cg—*Candida glabrata* ATCC2001. * $P < 0.05$; ** $P < 0.001$.

In addition to macrophages, dendritic cells (DC) play a major role in the induction of the T cell-mediated immune response to *Candida* spp. infections [86,87] and may determine the infection outcome [88,89]. DC are able to modulate adaptive responses, depending on the *Candida* spp. morphotype encountered [73,74,90]. DC can initiate and shape the antimicrobial immunity and, since candidiasis appears frequently in immunocompromised patients, these cells may hold the key to new antifungal strategies [91]. Accordingly, the numbers of splenic conventional DC, defined as CD11c^{high} cells, and surface maturation markers were evaluated upon *C. glabrata* systemic infection (Figure 4). A slight increase in splenic DC as compared to noninfected controls was observed in the infected mice, indicating that *C. glabrata* promoted the mobilization of these cells to the spleen or promoted their local proliferation. DC surface expression of the costimulatory molecule CD86, as evaluated by the mean fluorescence intensities (MFIs) due to antibody staining (Figure 4A,B), was elevated in infected mice, showing that *C. glabrata* induced the maturation of these cells. However, the stimulatory effect was not different among the treated and nontreated groups.

In contrast, the expression of MHC class II molecules on the surface of splenic DC of mice infected with this yeast was found to be below control levels, an effect that reached statistical difference in mice treated with caspofungin. As CD86 expression in infected mice was found to be elevated, it is unlikely that this could represent a suppressive mechanism and could just be subsequent to a previous stimulatory effect. A kinetic study would be necessary to elucidate this point.

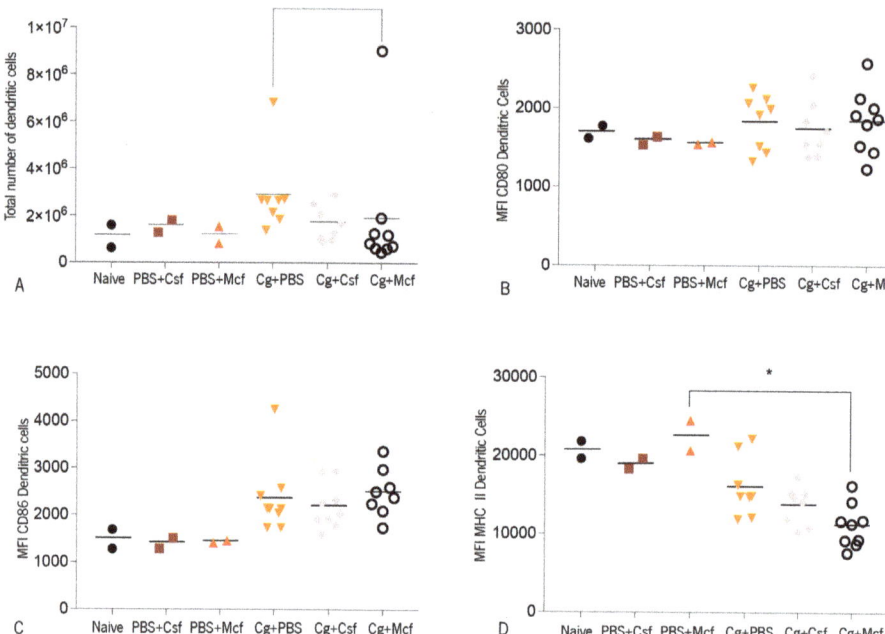

Figure 4. CD1 mice were challenged intravenously with 1×10^8 biofilm cells and then treated with PBS, caspofungin (Csf), or micafungin (Mcf). The obtained results are displayed as (**A**) total number of dendritic cells or mean fluorescence intensities (MFI) due to antibody staining against (**B**) CD80, (**C**) CD86, and (**D**) MHC class II on the surface of dendritic cells. The numbers of animals used were: controls (naïve; PBS + Csf; PBS + Mcf), $n = 2$; Cg + Csf, $n = 8$; Cg + Mcf, $n = 8$. Statistical differences among infected groups were evaluated using Kruskal–Wallis (overall ANOVA $P < 0.05$), post hoc Sidak's, and Dunn's multiple comparisons tests (* $P > 0.05$). Cg—*Candida glabrata* ATCC2001. * $P < 0.05$.

The expression of CD80, CD86, and MHC class II molecules on the surface of inflammatory monocytes was observed to be similar or slightly lower in the infected groups as compared to noninfected controls (Figure 5A–C). Likewise, and as observed on DC, no differences were observed among infected mouse groups, indicating that the treatment did not affect the expression of these activation markers on these innate immune cell populations. Finally, liver and kidney histopathologies were analyzed in infected mice, as these organs are preferred targets in i.v. *Candida* spp. infections [31,92]. As could be expected, no yeasts were found in the non-challenged control groups, and their organs presented no significant histological alterations.

Challenged mice showed inflammatory infiltrates in the liver. They were also shown, albeit less markedly, in the kidneys (nontreated and treated groups). The presence of polymorphonuclear cells was observed, but in general the infiltration remained mostly mononuclear. Yeasts were found in the liver, but not in the kidneys of treated and nontreated challenged groups. This fact corroborated the low CFU counts found in the kidneys.

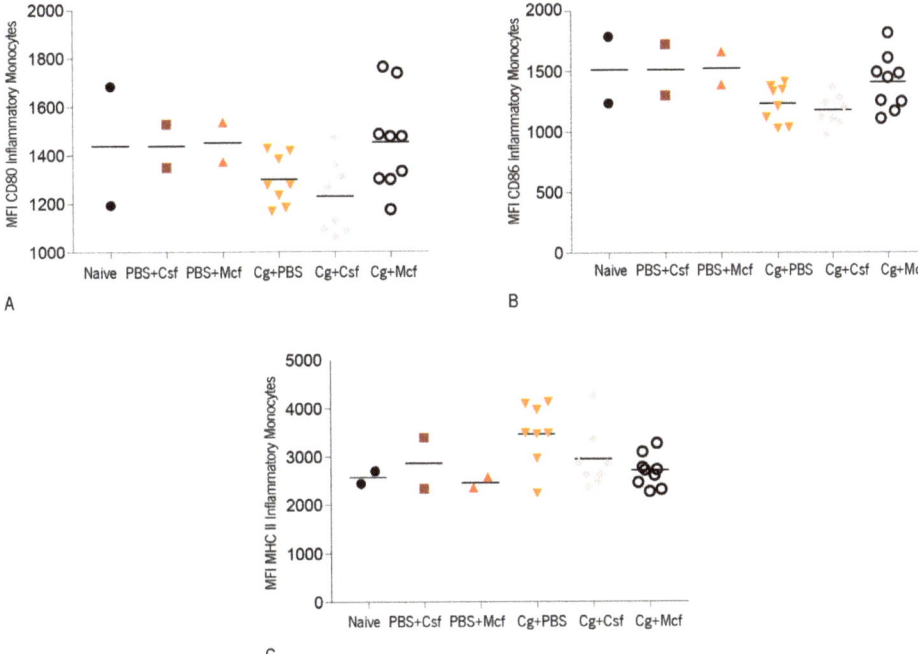

Figure 5. CD1 mice were challenged intravenously with 1×10^8 biofilm cells and then treated with PBS, caspofungin (Csf), or micafungin (Mcf). The obtained results are displayed as mean fluorescence intensities (MFI) due to antibody staining against (**A**) CD80, (**B**) CD86, and (**C**) MHC II on inflammatory monocytes. The numbers of animals per group were: controls (naïve; PBS + Csf; PBS + Mcf), $n = 2$; Cg + Csf, $n = 8$; Cg + Mcf, $n = 8$. Statistical differences among infected groups were evaluated using Kruskal–Wallis (Overall ANOVA $P < 0.05$) and post hoc Sidak's multiple comparison tests. Cg—*Candida glabrata* ATCC2001.

Together, these observations confirmed *C. glabrata* as a low inflammatory species and indicated that two-dose treatment with caspofungin and micafungin does not have a significant impact on liver and kidney fungal burden or recruited inflammatory infiltrate when mice are i.v. infected with *C. glabrata* biofilm-grown cells. These results confirm the biofilm in vitro outcome our group previously reported [93,94].

Finally, liver and kidney histopathologies were analyzed in infected mice, as these organs are preferred targets in i.v. *Candida* spp. infections [45,86]. As could be expected, no yeasts were found in the non-challenged control groups, and their organs presented no significant histological alterations (Figure 6). Challenged mice showed inflammatory infiltrates in the liver, and less markedly in the kidneys (nontreated and treated groups, data not shown). The presence of polymorphonuclear cells was observed, but in general the infiltration remained mostly mononuclear. Yeasts were found in the liver (Figure 6), but not in the kidneys (data not shown) of treated and nontreated challenged groups. This fact corroborated the low CFU counts found in the kidneys.

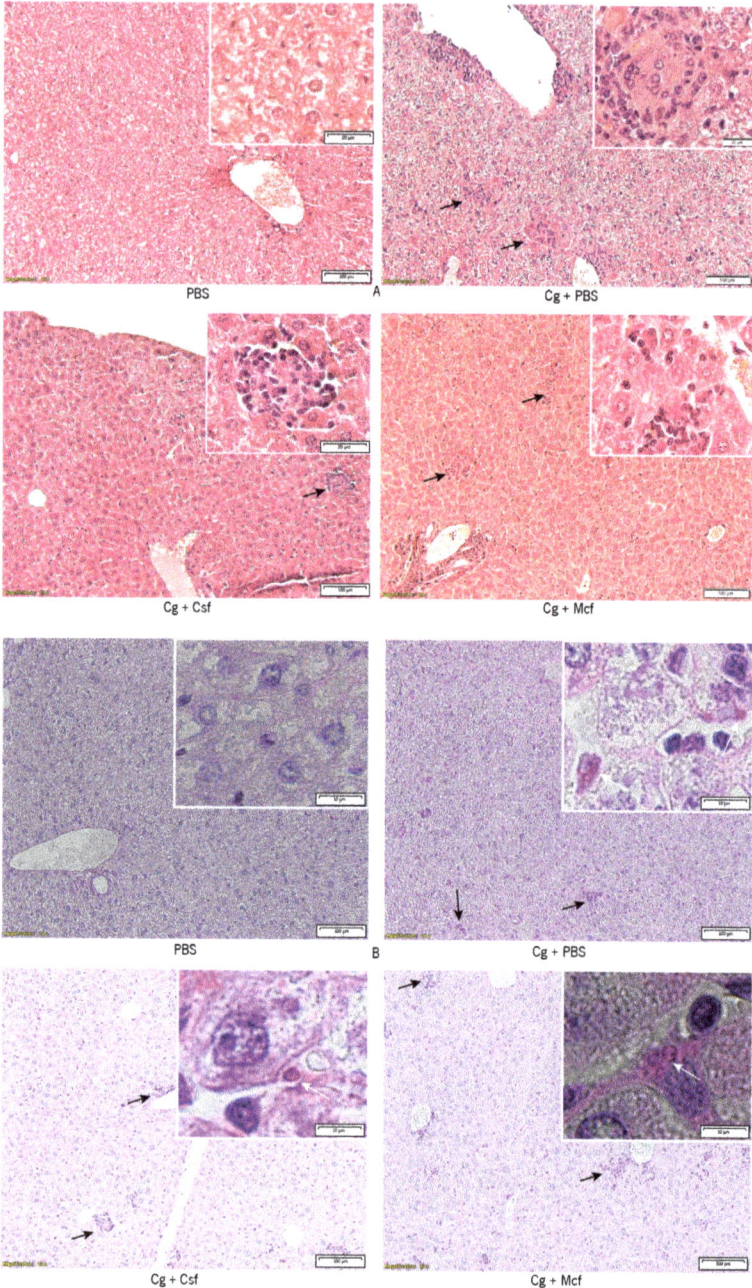

Figure 6. Analysis of liver histology in CD1 mice. (**A**) Representative hematoxylin-eosin and (**B**) periodic acid–Schiff (PAS)-stained examples of liver tissue from the indicated mouse groups. Black arrows denote inflammatory infiltrates that were mostly of the mononuclear type. Insets correspond to higher magnification micrographs. White arrows indicate PAS-stained *Candida glabrata* ATCC2001 cells. Scale bars are shown and apply to similar sized micrographs (100 µm) or insets (20 µm), as indicated.

4. Conclusions

In this work, a systemic infection exclusively originated from *C. glabrata* biofilm cells was simulated and a treatment evaluated. The observations here reported confirmed *C. glabrata* as a low inflammatory species and indicated that two-dose treatment with Csf and Mcf does not have a significant impact on liver and kidney fungal burden or recruited inflammatory infiltrate when mice are i.v. infected with *C. glabrata* biofilm-grown cells.

Author Contributions: C.F.R., A.C., M.H., and M.V. conceived and designed the experiments; C.F.R. and A.C. performed the experiments; C.F.R. and A.C. analyzed the data; M.H. and M.V. contributed to the reagents/materials; C.F.R., A.C., M.H., and M.V. wrote the paper.

Funding: This study was supported by the Portuguese Foundation for Science and Technology (FCT) under the scope of the strategic funding of UID/BIO/04469/2013 unit and COMPETE 2020 (POCI-01-0145-FEDER-006684) and BioTecNorte operation (NORTE-01-0145-FEDER-000004) funded by the European Regional Development Fund under the scope of the Norte2020-Programa Operacional Regional do Norte, financially supported by project UID/EQU/00511/2019—Laboratory for Process Engineering, Environment, Biotechnology and Energy (LEPABE) funded by national funds through FCT/MCTES (PIDDAC), Célia F. Rodrigues' (SFRH/BD/93078/20130) PhD grant and M. Elisa Rodrigues (SFRH/BPD/95401/2013) post-doc grant.

Acknowledgments: The authors would like to thank MSD® and Astellas® for the kind donation of Csf and Mcf, respectively.

Conflicts of Interest: The authors declare no conflict of interest.

References

1. Brunke, S.; Seider, K.; Fischer, D.; Jacobsen, I.D.; Kasper, L.; Jablonowski, N.; Wartenberg, A.; Bader, O.; Enache-Angoulvant, A.; Schaller, M.; et al. One Small Step for a Yeast -Microevolution within Macrophages Renders *Candida glabrata* Hypervirulent Due to a Single Point Mutation. *PLoS Pathog.* **2014**, *10*, e1004478. [CrossRef] [PubMed]
2. Rodrigues, C.F.; Rodrigues, M.; Silva, S.; Henriques, M. *Candida glabrata* Biofilms: How Far Have We Come? *J. Fungi* **2017**, *3*, 11. [CrossRef] [PubMed]
3. Archimedes, D.; Carolina, A.; Souza, R.; Colombo, A.L. Revisiting Species Distribution and Antifungal Susceptibility of Candida Bloodstream Isolates from Latin American Medical Centers. *J. Fungi* **2017**, *3*, 24.
4. Pfaller, M.A.; Diekema, D.J. Epidemiology of invasive candidiasis: A persistent public health problem. *Clin. Microbiol. Rev.* **2007**, *20*, 133–163. [CrossRef] [PubMed]
5. Fidel, P.L.P.; Vazquez, J.A.; Sobel, J. *Candida glabrata*: Review of Epidemiology, Pathogenesis, and Clinical Disease with Comparison to *C. albicans*. *Clin. Microbiol. Rev.* **1999**, *12*, 80–96. [CrossRef] [PubMed]
6. Arendrup, M.C. Candida and candidaemia. Susceptibility and epidemiology. *Dan. Med. J.* **2013**, *60*, B4698.
7. Shin, J.H.; Chae, M.J.; Song, J.W.; Jung, S.-I.; Cho, D.; Kee, S.J.; Kim, S.H.; Shin, M.G.; Suh, S.P.; Ryang, D.W. Changes in karyotype and azole susceptibility of sequential bloodstream isolates from patients with *Candida glabrata* candidemia. *J. Clin. Microbiol.* **2007**, *45*, 2385–2391. [CrossRef]
8. Bader, O.; Schwarz, A.; Kraneveld, E.A.; Tangwattanchuleeporn, M.; Schmidt, P.; Jacobsen, M.D.; Gross, U.; De Groot, P.W.J.; Weig, M. Gross Karyotypic and Phenotypic Alterations among Different Progenies of the *Candida glabrata* CBS138/ATCC2001 Reference Strain. *PLoS ONE* **2012**, *7*, e52218. [CrossRef]
9. Poláková, S.; Blume, C.; Zárate, J.A.; Mentel, M.; Jørck-Ramberg, D.; Stenderup, J.; Piskur, J. Formation of new chromosomes as a virulence mechanism in yeast *Candida glabrata*. *Proc. Natl. Acad. Sci. USA* **2009**, *106*, 2688–2693. [CrossRef]
10. Hachem, R.; Hanna, H.; Kontoyiannis, D.; Jiang, Y.; Raad, I. The changing epidemiology of invasive candidiasis: *Candida glabrata* and Candida krusei as the leading causes of candidemia in hematologic malignancy. *Cancer* **2008**, *112*, 2493–2499. [CrossRef]
11. Malani, A.; Hmoud, J.; Chiu, L.; Carver, P.L.; Bielaczyc, A.; Kauffman, C.A. *Candida glabrata* Fungemia: Experience in a Tertiary Care Center. *Clin. Infect. Dis.* **2005**, *41*, 975–981. [CrossRef]
12. Playford, E.G.; Marriott, D.; Nguyen, Q.; Chen, S.; Ellis, D.; Slavin, M.; Sorrell, T.C. Candidemia in nonneutropenic critically ill patients: Risk factors for non-albicans *Candida* spp. *Crit. Care Med.* **2008**, *36*, 2034–2039. [CrossRef] [PubMed]

13. Marriott, D.J.; Playford, E.G.; Chen, S.; Slavin, M.; Nguyen, Q.; Ellis, D.; Sorrell, T.C. Determinants of mortality in non-neutropenic ICU patients with candidaemia for the Australian Candidaemia Study. *Crit. Care* **2009**, *13*, 1–8. [CrossRef] [PubMed]
14. Sipsas, N.V.; Lewis, R.E.; Tarrand, J.; Hachem, R.; Rolston, K.V.; Raad, I.I.; Kontoyiannis, D.P. Candidemia in patients with hematologic malignancies in the era of new antifungal agents (2001–2007). *Cancer* **2009**, *115*, 4745–4752. [CrossRef] [PubMed]
15. Di Stasio, D.; Lauritano, D.; Minervini, G.; Paparella, R.S.; Petruzzi, M.; Romano, A.; Candotto, V.; Lucchese, A. Management of denture stomatitis: A narrative review. *J. Biol. Regul. Homeost. Agents* **2018**, *32*, 113–116. [PubMed]
16. Borst, A.; Raimer, M.T.; Warnock, D.W.; Morrison, C.J.; Arthington-Skaggs, B.A. Rapid Acquisition of Stable Azole Resistance by *Candida glabrata* Isolates Obtained before the Clinical Introduction of Fluconazole. *Antimicrob. Agents Chemother.* **2005**, *49*, 783–787. [CrossRef] [PubMed]
17. Sanglard, D.; Ischer, F.; Calabrese, D.; Majcherczyk, P.A.; Bille, J. The ATP binding cassette transporter gene CgCDR1 from *Candida glabrata* is involved in the resistance of clinical isolates to azole antifungal agents. *Antimicrob. Agents Chemother.* **1999**, *43*, 2753–2765. [CrossRef]
18. Akpan, A.; Morgan, R. Oral candidiasis. *Postgrad. Med. J.* **2002**, *78*, 455–459. [CrossRef]
19. Lott, T.J.; Holloway, B.P.; Logan, D.A.; Fundyga, R.; Arnold, J. Towards understanding the evolution of the human commensal yeast Candida albicans. *Microbiology* **1999**, *145*, 1137–1143. [CrossRef]
20. van der Meer, J.W.M.; van de Veerdonk, F.L.; Joosten, L.A.B.; Kullberg, B.-J.; Netea, M.G. Severe *Candida* spp. infections: New insights into natural immunity. *Int. J. Antimicrob. Agents* **2010**, *36*, S58–S62. [CrossRef]
21. Chandra, J.; Mukherjee, P.K. Candida Biofilms: Development, Architecture, and Resistance. *Microbiol. Spectr.* **2015**, *3*, 157–176. [CrossRef] [PubMed]
22. Kojic, E.M.E.M.; Darouiche, R.O.R.O. Candida infections of medical devices. *Clin. Microbiol. Rev.* **2004**, *17*, 255–267. [CrossRef] [PubMed]
23. Coenye, T.; Bjarnsholt, T. The complexity of microbial biofilm research—An introduction to the 3 rd Thematic Issue on Biofilms. *Pathog. Dis.* **2016**. [CrossRef] [PubMed]
24. Zarnowski, R.; Westler, W.M.; Lacmbouh, G.A.; Marita, J.M.; Bothe, J.R.; Bernhardt, J.; Sahraoui, A.L.H.; Fontainei, J.; Sanchez, H.; Hatfeld, R.D.; et al. Novel entries in a fungal biofilm matrix encyclopedia. *MBio* **2014**, *5*, 1–13. [CrossRef] [PubMed]
25. LaFleur, M.D.; Kumamoto, C.A.; Lewis, K. *Candida albicans* biofilms produce antifungal-tolerant persister cells. *Antimicrob. Agents Chemother.* **2006**, *50*, 3839–3846. [CrossRef] [PubMed]
26. Falagas, M.E.; Roussos, N.; Vardakas, K.Z. Relative frequency of albicans and the various non-albicans *Candida* spp. among candidemia isolates from inpatients in various parts of the world: A systematic review. *Int. J. Infect. Dis.* **2010**, *14*, e954–e966. [CrossRef] [PubMed]
27. Seneviratne, C.J.; Jin, L.; Samaranayake, L.P. Biofilm lifestyle of Candida: A mini review. *Oral Dis.* **2008**, *14*, 582–590. [CrossRef] [PubMed]
28. Douglas, L.J. Candida biofilms and their role in infection. *Trends Microbiol.* **2003**, *11*, 30–36. [CrossRef]
29. Mermel, L.A.; Allon, M.; Bouza, E.; Craven, D.E.; Flynn, P.; O'Grady, N.P.; Raad, I.I.; Rijnders, B.J.A.; Sherertz, R.J.; Warren, D.K. Clinical practice guidelines for the diagnosis and management of intravascular catheter-related infection: 2009 Update by the Infectious Diseases Society of America. *Clin. Infect. Dis.* **2009**, *49*, 1–45. [CrossRef]
30. Nucci, M.; Anaissie, E.; Betts, R.F.; Dupont, B.F.; Wu, C.; Buell, D.N.; Kovanda, L.; Lortholary, O. Early Removal of Central Venous Catheter in Patients with Candidemia Does Not Improve Outcome: Analysis of 842 Patients from 2 Randomized Clinical Trials. *Clin. Infect. Dis.* **2010**, *51*, 295–303. [CrossRef]
31. Jacobsen, I.D.; Brunke, S.; Seider, K.; Schwarzmüller, T.; Firon, A.; D'enfért, C.; Kuchler, K.; Hube, B. *Candida glabrata* Persistence in Mice Does Not Depend on Host Immunosuppression and Is Unaffected by Fungal Amino Acid Auxotrophy. *Infect. Immun.* **2010**, *78*, 1066–1077. [CrossRef] [PubMed]
32. McCarty, T.P.; Pappas, P.G. Invasive Candidiasis. *Infect. Dis. Clin. N. Am.* **2016**, *30*, 103–124. [CrossRef] [PubMed]
33. Lockhart, S.R.; Iqbal, N.; Cleveland, A.A.; Farley, M.M.; Harrison, L.H.; Bolden, C.B.; Baughman, W.; Stein, B.; Hollick, R.; Park, B.J.; et al. Species Identification and Antifungal Susceptibility Testing of Candida Bloodstream Isolates from Population-Based Surveillance Studies in Two U.S. Cities from 2008 to 2011. *J. Clin. Microbiol.* **2012**, *50*, 3435–3442. [CrossRef] [PubMed]

34. Pfaller, M.; Boyken, L.; Hollis, R.; Kroeger, J.; Messer, S.; Tendolkar, S.; Diekema, D. Use of Epidemiological Cutoff Values To Examine 9-Year Trends in Susceptibility of Candida Species to Anidulafungin, Caspofungin, and Micafungin. *J. Clin. Microbiol.* **2011**, *49*, 624–629. [CrossRef] [PubMed]
35. Cleary, J.D.; Garcia-Effron, G.; Chapman, S.W.; Perlin, D.S. Reduced *Candida glabrata* Susceptibility secondary to an FKS1 Mutation Developed during Candidemia Treatment. *Antimicrob. Agents Chemother.* **2008**, *52*, 2263–2265. [CrossRef] [PubMed]
36. Thompson, G.R.; Wiederhold, N.P.; Vallor, A.C.; Villareal, N.C.; Lewis, J.S.; Patterson, T.F. Development of caspofungin resistance following prolonged therapy for invasive candidiasis secondary to *Candida glabrata* infection. *Antimicrob. Agents Chemother.* **2008**, *52*, 3783–3785. [CrossRef] [PubMed]
37. Chapeland-Leclerc, F.; Hennequin, C.; Papon, N.; Noël, T.; Girard, A.; Socié, G.; Ribaud, P.; Lacroix, C. Acquisition of Flucytosine, Azole, and Caspofungin Resistance in *Candida glabrata* Bloodstream Isolates Serially Obtained from a Hematopoietic Stem Cell Transplant Recipient. *Antimicrob. Agents Chemother.* **2010**, *54*, 1360–1362. [CrossRef] [PubMed]
38. Durán-Valle, M.T.; Gago, S.; Gómez-López, A.; Cuenca-Estrella, M.; Jiménez Díez-Canseco, L.; Gómez-Garcés, J.L.; Zaragoza, O. Recurrent Episodes of Candidemia Due to *Candida glabrata* with a Mutation in Hot Spot 1 of the FKS2 Gene Developed after Prolonged Therapy with Caspofungin. *Antimcrob. Agents Chemoter.* **2012**, *56*, 3417–3419. [CrossRef]
39. Shields, R.K.; Nguyen, M.H.; Press, E.G.; Kwa, A.L.; Cheng, S.; Du, C.; Clancy, C.J. The presence of an FKS mutation rather than MIC is an independent risk factor for failure of echinocandin therapy among patients with invasive candidiasis due to *Candida glabrata*. *Antimicrob. Agents Chemother.* **2012**, *56*, 4862–4869. [CrossRef]
40. Pfeiffer, C.D.; Garcia-Effron, G.; Zaas, A.K.; Perfect, J.R.; Perlin, D.S.; Alexander, B.D. Breakthrough Invasive Candidiasis in Patients on Micafungin. *J. Clin. Microbiol.* **2010**, *48*, 2373–2380. [CrossRef]
41. Bizerra, F.C.; Jimenez-Ortigosa, C.; Souza, A.C.R.; Breda, G.L.; Queiroz-Telles, F.; Perlin, D.S.; Colombo, A.L. Breakthrough candidemia due to multidrug-resistant *Candida glabrata* during prophylaxis with a low dose of micafungin. *Antimicrob. Agents Chemoter.* **2014**, *58*, 2438–2440. [CrossRef] [PubMed]
42. Pham, C.D.; Iqbal, N.; Bolden, C.B.; Kuykendall, R.J.; Harrison, L.H.; Farley, M.M.; Schaffner, W.; Beldavs, Z.G.; Chiller, T.M.; Park, B.J.; et al. Role of FKS mutations in *Candida glabrata*: MIC values, echinocandin resistance, and multidrug resistance. *Antimicrob. Agents Chemother.* **2014**, *58*, 4690–4696. [CrossRef] [PubMed]
43. Park, S.; Kelly, R.; Kahn, J.N.N.; Robles, J.; Hsu, M.J.M.-J.; Register, E.; Li, W.; Vyas, V.; Fan, H.; Abruzzo, G.; et al. Specific substitutions in the echinocandin target Fks1p account for reduced susceptibility of rare laboratory and clinical Candida sp. isolates. *Antimicrob. Agents Chemother.* **2005**, *49*, 3264–3273. [CrossRef] [PubMed]
44. Perlin, D.S.; Teppler, H.; Donowitz, G.R.; Maertens, J.A.; Baden, L.R.; Milne, S.; Brown, A.J.; Gow, N.A. Resistance to echinocandin-class antifungal drugs. *Drug Resist. Updat.* **2007**, *10*, 121–130. [CrossRef] [PubMed]
45. Garcia-Effron, G.; Chua, D.J.; Tomada, J.R.; Dipersio, J.; Perlin, D.S.; Ghannoum, M.; Bonilla, H. Novel FKS Mutations Associated with Echinocandin Resistance in Candida Species. *Antimicrob. Agents Chemother.* **2010**, *54*, 2225–2227. [CrossRef] [PubMed]
46. Fonseca, E.; Silva, S.; Rodrigues, C.F.; Alves, C.; Azeredo, J.; Henriques, M. Effects of fluconazole on *Candida glabrata* biofilms and its relationship with ABC transporter gene expression. *Biofouling* **2014**, *30*, 447–457. [CrossRef] [PubMed]
47. Rodrigues, C.F.; Gonçalves, B.; Rodrigues, M.E.; Silva, S.; Azeredo, J.; Henriques, M. The Effectiveness of Voriconazole in Therapy of *Candida glabrata*'s Biofilms Oral Infections and Its Influence on the Matrix Composition and Gene Expression. *Mycopathologia* **2017**, *182*, 653–664. [CrossRef] [PubMed]
48. Rodrigues, C.F.; Henriques, M. Oral mucositis caused by *Candida glabrata* biofilms: Failure of the concomitant use of fluconazole and ascorbic acid. *Ther. Adv. Infect. Dis.* **2017**, *1*, 1–8. [CrossRef] [PubMed]
49. Arendrup, M.; Perlin, D.; Jensen, R.; Howard, S.; Goodwin, J.; Hopec, W. Differential in vivo activities of anidulafungin, caspofungin, and micafungin against *Candida glabrata* isolates with and without FSK resistance mutations. *Antimicrob. Agents Chemoter.* **2012**, 2435–2442. [CrossRef]

50. Andes, D.; Diekema, D.J.; Pfaller, M.A.; Bohrmuller, J.; Marchillo, K.; Lepak, A.; Andes, D.; Diekema, D.J.; Pfaller, M.A.; Bohrmuller, J.; et al. In Vivo comparison of the pharmacodynamic targets for echinocandin drugs against Candida species. *Antimicrob. Agents Chemother.* **2010**, *54*, 2497–2506. [CrossRef]
51. Teixeira, L.; Moreira, J.; Melo, J.; Bezerra, F.; Marques, R.M.; Fer-Reirinha, P.; Correia, A.; Monteiro, M.P.; Ferreira, P.G.; Vilanova, M. Immune response in the adipose tissue of lean mice infected with the protozoan parasite Neospora caninum. *Immunology* **2014**, *145*, 242–257. [CrossRef] [PubMed]
52. Kumar, R.; Saraswat, D.; Tati, S.; Edgerton, M. Novel Aggregation Properties of *Candida albicans* Secreted Aspartyl Proteinase Sap6 Mediate Virulence in Oral Candidiasis. *Infect. Immun.* **2015**, *83*, 2614–2626. [CrossRef] [PubMed]
53. Lockhart, S.R. Current Epidemiology of Candida Infection. *Clin. Microbiol. Newsl.* **2014**, *36*, 131–136. [CrossRef]
54. Silva, S.; Rodrigues, C.F.; Araújo, D.; Rodrigues, M.E.; Henriques, M. Candida Species Biofilms' Antifungal Resistance. *J. Fungi* **2017**, *3*, 8. [CrossRef] [PubMed]
55. Safdar, A.; Bannister, T.W.; Safdar, Z.; Ellis, M.; Ain, A. The predictors of outcome in immunocompetent patients with hematogenous candidasis. *Int. J. Infect. Dis.* **2004**, *8*, 180–186. [CrossRef] [PubMed]
56. Van Dijck, P.; Sjollema, J.; Camue, B.P.A.; Lagrou, K.; Berman, J.; d'Enfert, C.; Andes, D.R.; Arendrup, M.C.; Brakhage, A.A.; Calderone, R.; et al. Methodologies for in vitro and in vivo evaluation of efficacy of antifungal and antibiofilm agents and surface coatings against fungal biofilms. *Microb. Cell* **2018**, *5*, 300–326. [CrossRef] [PubMed]
57. Correia, A.; Lermann, U.; Teixeira, L.; Cerca, F.; Botelho, S.; Gil Da Costa, R.M.; Sampaio, P.; Gärtner, F.; Morschhäuser, J.; Vilanova, M.; et al. Limited Role of Secreted Aspartyl Proteinases Sap1 to Sap6 in *Candida albicans* Virulence and Host Immune Response in Murine Hematogenously Disseminated Candidiasis. *Infect. Immun.* **2010**, *78*, 4839–4849. [CrossRef]
58. Brieland, J.; Essig, D.; Jackson, C.; Frank, D.; Loebenberg, D.; Menzel, F.; Arnold, B.; DiDomenico, B.; Hare, R. Comparison of pathogenesis and host immune responses to *Candida glabrata* and *Candida albicans* in systemically infected immunocompetent mice. *Infect. Immun.* **2001**, *69*, 5046–5055. [CrossRef]
59. Kaur, R.; Ma, B.; Cormack, B.P. A family of glycosylphosphatidylinositol-linked aspartyl proteases is required for virulence of *Candida glabrata*. *Proc. Natl. Acad. Sci. USA* **2007**, *104*, 7628–7633. [CrossRef]
60. Srikantha, T.; Daniels, K.J.; Wu, W.; Lockhart, S.R.; Yi, S.; Sahni, N.; Ma, N.; Soll Correspondence, D.R.; Soll, D.R. Dark brown is the more virulent of the switch phenotypes of *Candida glabrata*. *Microbiology* **2008**, *154*, 3309–3318. [CrossRef]
61. Atkinson, B.A.; Bouthet, C.; Bocanegra, R.; Correa, A.; Luther, M.F.; Graybill, J.R. Comparison of fluconazole, amphotericin B and flucytosine in treatment of a murine model of disseminated infection with *Candida glabrata* in immunocompromised mice. *J. Antimicrob. Chemother.* **1995**, *35*, 631–640. [CrossRef] [PubMed]
62. Pfaller, M.A.; Moet, G.J.; Messer, S.A.; Jones, R.N.; Castanheira, M. Candida bloodstream infections: Comparison of species distributions and antifungal resistance patterns in community-onset and nosocomial isolates in the SENTRY Antimicrobial Surveillance Program, 2008-2009. *Antimicrob. Agents Chemother.* **2011**, *55*, 561–566. [CrossRef] [PubMed]
63. Healey, K.R.; Ortigosa, C.J.; Shor, E.; Perlin, D.S. Genetic Drivers of Multidrug Resistance in *Candida glabrata*. *Front. Microbiol.* **2016**, *7*, 1–9. [CrossRef] [PubMed]
64. Morio, F.; Jensen, R.H.; Le Pape, P.; Arendrup, M.C. Molecular basis of antifungal drug resistance in yeasts. *Int. J. Antimicrob. Agents* **2017**, *17*, 599–606. [CrossRef] [PubMed]
65. Perlin, D.S. Mechanisms of echinocandin antifungal drug resistance. *Ann. N. Y. Acad. Sci.* **2015**, *1354*, 1–11. [CrossRef] [PubMed]
66. Ferrari, S.; Sanguinetti, M.; De Bernardis, F.; Torelli, R.; Posteraro, B.; Vandeputte, P.; Sanglard, D. Loss of mitochondrial functions associated with azole resistance in *Candida glabrata* results in enhanced virulence in mice. *Antimicrob. Agents Chemother.* **2011**, *55*, 1852–1860. [CrossRef] [PubMed]
67. Al-fattani, M.A.; Douglas, L.J. Penetration of Candida Biofilms by Antifungal Agents. *Antimicrob. Agents Chemother.* **2004**, *48*, 3291–3297. [CrossRef]
68. De Luca, C.; Guglielminetti, M.; Ferrario, A.; Calabrò, M.; Casari, E. Candidemia: Species involved, virulence factors and antimycotic susceptibility. *New Microbiol.* **2012**, *35*, 459–468.
69. Grandesso, S.; Sapino, B.; Mazzuccato, S.; Solinas, M.; Bedin, M.; D'Angelo, M.; Gion, M. Study on in vitro susceptibility of *Candida* spp. isolated from blood culture. *Infect. Med.* **2012**, *20*, 25–30.

70. Lewis, R.; Kontoyiannis, D.; Darouiche, R.; Raad, I.; Prince, R. Antifungal activity of amphotericin B, fluconazole, and voriconazole in an in vitro model of Candida catheter-related bloodstream infection. *Antimicrob. Agents Chemother.* **2002**, *46*, 3499–3505. [CrossRef]
71. Donlan, R.; Costerton, J. Biofilms: Survival mechanisms of clinically relevant microorganisms. *Clin. Microbiol. Rev.* **2002**, *15*, 167–193. [CrossRef] [PubMed]
72. Basso, L.R.; Gast, C.E.; Mao, Y.; Wong, B. Fluconazole Transport into *Candida albicans* Secretory Vesicles by the Membrane Proteins Cdr1p, Cdr2p, and Mdr1p. *Eukaryot. Cell* **2010**, *9*, 960–970. [CrossRef] [PubMed]
73. Netea, M.G.; Joosten, L.A.; van der Meer, J.W.; Kullberg, B.J.; van de Veerdonk, F.L. Immune defence against Candida fungal infections. *Nat. Rev. Immunol.* **2015**, *15*, 630. [CrossRef] [PubMed]
74. Shoham, S.; Levitz, S.M. The immune response to fungal infections. *Br. J. Haematol.* **2005**, *129*, 569–582. [CrossRef] [PubMed]
75. V Zquez-torres, A.S.; Balish, E. Macrophages in Resistance to Candidiasis. *Microbiol. Mol. Biol. Rev.* **1997**, *61*, 170–192.
76. Ehrensaft, D.V.; Epstein, R.B.; Sarpel, S.; Andersen, B.R. Disseminated candidiasis in leukopenic dogs. *Proc. Soc. Exp. Biol. Med.* **1979**, *160*, 6–10. [CrossRef] [PubMed]
77. Elin, R.J.; Edelin, J.B.; Wolff, S.M. Infection and Immunoglobulin Concentrations in Chediak-Higashi Mice. *Infect. Immun.* **1974**, *10*, 88–91.
78. Holm, H.W.; Marwin, R.M. Effects of surface active agents on the susceptibility of Swiss mice to Candida albicans. *Mycopathol. Mycol. Appl.* **1967**, *33*, 186–192. [CrossRef]
79. Sharpe, H.; Romani Arlene Cenci, L.; Pitzurra, L.; Spreca, A.; Kopf, M.; Mencacci, A.; Montagnoli, C.; Bacci, A.; Cenci, E.; Sharpe, A.H.; et al. CD80+ Gr-1+ Myeloid Cells Inhibit Development of Antifungal Th1 Immunity in Mice with Candidiasis. *J. Immunol. Ref.* **2017**, *169*, 3180–3190.
80. Taylor, P.R.; Tsoni, S.V.; Willment, J.A.; Dennehy, K.M.; Rosas, M.; Findon, H.; Haynes, K.; Steele, C.; Botto, M.; Gordon, S.; et al. Dectin-1 is required for β-glucan recognition and control of fungal infection. *Nat. Immunol.* **2007**, *8*, 31–38. [CrossRef]
81. Taylor, P.R.; Brown, G.D.; Geldhof, A.B.; Martinez-Pomares, L.; Gordon, S. Pattern recognition receptors and differentiation antigens define murine myeloid cell heterogeneity ex vivo. *Eur. J. Immunol.* **2003**, *33*, 2090–2097. [CrossRef] [PubMed]
82. Westwater, C.; Schofield, D.A.; Nicholas, P.J.; Paulling, E.E.; Balish, E. *Candida glabrata* and *Candida albicans*: dissimilar tissue tropism and infectivity in a gnotobiotic model of mucosal candidiasis. *FEMS Immunol. Med. Microbiol.* **2007**, *51*, 134–139. [CrossRef] [PubMed]
83. Brunke, S.; Hube, B. Two unlike cousins: *Candida albicans* and *C. glabrata* infection strategies. *Cell. Microbiol.* **2013**, *15*, 701–708. [CrossRef] [PubMed]
84. Keppler-Ross, S.; Douglas, L.; Konopka, J.B.; Dean, N. Recognition of Yeast by Murine Macrophages Requires Mannan but Not Glucan. *Eukaryot. Cell* **2010**, *9*, 1776–1787. [CrossRef] [PubMed]
85. Seider, K.; Brunke, S.; Schild, L.; Jablonowski, N.; Wilson, D.; Majer, O.; Dagmar, B.; Haas, A.; Kuchler, K.; Schaller, M.; et al. The Facultative Intracellular Pathogen *Candida glabrata* Subverts Macrophage Cytokine Production and Phagolysosome Maturation. *J. Immunol.* **2011**, *187*, 3072–3086. [CrossRef] [PubMed]
86. Roetzer, A.; Gratz, N.; Kovarik, P.; Schüller, C. Autophagy supports *Candida glabrata* survival during phagocytosis. *Cell. Microbiol.* **2010**, *12*, 199–216. [CrossRef] [PubMed]
87. Jandric, Z.; Schuller, C. Stress response in *Candida glabrata*: Pieces of a fragmented picture. *Future Mirobiol.* **2011**, *6*, 1475–1484. [CrossRef]
88. Bonifazi, P.; Zelante, T.; D'Angelo, C.; De Luca, A.; Moretti, S.; Bozza, S.; Perruccio, K.; Iannitti, R.G.; Giovannini, G.; Volpi, C.; et al. Balancing inflammation and tolerance in vivo through dendritic cells by the commensal Candida albicans. *Mucosal Immunol.* **2009**, *2*, 362–374. [CrossRef]
89. Moraes Nicola, A.; Casadevall, A.; Goldman, D.L.; Nicola, A.M.; Casadevall, A.; Goldman, D.L. Fungal killing by mammalian phagocytic cells. *Curr. Opin. Microbiol.* **2008**, *11*, 313–317. [CrossRef]
90. Romani, L.; Montagnoli, C.; Bozza, S.; Perruccio, K.; Spreca, A.; Allavena, P.; Verbeek, S.; Calderone, R.A.; Bistoni, F.; Puccetti, P. The exploitation of distinct recognition receptors in dendritic cells determines the full range of host immune relationships with Candida albicans. *Int. Immunol.* **2004**, *16*, 149–161. [CrossRef]
91. Shi, D.; Li, D.; Qingxin, Y.; Qiu, Y.; Yan, H.; Shen, Y.; Guixia, L.; Liu, W. Silenced suppressor of cytokine signaling 1 (SOCS1) enhances the maturation and antifungal immunity of dendritic cells in response to *Candida albicans* in vitro. *Immunol. Res.* **2015**, *61*, 206–218. [CrossRef] [PubMed]

92. Ohno, N.; Uchiyama, M.; Tsuzuki, A.; Tokunaka, K.; Miura, N.N.; Adachi, Y.; Aizawa, M.W.; Tamura, H.; Tanaka, S.; Yadomae, T. Solubilization of yeast cell-wall β-(1→3)-D-glucan by sodium hypochlorite oxidation and dimethyl sulfoxide extraction. *Carbohydr. Res.* **1999**, *316*, 161–172. [CrossRef]
93. Rodrigues, C.F.; Boas, D.; Haynes, K.; Henriques, M. The MNN2 Gene Knockout Modulates the Antifungal Resistance of Biofilms of *Candida glabrata*. *Biomolecules* **2018**, *8*, 130. [CrossRef] [PubMed]
94. Rodrigues, C.F.; Rodrigues, M.E.; Henriques, M. Susceptibility of *Candida glabrata* biofilms to echinocandins: Alterations in the matrix composition. *Biofouling* **2018**, *34*, 892–7014. [CrossRef] [PubMed]

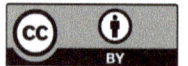

© 2019 by the authors. Licensee MDPI, Basel, Switzerland. This article is an open access article distributed under the terms and conditions of the Creative Commons Attribution (CC BY) license (http://creativecommons.org/licenses/by/4.0/).

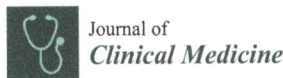

Review

Management of *Streptococcus mutans*-*Candida* spp. Oral Biofilms' Infections: Paving the Way for Effective Clinical Interventions

Bahare Salehi [1], Dorota Kregiel [2], Gail Mahady [3], Javad Sharifi-Rad [4,5,*], Natália Martins [6,7,*] and Célia F. Rodrigues [8,*]

1. Student Research Committee, School of Medicine, Bam University of Medical Sciences, Bam 44340847, Iran; bahar.salehi007@gmail.com
2. Department of Environmental Biotechnology, Lodz University of Technology, 90-924 Lodz, Wolczanska 171/173, Poland; dorota.kregiel@p.lodz.pl
3. Department of Pharmacy Practice, Clinical Pharmacognosy Laboratories, University of Illinois at Chicago, Chicago, IL 60612, USA; mahady@uic.edu
4. Phytochemistry Research Center, Shahid Beheshti University of Medical Sciences, Tehran 1991953381, Iran
5. Department of Chemistry, Richardson College for the Environmental Science Complex, The University of Winnipeg, 599 Portage Avenue, Winnipeg, MB R3B 2G3, Canada
6. Faculty of Medicine, University of Porto, Alameda Prof. Hernâni Monteiro, Porto 4200-319, Portugal
7. Institute for Research and Innovation in Health (i3S), University of Porto, Porto 4200-135, Portugal
8. LEPABE—Laboratory for Process Engineering, Environment, Biotechnology and Energy, Faculty of Engineering, University of Porto, Rua Dr. Roberto Frias, Porto 4200-465, Portugal
* Correspondence: c.fortunae@gmail.com (C.F.R.); javad.sharifirad@gmail.com (J.S.-R.); ncmartins@med.up.pt (N.M.)

Received: 6 January 2020; Accepted: 12 February 2020; Published: 14 February 2020

Abstract: Oral diseases are considered the most common noncommunicable diseases and are related to serious local and systemic disorders. Oral pathogens can grow and spread in the oral mucosae and frequently in biomaterials (e.g., dentures or prostheses) under polymicrobial biofilms, leading to several disorders such as dental caries and periodontal disease. Biofilms harbor a complex array of interacting microbes, increasingly unapproachable to antimicrobials and with dynamic processes key to disease pathogenicity, which partially explain the gradual loss of response towards conventional therapeutic regimens. New drugs (synthesized and natural) and other therapies that have revealed promising results for the treatment or control of these mixed biofilms are presented and discussed here. A structured search of bibliographic databases was applied to include recent research. There are several promising new approaches in the treatment of *Candida* spp.–*Streptococcus mutans* oral mixed biofilms that could be clinically applied in the near future. These findings confirm the importance of developing effective therapies for oral *Candida*–bacterial infections.

Keywords: oral biofilm; infection control; *Streptococcus mutans*; *Candida* spp.; natural compounds; antimicrobial resistance

1. Introduction

According to the World Health Organization (WHO), oral diseases are the most common noncommunicable diseases, causing discomfort, pain, disfigurement, and death [1,2]. Dental caries, the most prevalent condition, derives from microbial biofilms (plaque) formed on the tooth surface [1,2]. Presently, it is estimated that 2.4 billion people have caries of permanent teeth and 486 million children have caries of primary teeth [3]. Similarly, periodontal disease (which affects tissues that both surround and support the teeth), and dental caries are both related to bacterial/fungal infections and are significant causes of deciduous tooth decay in over 560 million children, involving hundreds of billions of dollars of expenses per year [1,4]. In low-income populations, the majority of dental caries are left untreated, and affected teeth are most often extracted due to pain and discomfort [1]. The pain and inflammation of severe dental caries can impair eating and sleeping, as well as the overall quality of life. Abscesses can occur and may result in pain and chronic systemic infection and diseases [1]. If not treated, these disorders can also lead to chronic diseases and serious systemic infections (e.g., Alzheimer's disease, cardiovascular disorders, oral cancer) [3,5].

Oral pathogens easily grow and propagate in the oral cavity, leading to the formation of dental plaque on both soft and hard tissue [6]. Dental plaque is formed by salivary molecules, proteins, bacterial/fungal debris, and sialic acid, which is then colonized by primary colonizers, including *Streptococcus sanguis* and *Actinomyces viscosus*. Their colonization is impacted by various food and environmental factors, including pH, carbon sources, and osmolarity [7–9]. Then, other bacterial species such as *Streptococcus mutans* adhere to the primary colonizers, and the tooth surface develops into a bacterial biofilm, known as dental plaque. Beyond dental plaque is dental calculus, which is a complex combination of dental plaque, salvia, and gingival crevicular fluid. The growth and invasiveness of oral pathogens are both regulated by an equilibrium between dental plaque bacteria and the innate immune system. The build-up of calcified dental plaque that extends into the subgingival layer can trigger inflammation due to perturbations of the immune system [7,8]. The calcified dental plaque can trap many biomolecules, viruses, and other bacteria and fungi, and alterations in the oral microbiome can lead to a wide range of diseases over a lifetime [8]. It has been suggested that the human oral microbiome is made up of over 2000 taxa of bacteria and fungi, including a wide range of opportunistic pathogens involved in cardiac, periodontal, respiratory, and other diseases, including cardiovascular and respiratory diseases, diabetes, and osteoporosis [8]. This review focuses on reports published in the last five years, related to one of the most important oral co-infections: *Streptococcus mutans–Candida* spp. biofilms.

Streptococcus mutans and Candida spp.: *Relevance in Oral Biofilms*

The colonization of teeth by cariogenic bacteria is one of the most important risk factors in the development of dental diseases, with *S. mutans* being the primary species associated with the early dental caries process [10]. *Streptococcus mutans* is a Gram-positive, facultative anaerobic bacteria, and the primary etiological agent of dental plaques and dental caries [11,12]. This species is closely related to the streptococci group that inhabits the mouth, pharynx, and intestine and is well adapted to form biofilms due to its ability to form amyloids, which are very prevalent in natural biofilms [12]. Also, it colonizes the dental surface, causing damage to the hard tooth structure in the presence of fermentable carbohydrates, since it is a recognized acid-producing bacterium (e.g., sucrose and fructose). Moreover, *S. mutans* can adhere to the enamel salivary pellicle and other plaque bacteria, where they produce acidic metabolites, build up glycogen stores, and synthesize extracellular polysaccharides (EPS), glucans, and fructans from dietary sugars, leading to increased dental caries. In fact, there are several acidogenic and aciduric species in dental plaque associated with dental caries development, but *S. mutans* is the primary producer of EPS, which makes these biofilms difficult to control [11].

Along with the thousands of *Streptococcus* spp., over 100 fungal phylotypes also colonize the oral cavity, including many *Candida* spp. [13]. They are often found in the oral cavity of healthy individuals, with *Candida albicans* being the most predominant species (~60%–70%), followed by *Candida tropicalis* and *Candida glabrata* [13,14]. Usually, *Candida* spp. are commensal; however, in specific situations, these fungi may become parasitic, causing oral candidiasis particularly in immunocompromised patients, such as those with HIV/AIDS [13,15,16]. These fungal species are present in coating surfaces, dentine, as well as in the cementum surface. Interestingly, *C. albicans* grows in enamel cracks, grooves and flows into the crevices of cavities, as well as deeply penetrating open dentinal tubules [13]. Several *Candida* spp. have been isolated from caries as well as from root and dentinal caries in both children and adults, with prevalence ranging from 66% to 97% in pediatric populations and 31% to 56% in adult populations [15]. Thus, *C. albicans* can contribute to dentine and root caries in both children and adults.

Remarkably, *Candida* spp. cannot effectively form plaque biofilms directly or bind to *S. mutans* unless sugar is present. In a 2017 study, it was found that an enzyme known as glucosyltransferase B (GftB, which promotes firm cell clustering, and increased cohesion of plaque), secreted by *S. mutans*, uses sugar from the diet to manufacture glue-like polymers called glucans. *Candida* spp. increases glucan formation, causing the formation of a sticky biofilm that allows the yeast to adhere to teeth and bind to *S. mutans* [17]. These researchers further showed that the outer portion of the *Candida* spp. cell wall, composed of molecules called mannans, was involved in binding GftB, and that mutant *Candida* strains that lacked the mannan components had impaired binding to *S. mutans* GftB and a reduced biofilm load [17]. They further tested this hypothesis on biofilm formation in a rodent model of early childhood caries. Rodents infected with both *S. mutans* and either the wild type or defective mutant *Candida* strains showed that animals infected with wild-type *Candida* spp. had abundant biofilm formation, while those infected with the mutant *Candida* strains had reduced biofilm formation by up to ~5-fold [17].

Glucosyltransferases (Gtfs)-derived EPS have been revealed to be a key mediator of co-species biofilm development and their co-existence with *C. albicans* induces the expression of virulence genes in *S. mutans*. In fact, water-soluble glucan synthesis is regulated by the *dexA* gene and affects biofilm aggregation and cariogenic pathogenicity in *S. mutans* [18]. The co-cultivation altered *S. mutans* signal transduction and the transcription of genes (*comC* and *ciaRH*) associated with fitness and virulence [19]. Arzmi and co-workers [20] suggested that polymicrobial biofilms differentially modulate oral microorganisms' phenotypes. Yang and co-workers [21] found that antigen I/II of *S. mutans* is important for *Candida* spp. incorporation into the biofilm and is also required for increased acid production. *S. mutans* not only modulates biofilm formation, but also attenuates *C. albicans* virulence [22,23]. Additionally, the possibility of a *quorum sensing* system stimulation of *S. mutans* by *C. albicans* was also demonstrated, consequently changing its virulence properties [24].

2. Research Methodology

A structured search of bibliographic databases (PubMed Central, Elsevier's ScienceDirect, SCOPUS, and Springer's SpringerLink) was undertaken. The keywords used were "streptococcus" + "mutans" + "candida" + "biofilms" + "resistance".

3. Compounds with Activity against Oral Infections

Oral microbial communities are some of the most complex microbial floras in the human body, consisting of thousands of bacterial and hundreds of fungal species [25]. Culture-independent molecular methods, such as proteomics and 16S rRNA sequencing, have demonstrated that *S. mutans* was the dominant species, with elevated levels of other streptococci including *Streptococcus sanguinis*, *Streptococcus mitis*, and *Streptococcus salivarius*. *Candida* spp. combined with *Streptococcus* spp. usually increases the virulence in invasive candidiasis, early childhood caries, or peri-implantitis [13,26,27]. The interactions between the various species in these mixed biofilms may be synergistic, in that the presence of one microorganism generates a niche for other pathogenic microorganisms, which serves to facilitate organisms' retention. Thus, *Streptococcus* spp. and *Candida* spp. create special synergistic consortia on solid oral surfaces [13,26].

Streptococcus mutans strains are considered the most cariogenic bacteria; however, *Candida* spp. can increase their cariogenicity. Bacterial and fungal cells are able to produce glucan as an extracellular polysaccharide that aids cariogenic biofilm formation [28]. Bacteria also convert dietary sucrose and free glucose or fructose into a diverse range of soluble and, particularly, insoluble extracellular polysaccharides (EPS) (e.g., water-insoluble glucans) through exoenzymes, such as Gtfs, and EPS, to build blocks of cariogenic biofilms. These structures promote the tooth surface colonization by *S. mutans* and additional microorganisms into dental plaque (e.g., *Porphyromonas gingivalis*, streptococci,

Fusobacterium spp., *Prevotella* spp.), while forming the scaffold core or matrix of the biofilm. In addition, the EPS matrix creates a special diffusion-limiting barrier, facilitating acidic microenvironments creation at the biofilm–tooth interface, which is critical for adjacent tooth enamel dissolution [29]. Furthermore, *S. mutans* displays many other virulence attributes, including its ability to produce acid and to tolerate an acidic environment.

Among *Candida* spp., *C. albicans* is the most prevalent on dental tissues, reaching 60%–70%, followed by *C. tropicalis* and *C. glabrata* [30]. As indicated earlier, these yeasts are usually commensal, but in some situations they can become parasitic, causing oral candidiasis [30,31]. The virulence attributes of *C. albicans* are the acidogenicity and aciduric nature, along with the ability to develop profuse biofilms, to ferment and assimilate dietary sugars, and to produce collagenolytic proteinases [15]. Also, *C. albicans* modulates the pH in dual-species biofilms to values above the critical pH where enamel dissolves. Although the species present low cariogenicity, biofilms formed by mixed populations of *C. albicans* and *S. mutans* are more voluminous [32]. The presence of *Candida* spp. enhances *S. mutans* growth, fitness, and accumulation within biofilms. It is documented that *C. albicans* growth stimulates *S. mutans* development via biofilm-derived metabolites [33]. Also, *C. albicans* mannans mediate *S. mutans* exoenzyme GtfB binding to modulate cross-kingdom biofilm development [17]. *Candida* spp.-derived β-1,3-glucans contribute to the EPS matrix structure, while fungal mannan and β-glucan provide sites for GtfB binding and activity; thus, the coexistence of *S. mutans* with *C. albicans* can cause dental caries progression or disease recurrence in the future [34]. It was also suggested that *S. mutans* co-cultivation with *C. albicans* influences carbohydrate utilization by bacterial cells [35,36], and the analysis of metabolites confirmed the increase in carbohydrate metabolism, with amounts of formate elevated by co-cultured biofilms [37]. Nonetheless, biofilm biomass and metabolic activity were both strain- and growth medium-dependent [37]. Liu and co-workers showed that nicotine promotes *S. mutans* attachment. The enhancement of the synergistic relationship may contribute to caries development in smokers [38,39]. On the other hand, there are contradictory reports in this matter. It was proposed that, by definition, *C. albicans* is not a cariogenic microorganism; it could prevent caries by actively increasing pH and preventing mineral loss [40]. Nonetheless, a study published in 2016 concluded that children with severe early childhood caries were likely infected by their mothers, as the mothers of these children were highly infected with *C. albicans* [41]. In fact, genetic testing of *Candida* strains from children and their mothers showed that most strains were genetically related [41].

Progress in understanding the etiology, epidemiology, and microbiology of periodontal pocket flora has called for new antimicrobial therapeutic schemes for oral diseases [42]. Distinctive means and compounds may be used to prevent oral infections. Biomolecules produced by *S. mutans*, lactoferrin, and probiotics, applying chemicals and photodynamic therapy, can support the management of oral candidiasis [43].

3.1. Chemical Compounds with Activity against Streptococcus mutans and Candida spp. Biofilms

Recently, a wide range of antimicrobial agents and methodologies have been reported to suppress the growth of dental *Streptococcus mutans*–*Candida* spp. biofilms (Table 1).

Table 1. Chemical compounds and their bioactivity against *Streptococcus* spp. and *Candida* spp.

Main Effect(s)	Compound	Targeted Species	Reference(s)
Pathogen toxicity	aPDT: chloroaluminium phthalocyanine (cationic nanoemulsion); hypericin-glucamine Rose Bengal in α-cyclodextrin; curcumin; methylene blue; toluidine blue O erythrosine with green light or Photodithazine®; rose Bengal, methylene blue and curcumin with white light	Mainly *C. albicans*, *C. glabrata*, *S. mutans*, and *S. sanguis*, but also other species	[44–55]
Antibiofilm	Chlorhexidine with low concentrations but with the addition of cis-2-decenoic acid	*S. mutans* and *C. albicans*, and bacterial–fungal dual-species consortia	[56]
	Chlorhexidine gluconate with tyrosol	Single and mixed-species oral biofilms	[57,58]
	Fluoride-releasing copolymer: methyl methacrylate, 2-hydroxyethyl methacrylate with polymethyl methacrylate (incorporating sodium fluoride)	Acidogenic mixed-species biofilms	[59]
Antimicrobial	2.5% sodium hypochlorite, 2% chlorhexidine, and ozonated water	Mono- and dual-species biofilms of *S. mutans* and *C. albicans*	[25]
	Chlorhexidine carrier nanosystem based on iron oxide magnetic nanoparticles and chitosan		[60]
	Chitosan, silver nanoparticles and ozonated olive oil	Several endodontic pathogens, including *S. mutans* and *C. albicans* mixed biofilms	[61]
	Chitosan and carboxymethyl chitosan	Biofilms of *Streptococcus* spp. and *Candida* spp.	[62–65]
	Materials containing silver nanoparticles alone or with polyphosphates	*C. albicans* and *S. mutans*	[66,67]
	Dimethylaminododecyl methacrylate modified denture base resin	Several microorganisms associated on the dental base	[68]
	Poly-(2-tert-butilaminoethyl) methacrylate	*S. mutans*	[69]
	Cetylpyridinium chloride and cetyltrimethylammonium bromide with plant terpinen-4-ol (Synthetic surfactants+)	*S. mutans* and *C. albicans*	[70]
	Nanoparticles of amphiphilic silanes with Chlorin e6	*Streptococcus* genus	[71]
Antimicrobial and antibiofilm	Hexagonal boron nitride nanoparticles	*S. mutans*, *Staphylococcus pasteuri*, *S. mutans*-*Candida* spp.	[72]
	Silver nanoparticles combined to calcium glycerophosphate or nanostructured silver vanadate (dental acrylic resins)	Several microorganisms associated with dental prostheses	[73,74]
	Modified pH-responsive cationic poly (ethylene glycol)-block-poly (2-(((2-aminoethyl) carbamoyl) oxy) ethyl methacrylate	Acidogenic mixed-species biofilms	[75]
Extracellular polysaccharides (EPS) inhibitors	Combination fluconazole with povidone iodine	*C. albicans* or mixed biofilm formation with *S. mutans*	[76]
	Thiazolidinediones, such as thiazolidinedione-8	Mixed biofilm formed by *Candida* spp. and bacterial strains (*S. mutans*)	[77]
	Lactams, such as γ-Alkylidene-γ-lactams solubilized in 3.5% dimethyl sulfoxide	*S. mutans* and *C. glabrata*	[78]

Photodynamic antimicrobial therapy (aPDT) is based on a photoactive dye—a chemical photosensitizer that binds to the target cell and is activated by a specific light wavelength. During this process, oxygen species such as singlet oxygen and free radicals are formed, exerting toxicity towards the cell [30]. The influence of pre-irradiation time employed in antimicrobial photodynamic therapy with a diode laser was recently checked [79]. It was found no effect due to *C. albicans* biofilm therapy; however, a pre-irradiation time of 1 min was effective against a microbial load of *S. mutans*. The effect of aPDT using chloroaluminium phthalocyanine in a cationic nanoemulsion was evaluated against multispecies biofilms of *C. albicans*, *C. glabrata*, and *S. mutans*. The technique led to photoinactivation of the biofilm and reduced colony count and metabolic activity [44]. Similar effects were obtained using hypericin–glucamine [45], Rose Bengal in α-cyclodextrin [46], curcumin [44,47–50], methylene blue [52], toluidine blue O [51], erythrosine with green light [55], or Photodithazine® obtained from the cyanobacterium *Spirulina platensis* [53,54]. Another study conducted by Soria-Lozano et al. [80], using Rose Bengal, methylene blue, and curcumin with white light, showed positive effects against the *S. mutans* and *S. sanguis* strains. Although methylene blue and Rose Bengal were the most efficient, *C. albicans* was the most resistant to all photosensitizers, and curcumin, in this case, was ineffective. Finally, aPDT embodies an important treatment as the photodynamic inactivation seems to be promising for biofilm-associated *S. mutans* and *Candida* spp. biofilm infection management, since there is no microbial resistance observed.

Chlorhexidine is the most commonly studied active agent [81,82]. It is widely used for preventing dental plaque or treating mouth yeast infections. Additionally, over the years, the number of studies on antibiofilm strategies using this compound or other chemicals has increased [83]. Chlorhexidine at low concentrations, but with the addition of cis-2-decenoic acid, was able to disperse single-species biofilms formed by *S. mutans* and *C. albicans*, as well as bacterial–fungal dual-species consortia [56]. Also, chlorhexidine gluconate with tyrosol was revealed to be effective against single and mixed-species oral biofilms [57,58]. A solution containing 2.5% sodium hypochlorite, 2% chlorhexidine, and ozonated water inhibited biofilms of *S. mutans* and *C. albicans* in mesiobuccal root canals after irrigation [25]. A chlorhexidine carrier nanosystem based on iron oxide magnetic nanoparticles and chitosan was synthesized, and its antimicrobial effect on mono- and dual-species biofilms of *C. albicans* and *S. mutans* was evaluated. The results confirmed the nanosystem potential as a preventive or therapeutic agent to fight biofilm-associated oral diseases [60]. The advantage of chlorhexidine is that its resistance is not as common as other chemicals'. Importantly, cases are being reported more often [84]. Hence, in order to reduce the number of cases, it is important to restrict its applications to indications with a strong patient benefit and to remove it from uses that are without any advantage or have doubtful value.

The antimicrobial activity of chitosan, silver nanoparticles, and ozonated olive oil was evaluated against endodontic pathogens, including *S. mutans* and *C. albicans*. This combination was characterized as novel, safe, and having the potential to eradicate mature mixed-species biofilms [61]. Chitosan and carboxymethyl chitosan were also active against *Candida* spp. and *Streptococcus* spp. biofilms [62–65]. Also, Kivanç and co-workers [72] investigated the antimicrobial and antibiofilm activities of hexagonal boron nitride nanoparticles against *S. mutans*, *Staphylococcus pasteuri*, *S. mutans* -*Candida* spp. Their results showed that, at an appropriate concentration (0.1 mg/mL), these nanoparticles could be considered a safe potential oral care product.

Similarly, EPS inhibitors may enhance antibiofilm activity [85,86]. A combination of the antifungal fluconazole with povidone iodine showed to completely inhibit *C. albicans* or mixed biofilm formation [76]. It was found that the inclusion of iodine derivative enhanced fluconazole efficacy by inhibiting α-glucan synthesis in *S. mutans*, which participates in protective bacterial EPS formation [76]. Moreover, thiazolidinediones have been found to act as effective *quorum sensing* quenchers, capable of preventing the mixed biofilm formed by *Candida* spp. and bacterial strains. These compounds can penetrate into deeper layers of the mixed biofilm, thereby increasing the antimicrobial activity. A small molecule, thiazolidinedione-8, has been revealed to be able to impair biofilm formation of various microbial pathogens. These compounds may disturb the symbiotic balance between *C. albicans* and *S. mutans* in a dual-species biofilm [77]. The inhibitory effects of lactams in mixed oral biofilms, including *S. mutans* and *C. glabrata*, have been assessed [78]. γ-Alkylidene-γ-lactams solubilized in 3.5% dimethyl sulfoxide led to a marked reduction in biofilm biomass. Furthermore, the total protein content and the quantity of EPS declined significantly. Hence, these compounds show important antibiomass activity, which can be important for promoting the diffusion of a second drug into oral biofilms, for its total eradication.

Several materials containing silver nanoparticles, alone or with polyphosphates, were evaluated as antimicrobials against *C. albicans* and *S. mutans*. These composites demonstrated significant antimicrobial activity, especially against *S. mutans*, which might make them a possible alternative for new dental materials [66,67]. Silver nanoparticles, combined with calcium glycerophosphate as well as nanostructured silver vanadate in dental acrylic resins, have also been shown to have antimicrobial and antibiofilm activities against dental prostheses-associated microorganisms [73,74]. Silver has found several uses since its toxicity toward human cells is considerably lower than toward bacteria; thus, this application is promising.

Base resins have also shown promising bioactive responses against *C. albicans* and *S. mutans*. Dimethylaminododecyl methacrylate-modified denture base resin proved to be a favorable therapeutic system against problems triggered by denture base microbes (e.g., denture stomatitis) [68]. Likewise, poly-(2-tert-butilaminoethyl) methacrylate decreased *S. mutans'* adhesion to the material surface, but did not exhibit an antimicrobial effect against *C. albicans* [69]. Furthermore, a novel fluoride-releasing copolymer composed of methyl methacrylate, 2-hydroxyethyl methacrylate with polymethyl methacrylate was developed by incorporating sodium fluoride. This copolymer inhibited acidogenic mixed-species biofilms, showing potential to control these diseases by limiting biofilm growth [59]. Finally, a modified pH-responsive cationic poly (ethylene glycol)-block-poly (2-(((2-aminoethyl) carbamoyl) oxy) ethyl methacrylate has been revealed to be a promising agent for dental caries therapy and provided guidelines for drug delivery system design in other acidic pathologic systems [75].

Regarding synthetic surfactants, several compounds have also shown great potential. Cetylpyridinium chloride and cetyltrimethylammonium bromide with plant terpinen-4-ol revealed antimicrobial activity against *S. mutans* and *C. albicans* [70]. Nanoparticles of amphiphilic silanes with Chlorin e6 exhibited strong antibiofilm activity against periodontitis-related pathogens belonging to the *Streptococcus* genus [71]. These compounds have good prospects in antimicrobial applications to inhibit both oral disease occurrence and progression, namely periodontitis, one of the most relevant oral diseases.

3.2. Natural Compounds with Bioactivity Against Streptococcus mutans and Candida spp. Biofilms

Due to the incidence of oral disease, increased resistance by bacteria and fungi to antimicrobials, and the adverse effects of some drugs currently used in dentistry (and general medicine), there is a great need for alternative prophylaxis and treatment options that are not only safer but also cost-effective. While several antimicrobial agents are commercially available, these chemicals can alter the oral microbiota and have undesirable side effects (e.g., nausea, diarrhea, vomiting, tooth staining). Henceforth, traditional medicine and the search for alternative products are still important. In fact, natural products offer an assortment of chemical structures and possess an extensive variety of biological properties; thus, they are a source for new pharmaceuticals. Bioactive secondary metabolites have been revealed to be useful as new antimicrobial and antibiofilm drugs, such as numerous furanones, alkaloids, and flavonoids, from many plants and marine organisms [87]. Table 2 presents natural compounds and plant extracts with antimicrobial potential, particularly focused on anti-*Streptococcus* spp. anti-*Candida* spp. activities.

Table 2. Natural compounds/extracts and their in vitro bioactivity against *Streptococcus* spp. and *Candida* spp.

Year	In vitro Assays	Natural Compound/Extract	Effect	Reference(s)
2018	Antibacterial and antifungal bioactivity	*Acacia arabica* (extract)	Antibacterial source of anticariogenic agents	[88]
2018	Antibacterial and antifungal bioactivity	*Myracrodruon urundeuva* and *Qualea grandiflora* (hydroalcoholic extracts)	Activity against *S. mutans* biofilm	[89]
2018	Antibacterial and antifungal bioactivity	*Cissampelos torulosa*, *Spirostachys africana*, *Clematis brachiata*, *Englerophytum magalismonatanum* (extracts)	Activity against both *Streptococcus* spp. and *Candida* spp.	[90]
2017	Antibacterial and antifungal bioactivity Cytotoxicity and genotoxicity: murine macrophages (RAW 264.7), human gingival fibroblasts (FMM-1), human breast carcinoma cells (MCF-7), and cervical carcinoma cells (HeLa)	*Thymus vulgaris* and *Rosmarinus officinalis* (extracts)	Antimicrobial and anti-inflammatory effects against oral pathogens	[91,92]
2017	Antibacterial and antifungal bioactivity Antibacterial, antifungal, and antiadhesion in a tissue conditioner	*Azadirachta indica* (leaf extract)	Potential antimicrobial agent against both *S. mutans* and *C. albicans*	[93]
2017	Antibacterial and antifungal, antibiofilm and antioxidant bioactivity	*Camellia japonica* and *Thuja orientalis*	Significantly inhibited the microbial grow of oral pathogens	[94]
2016	Antibacterial and antifungal, antibiofilm bioactivity Cytotoxicity and anti-inflammatory effects: human oral epithelial cells	*Houttuynia cordata* (herbal tea)	Antibiofilm effects against *S. mutans* and *C. albicans*	[95]
2015	Antibacterial and antifungal bioactivity	*Ricinus communis* and sodium hypochlorite (cleanser solutions)	Effective in controlling denture biofilms	[96]
2014	Anti-adherent properties (antibiofilm)	*Schinus terebinthifolius* and *Croton urucurana* (methanol and acetate methanol extract fractions in hydroalcoholic and dimethylsulfoxide)	Antibiofilm activity against *S. mutans* and *C. albicans*	[97]

Plant-derived compounds are a good source of therapeutic agents and inhibitors of dental caries, periodontal diseases, and candidiasis. For example, α-mangostin or lawsone methyl ether showed antimicrobial, antibiofilm, and anti-inflammatory activities. Indeed, an oral spray containing these natural chemicals was effective against common oral pathogens [98]. Lupinifolin from *Albizia myriophylla* wood exhibits good anti-*S. mutans* activity by damaging bacterial membranes, resulting in cell leakage [99]. Essential oils and bioactive fractions from *Aloysia gratissima*, *Baccharis dracunculifolia*, *Coriandrum sativum*, *Cyperus articulatus*, and *Lippia sidoides* were also evaluated as antimicrobials against *S. mutans* and *Candida* spp. A significant reduction in extracellular polysaccharides and bacteria was observed for *A. gratissima* and *L. sidoides*, indicating that these fractions disrupted biofilm integrity.

Plus, *C. sativum* oils drastically affected *C. albicans* viability [100], and might be considered as alternative anticaries agents. In turn, quercetin and kaempferol or farnesol with myricetin showed favorable properties in terms of controlling some virulence factors of *S. mutans* and *C. albicans* biofilms [101–104]. It was suggested that tyrosol decreased the metabolic activity and number of viable cells in single and mixed-species biofilms [105]. Correspondingly, β-caryophyllene—a bicyclic sesquiterpene of numerous essential oils—may inhibit cariogenic biofilms and may be a candidate agent for the prevention of dental caries [28]. These results highlight the promising antimicrobial activity of plants for the treatment of dental caries and oral candidiasis.

Propolis, rich in flavonoids, has a long history of use as a natural treatment for a host of health problems. It is also used as an ingredient in certain medicinal products applied directly to the skin, or in mouthwash and toothpaste. Propolis is under preliminary research for the potential development of new drugs associated with the control of *C. albicans* and immunomodulatory effects. Propolis and miswak (*Salvadora persica* tree), used in toothpaste, dental varnishes, and mouthwash, led to a significant reduction in the colony-forming units of oral biofilms [106,107].

Antimicrobial peptides have also been widely tested for controlling bacterial biofilms. Shang and colleagues [108] tested the efficacy of peptides from *Rana chensinensis* skin secretions in preventing biofilm formation by cariogenic and periodontic pathogens. Peptide L-K6, a temporin-1CEb analog, exhibited high antimicrobial activity against tested oral pathogens and was able to inhibit *S. mutans* biofilm formation. This peptide significantly reduced cell viability within oral biofilms. Its anti-inflammatory activity was correlated with L-K6 binding to LPS and dissociating LPS aggregates. Likewise, cyclic dipeptides (CDPs) are common metabolites widely biosynthesized by cyclodipeptide synthases or nonribosomal peptide synthetases by both prokaryotic and eukaryotic cells. Examples of CDPs that inhibit biofilm formation by *Streptococcus epidermidis* include cyclo-(l-Leucyl-l-Tyrosyl) isolated from mold *Penicillium* sp. and cyclo-(l-Leucyl-l-Prolyl) isolated from *Bacillus amyoliquefaciens*. The antibiofilm activity of 75 synthetic CDPs was assessed against oral pathogens, allowing for the identification of five novel CDPs that inhibit biofilm formation and adherence properties. Among them, five new active compounds were identified as preventing biofilm formation by *S. mutans* and *C. albicans* on the hydroxylapatite surface [109].

Similarly, the application of probiotics and antagonistic microorganisms for oral pathogens can bring about tangible benefits, namely boosting host immunity and disturbing the pathogen's environment via competition for space and nutrients. Krzyściak et al. [35] evaluated the anticariogenic effects of *Lactobacillus salivarius* by reducing pathogenic species in biofilm models. This microorganism has demonstrated the ability to secrete intermediates capable of inhibiting the formation of cariogenic *S. mutans* and *C. albicans* biofilms. In other studies, single and mixed biofilms were inhibited by probiotic lactobacilli [110,111]. Therefore, they seem to be useful as an adjunctive therapeutic mode against oral *Candida* spp. infections. Another study reported that the *Candida sorbosivorans* SSE-24 strain was used to stimulate erythritol production at a level of 60 g/L. It was detected a significant inhibitory effect of erythritol on the growth and biofilm formation of *S. mutans* [112]. Interestingly, a novel phage (ΦAPCM01) with activity against *S. mutans* biofilms was recently isolated from human saliva [113], and the inhibition of *S. mutans* biofilms was also found by the use of liamocins from *Aureobasidium pullulans* [114]. Chemically, liamocins are mannitol oils specific to *Streptococcus* spp., having the potential to act as new inhibitors of oral streptococcal biofilms that should not affect normal oral microflora.

4. Conclusions and Future Prospects

Oral diseases continue to increase despite the best efforts of the medical and scientific communities. The most complicated pathologies derive from microbial biofilms (plaque), formed by a consortium of microorganisms, which are protected by a net of polymers (e.g., EPS, DNA). The biofilm matrix delays or blocks the antimicrobials' diffusion, making treatment much more difficult or even unsuccessful. The oral *S. mutans*–*Candida* spp. mixed biofilm has been subject to various studies involving alternative therapeutics (e.g., aPDT), new chemical structures (natural and synthetic) with antimicrobial and antibiofilm activities, and nanotechnology, revealing different but promising antimicrobial properties. Nonetheless, more and deeper studies involving in vivo and clinical approaches are still needed.

Author Contributions: Conceptualization, methodology, and validation: C.F.R. and N.M.; investigation and data curation: B.S., D.K., G.M., J.S.-R., N.M., and C.F.R.; writing—original draft preparation: B.S., D.K., G.M., J.S.-R., N.M., and C.F.R.; writing—review and editing: C.F.R. and N.M. All authors have read and agreed to the published version of the manuscript.

Funding: This research received no external funding.

Acknowledgments: C.F.R. would like to acknowledge the UID/EQU/00511/2019 Project—Laboratory of Process Engineering, Environment, Biotechnology and Energy (LEPABE), financed by national funds through FCT/MCTES (PIDDAC). N.M. would like to thank the Portuguese Foundation for Science and Technology (FCT-Portugal) for the Strategic project ref. UID/BIM/04293/2013 and "NORTE2020—Northern Regional Operational Program" (NORTE-01-0145-FEDER-000012).

Conflicts of Interest: The authors declare no conflict of interest.

References

1. WHO Oral Health—WHO Fact Sheets. Available online: https://www.who.int/news-room/fact-sheets/detail/oral-health (accessed on 15 January 2019).
2. Tonetti, M.S.; Jepsen, S.; Jin, L.; Otomo-Corgel, J. Impact of the global burden of periodontal diseases on health, nutrition and wellbeing of mankind: A call for global action. *J. Clin. Periodontol.* **2017**, *44*, 456–462. [CrossRef] [PubMed]
3. Vos, T.; Abajobir, A.A.; Abate, K.H.; Abbafati, C.; Abbas, K.M.; Abd-Allah, F.; Abdulkader, R.S.; Abdulle, A.M.; Abebo, T.A.; Abera, S.F.; et al. Global, regional, and national incidence, prevalence, and years lived with disability for 328 diseases and injuries for 195 countries, 1990–2016: A systematic analysis for the Global Burden of Disease Study 2016. *Lancet* **2017**, *390*, 1211–1259. [CrossRef]
4. Listl, S.; Galloway, J.; Mossey, P.A.; Marcenes, W. Global Economic Impact of Dental Diseases. *J. Dent. Res.* **2015**, *94*, 1355–1361. [CrossRef] [PubMed]
5. Petersen, P.E.; Bourgeois, D.; Ogawa, H.; Estupinan-Day, S.; Ndiaye, C. The global burden of oral diseases and risks to oral health. *Bull. World Health Organ.* **2005**, *83*, 661–669. [PubMed]
6. Pihlstrom, B.L.; Michalowicz, B.S.; Johnson, N.W. Periodontal diseases. *Lancet* **2005**, *366*, 1809–1820. [CrossRef]
7. Dewhirst, F.E.; Chen, T.; Izard, J.; Paster, B.J.; Tanner, A.C.R.; Yu, W.-H.; Lakshmanan, A.; Wade, W.G. The Human Oral Microbiome. *J. Bacteriol.* **2010**, *192*, 5002–5017. [CrossRef]
8. Kuo, L.-C.; Polson, A.M.; Kang, T. Associations between periodontal diseases and systemic diseases: A review of the inter-relationships and interactions with diabetes, respiratory diseases, cardiovascular diseases and osteoporosis. *Public Health* **2008**, *122*, 417–433. [CrossRef]
9. Huttenhower, C.; Gevers, D.; Knight, R.; Abubucker, S.; Badger, J.H.; Chinwalla, A.T.; Creasy, H.H.; Earl, A.M.; FitzGerald, M.G.; Fulton, R.S.; et al. Structure, function and diversity of the healthy human microbiome. *Nature* **2012**, *486*, 207–214.
10. Loesche, W.J. Role of Streptococcus mutans in human dental decay. *Microbiol. Rev.* **1986**, *50*, 353–380. [CrossRef]
11. Forssten, S.D.; Björklund, M.; Ouwehand, A.C. Streptococcus mutans, Caries and Simulation Models. *Nutrients* **2010**, *2*, 290–298. [CrossRef]
12. Larsen, P.; Nielsen, J.L.; Otzen, D.; Nielsen, P.H. Amyloid-Like Adhesins Produced by Floc-Forming and Filamentous Bacteria in Activated Sludge. *Appl. Environ. Microbiol.* **2008**, *74*, 1517–1526. [CrossRef]
13. Chevalier, M.; Ranque, S.; Prêcheur, I. Oral fungal-bacterial biofilm models in vitro: A review. *Med. Mycol.* **2017**, *56*, 653–667. [CrossRef]
14. Rodrigues, C.F.; Rodrigues, M.; Silva, S.; Henriques, M. Candida glabrata Biofilms: How Far Have We Come? *J. Fungi* **2017**, *3*, 11. [CrossRef]
15. Pereira, D.F.A.; Seneviratne, C.J.; Koga-Ito, C.Y.; Samaranayake, L.P. Is the oral fungal pathogen Candida albicans a cariogen? *Oral Dis.* **2017**, *24*, 518–526. [CrossRef]

16. Rodrigues, C.F.; Henriques, M. Oral mucositis caused by Candida glabrata biofilms: Failure of the concomitant use of fluconazole and ascorbic acid. *Ther. Adv. Infect. Dis.* **2017**, *4*, 10–17.
17. Hwang, G.; Liu, Y.; Kim, D.; Li, Y.; Krysan, D.J.; Koo, H. Candida albicans mannans mediate Streptococcus mutans exoenzyme GtfB binding to modulate cross-kingdom biofilm development in vivo. *PLOS Pathog.* **2017**, *13*, e1006407. [CrossRef]
18. Yang, Y.; Mao, M.; Lei, L.; Li, M.; Yin, J.; Ma, X.; Tao, X.; Yang, Y.; Hu, T. Regulation of water-soluble glucan synthesis by the Streptococcus mutans dexA gene effects biofilm aggregation and cariogenic pathogenicity. *Mol. Oral Microbiol.* **2019**, *34*, 51–63. [CrossRef]
19. He, J.; Kim, D.; Zhou, X.; Ahn, S.-J.; Burne, R.A.; Richards, V.P.; Koo, H. RNA-Seq Reveals Enhanced Sugar Metabolism in Streptococcus mutans Co-cultured with Candida albicans within Mixed-Species Biofilms. *Front. Microbiol.* **2017**. [CrossRef]
20. Arzmi, M.H.; Cirillo, N.; Lenzo, J.C.; Catmull, D.V.; O'Brien-Simpson, N.; Reynolds, E.C.; Dashper, S.; McCullough, M. Monospecies and polymicrobial biofilms differentially regulate the phenotype of genotype-specific oral cancer cells. *Carcinogenesis* **2018**, *40*, 184–193. [CrossRef]
21. Yang, C.; Scoffield, J.; Wu, R.; Deivanayagam, C.; Zou, J.; Wu, H. Antigen I/II mediates interactions between Streptococcus mutans and Candida albicans. *Mol. Oral Microbiol.* **2018**, *33*, 283–291. [CrossRef]
22. Barbosa, J.O.; Rossoni, R.D.; Vilela, S.F.G.; de Alvarenga, J.A.; dos Santos Velloso, M.; de Azevedo Prata, M.C.; Jorge, A.O.C.; Junqueira, J.C. Streptococcus mutans Can Modulate Biofilm Formation and Attenuate the Virulence of Candida albicans. *PLoS ONE* **2016**, *11*, e0150457. [CrossRef]
23. Cavalcanti, Y.W.; Wilson, M.; Lewis, M.; Del-Bel-Cury, A.A.; da Silva, W.J.; Williams, D.W. Modulation of Candida albicans virulence by bacterial biofilms on titanium surfaces. *Biofouling* **2016**, *32*, 123–134. [CrossRef]
24. Sztajer, H.; Szafranski, S.P.; Tomasch, J.; Reck, M.; Nimtz, M.; Rohde, M.; Wagner-Döbler, I. Cross-feeding and interkingdom communication in dual-species biofilms of Streptococcus mutans and Candida albicans. *ISME J.* **2014**. [CrossRef]
25. Pinheiro, S.; da Silva, C.; da Silva, L.; Cicotti, M.; da Silveira Bueno, C.; Fontana, C.; Pagrion, L.; Dalmora, N.; Daque, T.; de Campos, F. Antimicrobial efficacy of 2.5% sodium hypochlorite, 2% chlorhexidine, and ozonated water as irrigants in mesiobuccal root canals with severe curvature of mandibular molars. *Eur. J. Dent.* **2018**, *12*, 94. [CrossRef]
26. Bourgeois, D.; David, A.; Inquimbert, C.; Tramini, P.; Molinari, N.; Carrouel, F. Quantification of carious pathogens in the interdental microbiota of young caries-free adults. *PLoS ONE* **2017**, *12*, e0185804. [CrossRef]
27. Hertel, S.; Wolf, A.; Basche, S.; Viergutz, G.; Rupf, S.; Hannig, M.; Hannig, C. Initial microbial colonization of enamel in children with different levels of caries activity: An in situ study. *Am. J. Dent.* **2017**, *30*, 171–176.
28. Yoo, H.-J.; Jwa, S.-K. Inhibitory effects of upbeta-caryophyllene on Streptococcus mutans biofilm. *Arch. Oral Biol.* **2018**, *88*, 42–46. [CrossRef]
29. Koo, H.; Bowen, W.H. Candida albicans and Streptococcus mutans: A potential synergistic alliance to cause virulent tooth decay in children. *Future Microbiol.* **2014**, *9*, 1295–1297. [CrossRef]
30. Fumes, A.C.; da Silva Telles, P.D.; Corona, S.A.M.; Borsatto, M.C. Effect of aPDT on Streptococcus mutans and Candida albicans present in the dental biofilm: Systematic review. *Photodiagn. Photodyn. Ther.* **2018**, *21*, 363–366. [CrossRef]
31. Rodrigues, C.F.; Rodrigues, M.; Henriques, M.; Candida, S.P. Infections in Patients with Diabetes Mellitus. *J. Clin. Med.* **2019**, *8*, 76. [CrossRef]
32. Sampaio, A.; Souza, S.; Ricomini-Filho, A.; Del Bel Cury, A.; Cavalcanti, Y.; Cury, J. Candida albicans Increases Dentine Demineralization Provoked by Streptococcus mutans Biofilm. *Caries Res.* **2018**, *53*, 322–331. [CrossRef]
33. Kim, D.; Sengupta, A.; Niepa, T.H.R.; Lee, B.-H.; Weljie, A.; Freitas-Blanco, V.S.; Murata, R.M.; Stebe, K.J.; Lee, D.; Koo, H. Candida albicans stimulates Streptococcus mutans microcolony development via cross-kingdom biofilm-derived metabolites. *Sci. Rep.* **2017**, *7*, 41332. [CrossRef]
34. Falsetta, M.L.; Klein, M.I.; Colonne, P.M.; Scott-Anne, K.; Gregoire, S.; Pai, C.-H.H.; Gonzalez-Begne, M.; Watson, G.; Krysan, D.J.; Bowen, W.H.; et al. Symbiotic Relationship between Streptococcus mutans and Candida albicans Synergizes Virulence of Plaque Biofilms In Vivo. *Infect. Immun.* **2014**, *82*, 1968–1981. [CrossRef]

35. Krzyściak, W.; Kościelniak, D.; Papież, M.; Vyhouskaya, P.; Zagórska-Świeży, K.; Kołodziej, I.; Bystrowska, B.; Jurczak, A. Effect of a Lactobacillus Salivarius Probiotic on a Double-Species Streptococcus Mutans and Candida Albicans Caries Biofilm. *Nutrients* **2017**, *9*, 1242. [CrossRef]
36. Ellepola, K.; Liu, Y.; Cao, T.; Koo, H.; Seneviratne, C.J. Bacterial GtfB Augments Candida albicans Accumulation in Cross-Kingdom Biofilms. *J. Dent. Res.* **2017**, *96*, 1129–1135. [CrossRef]
37. Arzmi, M.H.; Alnuaimi, A.D.; Dashper, S.; Cirillo, N.; Reynolds, E.C.; McCullough, M. Polymicrobial biofilm formation byCandida albicans, Actinomyces naeslundii, and Streptococcus mutans is Candida albicansstrain and medium dependent. *Med. Mycol.* **2016**, *54*, 856–864. [CrossRef]
38. Liu, S.; Qiu, W.; Zhang, K.; Zhou, X.; Ren, B.; He, J.; Xu, X.; Cheng, L.; Li, M. Nicotine Enhances Interspecies Relationship between Streptococcus mutans and Candida albicans. *BioMed Res. Int.* **2017**, *2017*, 7953920. [CrossRef]
39. Liu, S.; Qiu, W.; Zhang, K.; Zhou, X.; Ren, B.; He, J.; Xu, X.; Cheng, L.; Li, M. Corrigendum to Nicotine Enhances Interspecies Relationship between Streptococcus mutans and Candida albicans. *BioMed Res. Int.* **2017**, *2017*, 5803246. [CrossRef]
40. Willems, M.; Kos, K.; Jabra-rizk, M.A.; Krom, B.P. Candida albicans in oral biofilms could prevent caries. *Pathog. Dis.* **2016**, *74*, 1–6. [CrossRef]
41. Xiao, J.; Moon, Y.; Li, L.; Rustchenko, E.; Wakabayashi, H.; Zhao, X.; Feng, C.; Gill, S.R.; McLaren, S.; Malmstrom, H.; et al. Candida albicans Carriage in Children with Severe Early Childhood Caries (S-ECC) and Maternal Relatedness. *PLoS ONE* **2016**, *11*, e0164242. [CrossRef]
42. Chi, M.; Qi, M.; A, L.; Wang, P.; Weir, M.; Melo, M.; Sun, X.; Dong, B.; Li, C.; Wu, J.A.; et al. Novel Bioactive and Therapeutic Dental Polymeric Materials to Inhibit Periodontal Pathogens and Biofilms. *Int. J. Mol. Sci.* **2019**, *20*, 278. [CrossRef]
43. Chanda, W.; Joseph, T.P.; Wang, W.; Padhiar, A.A.; Zhong, M. The potential management of oral candidiasis using anti-biofilm therapies. *Med. Hypotheses* **2017**, *106*, 15–18. [CrossRef]
44. Trigo-Gutierrez, J.K.; Sanitá, P.V.; Tedesco, A.C.; Pavarina, A.C.; de Oliveira Mima, E.G. Effect of Chloroaluminium phthalocyanine in cationic nanoemulsion on photoinactivation of multispecies biofilm. *Photodiagn. Photodyn. Ther.* **2018**, *24*, 212–219. [CrossRef]
45. Macedo, P.D.; Corbi, S.T.; de Oliveira, G.J.P.L.; Perussi, J.R.; Ribeiro, A.O.; Marcantonio, R.A.C. Hypericin-glucamine antimicrobial photodynamic therapy in the progression of experimentally induced periodontal disease in rats. *Photodiagn. Photodyn. Ther.* **2019**, *25*, 43–49. [CrossRef]
46. Alexandrino, F.J.; Bezerra, E.M.; Da Costa, R.F.; Cavalcante, L.R.; Sales, F.A.; Francisco, T.S.; Rodrigues, L.K.; de Brito, D.A.; Ricardo, N.M.; Costa, S.N.; et al. Rose Bengal incorporated to alpha-cyclodextrin microparticles for photodynamic therapy against the cariogenic microorganism Streptococcus mutans. *Photodiagn. Photodyn. Ther.* **2019**, *25*, 111–118. [CrossRef]
47. Méndez, D.A.C.; Gutierres, E.; Dionisio, E.J.; Buzalaf, M.A.R.; Oliveira, R.C.; Machado, M.A.A.M.; Cruvinel, T. Curcumin-mediated antimicrobial photodynamic therapy reduces the viability and vitality of infected dentin caries microcosms. *Photodiagn. Photodyn. Ther.* **2018**, *24*, 102–108. [CrossRef]
48. Quishida, C.C.C.; Mima, E.G.D.O.; Jorge, J.H.; Vergani, C.E.; Bagnato, V.S.; Pavarina, A.C. Photodynamic inactivation of a multispecies biofilm using curcumin and {LED} light. *Lasers Med. Sci.* **2016**, *31*, 997–1009. [CrossRef]
49. Sakima, V.; Barbugli, P.; Cerri, P.; Chorilli, M.; Carmello, J.; Pavarina, A.; Mima, E. Antimicrobial Photodynamic Therapy Mediated by Curcumin-Loaded Polymeric Nanoparticles in a Murine Model of Oral Candidiasis. *Molecules* **2018**, *23*, 2075. [CrossRef]
50. Oda, D.F.; Duarte, M.A.H.; Andrade, F.B.; Moriyama, L.T.; Bagnato, V.S.; de Moraes, I.G. Antimicrobial action of photodynamic therapy in root canals using LED curing light, curcumin and carbopol gel. *Int. Endod. J.* **2019**, *52*, 1010–1019. [CrossRef]
51. Pinto, A.P.; Rosseti, I.B.; Carvalho, M.L.; da Silva, B.G.M.; Alberto-Silva, C.; Costa, M.S. Photodynamic Antimicrobial Chemotherapy ({PACT}), using Toluidine blue O inhibits the viability of biofilm produced by Candida albicans at different stages of development. *Photodiagn. Photodyn. Ther.* **2018**, *21*, 182–189. [CrossRef]
52. de Freitas-Pontes, K.M.; de Albuquerque Gomes, C.E.; de Carvalho, B.M.D.F.; de Sousa Carvalho Sabóia, R.; Garcia, B.A. Photosensitization of in vitro biofilms formed on denture base resin. *J. Prosthet. Dent.* **2014**, *112*, 632–637. [CrossRef]

53. Quishida, C.C.C.; de Oliveira Mima, E.G.; Dovigo, L.N.; Jorge, J.H.; Bagnato, V.S.; Pavarina, A.C. Photodynamic inactivation of a multispecies biofilm using Photodithazine® and {LED} light after one and three successive applications. *Lasers Med. Sci.* **2015**, *30*, 2303–2312. [CrossRef]
54. Carmello, J.C.; Alves, F.; de Oliveira Mima, E.G.; Jorge, J.H.; Bagnato, V.S.; Pavarina, A.C. Photoinactivation of single and mixed biofilms of Candida albicans and non- albicans Candida species using Photodithazine®. *Photodiagn. Photodyn. Ther.* **2017**, *17*, 194–199. [CrossRef]
55. Tomé, F.M.; Ramos, L.D.P.; Freire, F.; Pereira, C.A.; de Oliveira, I.C.B.; Junqueira, J.C.; Jorge, A.O.C.; de Oliveira, L.D. Influence of sucrose on growth and sensitivity of Candida albicans alone and in combination with Enterococcus faecalis and Streptococcus mutans to photodynamic therapy. *Lasers Med. Sci.* **2017**, *32*, 1237–1243. [CrossRef]
56. Rahmani-Badi, A.; Sepehr, S.; Babaie-Naiej, H. A combination of cis-2-decenoic acid and chlorhexidine removes dental plaque. *Arch. Oral Biol.* **2015**, *60*, 1655–1661. [CrossRef]
57. Monteiro, D.R.; Arias, L.S.; Fernandes, R.A.; Straioto, F.G.; Barros Barbosa, D.; Pessan, J.P.; Delbem, A.C.B. Role of tyrosol on Candida albicans, Candida glabrata and Streptococcus mutans biofilms developed on different surfaces. *Am. J. Dent.* **2017**, *30*, 35–39.
58. do Vale, L.R.; Delbem, A.C.B.; Arias, L.S.; Fernandes, R.A.; Vieira, A.P.M.; Barbosa, D.B.; Monteiro, D.R. Differential effects of the combination of tyrosol with chlorhexidine gluconate on oral biofilms. *Oral Dis.* **2017**, *23*, 537–541. [CrossRef]
59. Yassin, S.A.; German, M.J.; Rolland, S.L.; Rickard, A.H.; Jakubovics, N.S. Inhibition of multispecies biofilms by a fluoride-releasing dental prosthesis copolymer. *J. Dent.* **2016**, *48*, 62–70. [CrossRef]
60. Vieira, A.P.M.; Arias, L.S.; de Souza Neto, F.N.; Kubo, A.M.; Lima, B.H.R.; de Camargo, E.R.; Pessan, J.P.; Delbem, A.C.B.; Monteiro, D.R. Antibiofilm effect of chlorhexidine-carrier nanosystem based on iron oxide magnetic nanoparticles and chitosan. *Colloids Surf. B Biointerfaces* **2019**, *174*, 224–231. [CrossRef]
61. Elshinawy, M.I.; Al-Madboly, L.A.; Ghoneim, W.M.; El-Deeb, N.M. Synergistic Effect of Newly Introduced Root Canal Medicaments Ozonated Olive Oil and Chitosan Nanoparticles, Against Persistent Endodontic Pathogens. *Front. Microbiol.* **2018**, *9*, 1371. [CrossRef]
62. Tan, Y.; Leonhard, M.; Moser, D.; Schneider-Stickler, B. Antibiofilm activity of carboxymethyl chitosan on the biofilms of non-Candida albicans Candida species. *Carbohydr. Polym.* **2016**, *149*, 77–82. [CrossRef]
63. Tan, Y.; Leonhard, M.; Moser, D.; Ma, S.; Schneider-Stickler, B. Inhibition of mixed fungal and bacterial biofilms on silicone by carboxymethyl chitosan. *Colloids Surf. B Biointerfaces* **2016**, *148*, 193–199. [CrossRef]
64. Costa, E.; Silva, S.; Tavaria, F.; Pintado, M. Antimicrobial and Antibiofilm Activity of Chitosan on the Oral Pathogen Candida albicans. *Pathogens* **2014**, *3*, 908–919. [CrossRef]
65. Tan, Y.; Leonhard, M.; Ma, S.; Moser, D.; Schneider-Stickler, B. Efficacy of carboxymethyl chitosan against Candida tropicalis and Staphylococcus epidermidis monomicrobial and polymicrobial biofilms. *Int. J. Biol. Macromol.* **2018**, *110*, 150–156. [CrossRef]
66. Mendes-Gouvêa, C.C.; do Amaral, J.G.; Fernandes, R.A.; Fernandes, G.L.; Gorup, L.F.; Camargo, E.R.; Delbem, A.C.B.; Barbosa, D.B. Sodium trimetaphosphate and hexametaphosphate impregnated with silver nanoparticles: Characteristics and antimicrobial efficacy. *Biofouling* **2018**, *34*, 299–308. [CrossRef]
67. Panpaliya, N.P.; Dahake, P.T.; Kale, Y.J.; Dadpe, M.V.; Kendre, S.B.; Siddiqi, A.G.; Maggavi, U.R. In vitro evaluation of antimicrobial property of silver nanoparticles and chlorhexidine against five different oral pathogenic bacteria. *Saudi Dent. J.* **2019**, *31*, 76–83. [CrossRef]
68. Zhang, K.; Ren, B.; Zhou, X.; Xu, H.; Chen, Y.; Han, Q.; Li, B.; Weir, M.; Li, M.; Feng, M.; et al. Effect of Antimicrobial Denture Base Resin on Multi-Species Biofilm Formation. *Int. J. Mol. Sci.* **2016**, *17*, 1033. [CrossRef]
69. Toda, C.; Marin, D.O.M.; Rodriguez, L.S.; Paleari, A.G.; Pero, A.C.; Compagnoni, M.A. Antimicrobial Activity of a Tissue Conditioner Combined with a Biocide Polymer. *J. Contemp. Dent. Pract.* **2015**, *16*, 101–106.
70. Bucci, A.R.; Marcelino, L.; Mendes, R.K.; Etchegaray, A. The antimicrobial and antiadhesion activities of micellar solutions of surfactin, CTAB and CPCl with terpinen-4-ol: Applications to control oral pathogens. *World J. Microbiol. Biotechnol.* **2018**, *34*, 86. [CrossRef]
71. Sun, X.; Wang, L.; Lynch, C.D.; Sun, X.; Li, X.; Qi, M.; Ma, C.; Li, C.; Dong, B.; Zhou, Y.; et al. Nanoparticles having amphiphilic silane containing Chlorin e6 with strong anti-biofilm activity against periodontitis-related pathogens. *J. Dent.* **2019**, *81*, 70–84. [CrossRef]

72. Kıvanç, M.; Barutca, B.; Koparal, A.T.; Göncü, Y.; Bostanci, S.H.; Ay, N. Effects of hexagonal boron nitride nanoparticles on antimicrobial and antibiofilm activities, cell viability. *Mater. Sci. Eng. C* **2018**, *91*, 115–124. [CrossRef] [PubMed]
73. Souza, J.A.S.; Barbosa, D.B.; Berretta, A.A.; do Amaral, J.G.; Gorup, L.F.; de Souza Neto, F.N.; Fernandes, R.A.; Fernandes, G.L.; Camargo, E.R.; Agostinho, A.M.; et al. Green synthesis of silver nanoparticles combined to calcium glycerophosphate: Antimicrobial and antibiofilm activities. *Future Microbiol.* **2018**, *13*, 345–357. [CrossRef] [PubMed]
74. de Castro, D.T.; Valente, M.L.C.; da Silva, C.H.L.; Watanabe, E.; Siqueira, R.L.; Schiavon, M.A.; Alves, O.L.; dos Reis, A.C. Evaluation of antibiofilm and mechanical properties of new nanocomposites based on acrylic resins and silver vanadate nanoparticles. *Arch. Oral Biol.* **2016**, *67*, 46–53. [CrossRef] [PubMed]
75. Zhao, Z.; Ding, C.; Wang, Y.; Tan, H.; Li, J. pH-Responsive polymeric nanocarriers for efficient killing of cariogenic bacteria in biofilms. *Biomater. Sci.* **2019**, *7*, 1643–1651. [CrossRef]
76. Kim, D.; Liu, Y.; Benhamou, R.I.; Sanchez, H.; Simón-Soro, Á.; Li, Y.; Hwang, G.; Fridman, M.; Andes, D.R.; Koo, H. Bacterial-derived exopolysaccharides enhance antifungal drug tolerance in a cross-kingdom oral biofilm. *ISME J.* **2018**, *12*, 1427–1442. [CrossRef]
77. Feldman, M.; Shenderovich, J.; Lavy, E.; Friedman, M.; Steinberg, D. A Sustained-Release Membrane of Thiazolidinedione-8: Effect on Formation of a Candida/Bacteria Mixed Biofilm on Hydroxyapatite in a Continuous Flow Model. *BioMed Res. Int.* **2017**, *2017*, 1–9. [CrossRef]
78. de Almeida, J.; Pimenta, A.L.; Pereira, U.A.; Barbosa, L.C.A.; Hoogenkamp, M.A.; van der Waal, S.V.; Crielaard, W.; Felippe, W.T. Effects of three gamma-alkylidene-gamma-lactams on the formation of multispecies biofilms. *Eur. J. Oral Sci.* **2018**, *126*, 214–221. [CrossRef]
79. Fumes, A.C.; Romualdo, P.C.; Monteiro, R.M.; Watanabe, E.; Corona, S.A.M.; Borsatto, M.C. Influence of pre-irradiation time employed in antimicrobial photodynamic therapy with diode laser. *Lasers Med. Sci.* **2017**, *33*, 67–73. [CrossRef]
80. Soria-Lozano, P.; Gilaberte, Y.; Paz-Cristobal, M.P.; Pérez-Artiaga, L.; Lampaya-Pérez, V.; Aporta, J.; Pérez-Laguna, V.; García-Luque, I.; Revillo, M.J.; Rezusta, A. In vitro effect photodynamic therapy with differents photosensitizers on cariogenic microorganisms. *BMC Microbiol.* **2015**, *15*. [CrossRef]
81. Duque, C.; Aida, K.L.; Pereira, J.A.; Teixeira, G.S.; Caldo-Teixeira, A.S.; Perrone, L.R.; Caiaffa, K.S.; de Cássia Negrini, T.; de Castilho, A.R.F.; de Souza Costa, C.A. In vitro and in vivo evaluations of glass-ionomer cement containing chlorhexidine for Atraumatic Restorative Treatment. *J. Appl. Oral Sci.* **2017**, *25*, 541–550. [CrossRef]
82. D'Ercole, S.; Tieri, M.; Fulco, D.; Martinelli, D.; Tripodi, D. The use of chlorhexidine in mouthguards. *J. Biol. Regul. Homeost. Agents* **2017**, *31*, 487–493.
83. Takenaka, S.; Ohsumi, T.; Noiri, Y. Evidence-based strategy for dental biofilms: Current evidence of mouthwashes on dental biofilm and gingivitis. *Jpn. Dent. Sci. Rev.* **2019**, *55*, 33–40. [CrossRef]
84. Shen, Y.; Zhao, J.; De La Fuente-Núñez, C.; Wang, Z.; Hancock, R.E.; Roberts, C.R.; Ma, J.; Li, J.; Haapasalo, M.; Wang, Q. Experimental and Theoretical Investigation of Multispecies Oral Biofilm Resistance to Chlorhexidine Treatment. *Sci. Rep.* **2016**, *6*, 27537. [CrossRef]
85. Rodrigues, C.F.; Boas, D.; Haynes, K.; Henriques, M. The MNN2 Gene Knockout Modulates the Antifungal Resistance of Biofilms of Candida glabrata. *Biomolecules* **2018**, *8*, 130. [CrossRef]
86. Ivanova, K.; Ramon, E.; Hoyo, J.; Tzanov, T. Innovative Approaches for Controlling Clinically Relevant Biofilms: Current Trends and Future Prospects. *Curr. Top. Med. Chem.* **2017**, *17*, 1–18. [CrossRef]
87. Buommino, E.; Scognamiglio, M.; Donnarumma, G.; Fiorentino, A.; D'Abrosca, B. Recent Advances in Natural Product-Based Anti-Biofilm Approaches to Control Infections. *Mini-Rev. Med. Chem.* **2015**, *14*, 1169–1182. [CrossRef]
88. Ramalingam, K.; Amaechi, B.T. Antimicrobial effect of herbal extract of Acacia arabica with triphala on the biofilm forming cariogenic microorganisms. *J. Ayurveda Integr. Med.* **2018**. [CrossRef]
89. Pires, J.G.; Zabini, S.S.; Braga, A.S.; de Cássia Fabris, R.; de Andrade, F.B.; de Oliveira, R.C.; Magalhães, A.C. Hydroalcoholic extracts of Myracrodruon urundeuva All. and Qualea grandiflora Mart. leaves on Streptococcus mutans biofilm and tooth demineralization. *Arch. Oral Biol.* **2018**, *91*, 17–22. [CrossRef]
90. Akhalwaya, S.; van Vuuren, S.; Patel, M. An in vitro investigation of indigenous South African medicinal plants used to treat oral infections. *J. Ethnopharmacol.* **2018**, *210*, 359–371. [CrossRef]

91. de Oliveira, J.R.; de Jesus Viegas, D.; Martins, A.P.R.; Carvalho, C.A.T.; Soares, C.P.; Camargo, S.E.A.; Jorge, A.O.C.; de Oliveira, L.D. Thymus vulgaris L. extract has antimicrobial and anti-inflammatory effects in the absence of cytotoxicity and genotoxicity. *Arch. Oral Biol.* **2017**, *82*, 271–279. [CrossRef]
92. de Oliveira, J.R.; de Jesus, D.; Figueira, L.W.; de Oliveira, F.E.; Soares, C.P.; Camargo, S.E.A.; Jorge, A.O.C.; de Oliveira, L.D. Biological activities of Rosmarinus officinalis L. (rosemary) extract as analyzed in microorganisms and cells. *Exp. Biol. Med.* **2017**, *242*, 625–634. [CrossRef] [PubMed]
93. Barua, D.R. Efficacy of Neem Extract and Three Antimicrobial Agents Incorporated into Tissue Conditioner in Inhibiting the Growth of C. Albicans and S. Mutans. *J. Clin. Diagn. Res.* **2017**, *11*, ZC97–ZC101. [CrossRef] [PubMed]
94. Choi, H.-A.; Cheong, D.-E.; Lim, H.-D.; Kim, W.-H.; Ham, M.-H.; Oh, M.-H.; Wu, Y.; Shin, H.-J.; Kim, G.-J. Antimicrobial and Anti-Biofilm Activities of the Methanol Extracts of Medicinal Plants against Dental Pathogens Streptococcus mutans and Candida albicans. *J. Microbiol. Biotechnol.* **2017**, *27*, 1242–1248. [CrossRef] [PubMed]
95. Sekita, Y.; Murakami, K.; Yumoto, H.; Amoh, T.; Fujiwara, N.; Ogata, S.; Matsuo, T.; Miyake, Y.; Kashiwada, Y. Preventive Effects of Houttuynia cordata Extract for Oral Infectious Diseases. *BioMed Res. Int.* **2016**, *2016*, 2581876. [CrossRef] [PubMed]
96. Salles, M.M.; Badaró, M.M.; de Arruda, C.N.F.; Leite, V.M.F.; da Silva, C.H.L.; Watanabe, E.; de Cássia Oliveira, V.; de Freitas Oliveira Paranhos, H. Antimicrobial activity of complete denture cleanser solutions based on sodium hypochlorite and Ricinus communis a randomized clinical study. *J. Appl. Oral Sci.* **2015**, *23*, 637–642. [CrossRef]
97. Barbieri, D.S.V.; Tonial, F.; Lopez, P.V.A.; Maia, B.H.L.N.S.; Santos, G.D.; Ribas, M.O.; Glienke, C.; Vicente, V.A. Antiadherent activity of Schinus terebinthifolius and Croton urucurana extracts on in vitro biofilm formation of Candida albicans and Streptococcus mutans. *Arch. Oral Biol.* **2014**, *59*, 887–896. [CrossRef]
98. Nittayananta, W.; Limsuwan, S.; Srichana, T.; Sae-Wong, C.; Amnuaikit, T. Oral spray containing plant-derived compounds is effective against common oral pathogens. *Arch. Oral Biol.* **2018**, *90*, 80–85. [CrossRef]
99. Limsuwan, S.; Moosigapong, K.; Jarukitsakul, S.; Joycharat, N.; Chusri, S.; Jaisamut, P.; Voravuthikunchai, S.P. Lupinifolin from Albizia myriophylla wood: A study on its antibacterial mechanisms against cariogenic Streptococcus mutans. *Arch. Oral Biol.* **2018**, *93*, 195–202. [CrossRef]
100. Freires, I.A.; Bueno-Silva, B.; de Carvalho Galvão, L.C.; Duarte, M.C.T.; Sartoratto, A.; Figueira, G.M.; de Alencar, S.M.; Rosalen, P.L. The Effect of Essential Oils and Bioactive Fractions on Streptococcus mutans and Candida albicans Biofilms: A Confocal Analysis. *Evid.-Based Complement. Altern. Med.* **2015**, *2015*, 871316. [CrossRef]
101. Fernandes, R.A.; Monteiro, D.R.; Arias, L.S.; Fernandes, G.L.; Delbem, A.C.B.; Barbosa, D.B. Biofilm formation byCandida albicansandStreptococcus mutansin the presence of farnesol: A quantitative evaluation. *Biofouling* **2016**, *32*, 329–338. [CrossRef]
102. Fernandes, R.A.; Monteiro, D.R.; Arias, L.S.; Fernandes, G.L.; Delbem, A.C.B.; Barbosa, D.B. Virulence Factors in Candida albicans and Streptococcus mutans Biofilms Mediated by Farnesol. *Indian J. Microbiol.* **2018**, *58*, 138–145. [CrossRef] [PubMed]
103. Rocha, G.R.; Salamanca, E.J.F.; de Barros, A.L.; Lobo, C.I.V.; Klein, M.I. Effect of tt-farnesol and myricetin on in vitro biofilm formed by Streptococcus mutans and Candida albicans. *BMC Complement. Altern. Med.* **2018**, *18*, 61. [CrossRef] [PubMed]
104. Zeng, Y.; Nikitkova, A.; Abdelsalam, H.; Li, J.; Xiao, J. Activity of quercetin and kaemferol against Streptococcus mutans biofilm. *Arch. Oral Biol.* **2019**, *98*, 9–16. [CrossRef] [PubMed]
105. Arias, L.S.; Delbem, A.C.B.; Fernandes, R.A.; Barbosa, D.B.; Monteiro, D.R. Activity of tyrosol against single and mixed-species oral biofilms. *J. Appl. Microbiol.* **2016**, *120*, 1240–1249. [CrossRef] [PubMed]
106. Waldner-Tomic, N.; Vanni, R.; Belibasakis, G.; Thurnheer, T.; Attin, T.; Schmidlin, P. The in Vitro Antimicrobial Efficacy of Propolis against Four Oral Pathogens: A Review. *Dent. J.* **2014**, *2*, 85–97. [CrossRef]
107. Wassel, M.O.; Khattab, M.A. Antibacterial activity against Streptococcus mutans and inhibition of bacterial induced enamel demineralization of propolis, miswak, and chitosan nanoparticles based dental varnishes. *J. Adv. Res.* **2017**, *8*, 387–392. [CrossRef]
108. Shang, D.; Liang, H.; Wei, S.; Yan, X.; Yang, Q.; Sun, Y. Effects of antimicrobial peptide L-K6, a temporin-1CEb analog on oral pathogen growth, Streptococcus mutans biofilm formation, and anti-inflammatory activity. *Appl. Microbiol. Biotechnol.* **2014**, *98*, 8685–8695. [CrossRef]

109. Simon, G.; Bérubé, C.; Voyer, N.; Grenier, D. Anti-biofilm and anti-adherence properties of novel cyclic dipeptides against oral pathogens. *Bioorg. Med. Chem.* **2019**, *27*, 2223–2231. [CrossRef]
110. Jiang, Q.; Stamatova, I.; Kainulainen, V.; Korpela, R.; Meurman, J.H. Interactions between Lactobacillus rhamnosus and oral micro-organisms in an in vitro biofilm model. *BMC Microbiol.* **2016**, *16*, 149. [CrossRef]
111. Tan, Y.; Leonhard, M.; Moser, D.; Ma, S.; Schneider-Stickler, B. Inhibitory effect of probiotic lactobacilli supernatants on single and mixed non- albicans Candida species biofilm. *Arch. Oral Biol.* **2018**, *85*, 40–45. [CrossRef]
112. Saran, S.; Mukherjee, S.; Dalal, J.; Saxena, R.K. High production of erythritol from Candida sorbosivorans (SSE)-24 and its inhibitory effect on biofilm formation of Streptococcus mutans. *Bioresour. Technol.* **2015**, *198*, 31–38. [CrossRef] [PubMed]
113. Dalmasso, M.; de Haas, E.; Neve, H.; Strain, R.; Cousin, F.J.; Stockdale, S.R.; Ross, R.P.; Hill, C. Isolation of a Novel Phage with Activity against Streptococcus mutans Biofilms. *PLoS ONE* **2015**, *10*, e0138651. [CrossRef] [PubMed]
114. Leathers, T.D.; Rich, J.O.; Bischoff, K.M.; Skory, C.D.; Nunnally, M.S. Inhibition of Streptococcus mutans and S. sobrinus biofilms by liamocins from Aureobasidium pullulans. *Biotechnol. Rep.* **2019**, *21*, e00300. [CrossRef] [PubMed]

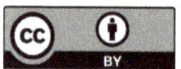

© 2020 by the authors. Licensee MDPI, Basel, Switzerland. This article is an open access article distributed under the terms and conditions of the Creative Commons Attribution (CC BY) license (http://creativecommons.org/licenses/by/4.0/).

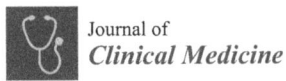

Review
Candida sp. Infections in Patients with Diabetes Mellitus

Célia F. Rodrigues [1,2,*], Maria Elisa Rodrigues [1] and Mariana Henriques [1]

1. CEB, Centre of Biological Engineering, LIBRO-Laboratório de Investigação em Biofilmes Rosário Oliveira, University of Minho, 4710-057 Braga, Portugal; elisarodrigues@deb.uminho.pt (M.E.R.); mcrh@deb.uminho.pt (M.H.)
2. LEPABE—Department of Chemical Engineering, Faculty of Engineering, University of Porto, Rua Dr. Roberto Frias, s/n, 4200-465 Porto, Portugal
* Correspondence: c.fortunae@gmail.com; Tel.: +351-22-041-4859

Received: 14 December 2018; Accepted: 3 January 2019; Published: 10 January 2019

Abstract: Candidiasis has increased substantially worldwide over recent decades and is a significant cause of morbidity and mortality, especially among critically ill patients. Diabetes mellitus (DM) is a metabolic disorder that predisposes individuals to fungal infections, including those related to *Candida* sp., due to a immunosuppressive effect on the patient. This review aims to discuss the latest studies regarding the occurrence of candidiasis on DM patients and the pathophysiology and etiology associated with these co-morbidities. A comprehensive review of the literature was undertaken. PubMed, Scopus, Elsevier's ScienceDirect, and Springer's SpringerLink databases were searched using well-defined search terms. Predefined inclusion and exclusion criteria were applied to classify relevant manuscripts. Results of the review show that DM patients have an increased susceptibility to *Candida* sp. infections which aggravates in the cases of uncontrolled hyperglycemia. The conclusion is that, for these patients, the hospitalization periods have increased and are commonly associated with the prolonged use of indwelling medical devices, which also increase the costs associated with disease management.

Keywords: *Candida*; biofilms; diabetes; medical devices; candidiasis; metabolic disorder; hyperglycemia; infection

---

1. Introduction

Diabetes mellitus (DM) is a chronic metabolic and degenerative disorder that is characterized by chronic hyperglycemia and causes long-term complications like retinopathy, neuropathy, and nephropathy, generally accelerating macro- and micro-vascular changes. It is becoming one of the largest emerging threats to public health in the 21st century [1,2]. Several immune alterations have been described in diabetes with cellular immunity being more compromised and with changes in polymorphonuclear cells, monocytes, and lymphocytes [3]. DM individuals have higher glucose serum concentrations than healthy individuals (between 4.0 to 5.4 mmol/L or 72 to 99 mg/dL when fasting and up to 7.8 mmol/L or 140 mg/dL two hours after eating [4]; hemoglobin A1c (glycohemoglobin) ≤5.7%). In type 1 DM, the pathogenesis is multifactorial because of antibody-mediated autoimmunity, environmental toxins exposure, and major histocompatibility complex (MHC) Class II histocompatibility complex HLA-DR/DQ genetic polymorphisms. These features create an increased susceptibility to disease onset due to a continuous loss of insulin-producing β-cells in the pancreas, which is due to the T-cells' infiltration through mitochondrial-driven apoptosis [5]. On the other hand, in type 2 DM, there is an insulin resistance that is associated with changes in the mitochondrial metabolism with reduced mitochondrial density, ATP production, and mitochondrial RNA (mtRNA) levels, as well as increased markers for oxidative stress. The chronic exposure of the circular mtDNA to these effects might trigger significant tissue modifications found in the pancreas and endothelial cells, leading to secondary vascular disease and causing cardiac, renal, ophthalmic, and neurological complications [5–7] (Figure 1).

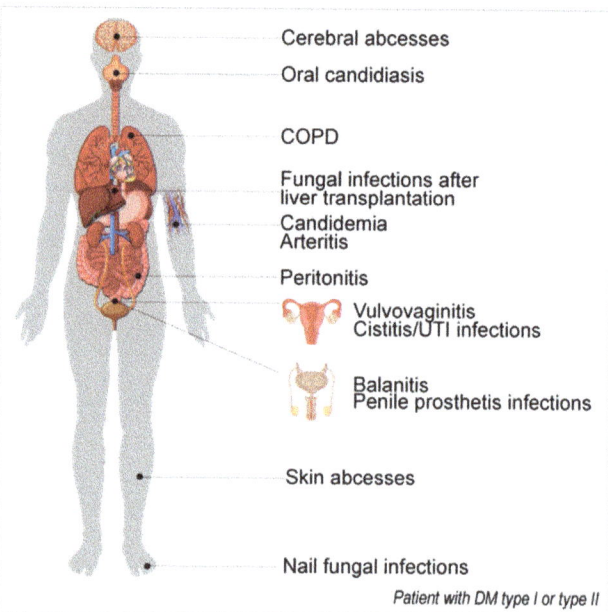

Figure 1. Main diseases related to *Candida* sp. occurring with higher incidence in patients with diabetes mellitus type 1 or type 2 (adapted image from GraphicsRF on stock.adobe.com).

In 2017, the worldwide prevalence of adult-onset diabetes (20–79 years) was nearly 425 million, and the World Health Organization and the International Diabetes Federation predicted that the number of adults in the world with diabetes will rise near 629 million by the year 2045 [8,9] (Figure 2). A higher prevalence of DM, cardiac, and pulmonary diseases can be found in senior patients with candidemia [10–13]. The relationship between diabetes and candidiasis has been widely studied [13–16], particularly due to the increased susceptibility of diabetic patients to fungal infections compared to those without DM [14,15,17,18].

Several mechanisms are attributed to higher *Candida* sp. predisposition among DM patients depending on the local or systemic infection. Among the recognized host conditions for candidal colonization and subsequent infection are yeast adhesion to epithelial cell surfaces [19], higher salivary glucose levels [15,20], reduced salivary flow [21], microvascular degeneration, and impaired candidacidal activity of neutrophils. These conditions are particularly serious in the presence of glucose [22,23], secretion of several degradative enzymes [24–26], or even a generalized immunosuppression state of the patient [8,27–31]. These factors have a major influence on the balance between host and yeasts, favoring the transition of *Candida* sp. from commensal to pathogen and causing infection. In fact, in a very recent study, Gürsoy et al. [32] suggested that there is a higher presence of intestinal *Candida albicans* colonization in diabetic patients. In fact, there may be a tendency of type 1 DM in patients with a high prevalence of intestinal *C. albicans*. *C. albicans* is also known to wait for a change in some aspect of the host physiology that normally suppress growth and invasiveness through a phenomenon called phenotypic switch system or white-opaque transition, described in 1987.

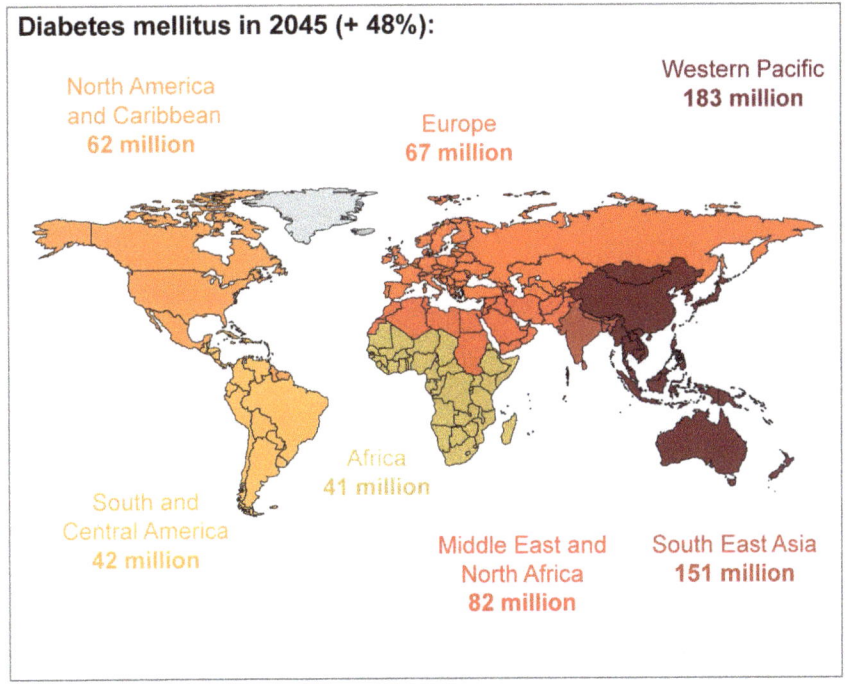

Figure 2. The estimated number of people with diabetes worldwide and per region in 2045 between 20–79 years in age, with a total of 629 million (source: International Diabetes Federation) (adapted image from GraphicsRF on stock.adobe.com).

This involves reversible and heritable switching between alternative cellular phenotypes. It occurs at sites of infection and recurrently in episodes of infection in certain cases in diabetic patients [33].

Yeasts are part of the normal gut microflora, but cell counts do not normally surpass 10 colony forming units (CFU)/g feces [34,35]. Nevertheless, it has been described that *Candida* sp. is more widespread in the feces of patients with type 1 and type 2 DM with poor glycemic control as opposed to healthy subjects [36]. The main reasons for this colonization seem to be altered functions of the immune system in diabetic patients with poor glycemic control or a direct effect of elevated blood glucose levels, creating specific conditions for intensive fungal colonization [36]. In fact, another report [37] showed that in patients with type 1 DM, the total gut CFUs significantly rise up to 40% in *C. albicans* colonization compared to 14.3% in healthy individuals. This may be related to the decrease in commensal bacteria-probably the result of yeast-bacterial competition. Also, this higher growth may disrupt the ecological balance of intestinal flora, which occurs in type 1 DM [37]. Regarding the gastrointestinal colonization, Kowalewska et al. [38] studied the serum levels of interleukin-12 (IL12) in relation to the percentage of yeast-like fungi colonies residing in the gastrointestinal tract in children and adolescents with DM type 1. Results showed that high IL12 levels can inhibit infection with yeast-like fungal colonizing the gastrointestinal tract in children and adolescents with type 1 DM. However, further studies are needed to confirm the antifungal activity of IL12 [38].

The development of drug resistance among *Candida* sp. isolates allied to epidemiologic variations in *Candida* sp. natural flora has significant implications for morbidity and mortality [39–42]. The extensive use of medications, especially azoles, has promoted the selection of resistant species by shifting colonization to more naturally resistant *Candida* sp., such as *C. glabrata*, *C. dubliniensis*, and *C. krusei* [43–46]. Presently, the world distribution of *Candida* sp. is a feature of the epidemiology in the area, but it indicates a predominance of *C. albicans*, *C. glabrata*, *C. tropicalis*, *C. parapsilosis*, and *C. krusei* [45,47]. It has been confirmed that 90% of fungemia cases are attributed to *Candida* sp. [39,40], and the mortality has ranged from 40% to 80% in immunocompromised hosts [39,40,48]. Furthermore, a high mortality rate was also detected among non-immunocompromised patients (60%) [49] and those with diabetes (67%) [41].

The main pathophysiologic and nutritionally relevant sugars in diabetic patients are glucose and fructose, but other simple carbon sources also play an important part in the growth of *Candida* sp. in DM patients. Man et al. [50] evaluated the growth rate of *C. albicans* in the presence of different concentrations of glucose and fructose to obtain a better understanding of the nutrient acquisition strategy and its possible relation to the hyperglycemic status of diabetic patients. The authors determined that the glucose concentration is directly related to *C. albicans* growth, which may be linked to the frequent yeast infections that occur in non-controlled diabetic patients. Interestingly, fructose showed *C. albicans* inhibition capacities. This implies fructose-containing food may prevent the development of candidiasis. This is an important outcome in oral *Candida* sp. biofilms, especially for patients who use prosthesis [50]. In fact, other carbon compounds such as sucrose, maltose, and lactose increase the fungal population density [43,51,52] and decrease the activity of antifungal agents. A recent report explored the effects of glucose in diabetic mice on the susceptibility of *Candida* sp. to antifungal agents [53]. In that work, Mandal et al. [53] revealed that voriconazole (Vcz) has the greatest reduction in antifungal drug efficacy followed by amphotericin B (AmB). Glucose displayed a higher affinity to bind to Vcz through hydrogen bonding, decreasing the susceptibility of antifungal agents during chemotherapy. Additionally, Mandal et al. [53] confirmed that Vcz presented three important hydrogen bonds and AmB presented two hydrogen bonds that stabilized the glucose. In vivo results of the same study proposed that the physiologically relevant higher glucose level in the bloodstream of mice with DM might interact with the available selective agents during antifungal therapy, decreasing glucose activity by complex formation. Vcz-glucose and AmB-glucose complexes seem to present less effectiveness as their pure molecule. Accordingly, a proper selection of drugs for DM patients is important if we are to control infectious diseases [53]. Similarly, Rodaki et al. [54] studied the impact of glucose on *C. albicans* transcriptome for the modulation of carbon assimilatory pathways during pathogenesis. The elevated resistance to oxidative and cationic stresses and resistance to miconazole uncovered that glucose concentrations in the bloodstream have a significant impact upon *C. albicans* gene regulation. No significant susceptibility level was perceived for anidulafungin, while Vcz and AmB became less effective [54]. In another study, Rodrigues et al. [52] demonstrated that *C. glabrata* decreases its susceptibility to fluconazole when cultured in a medium enriched with glucose [52].

Accordingly, the aim of this review is to analyze the literature related to the occurrence of candidiasis in diabetic patients by discussing specific features of *Candida* sp. that relate directly to the occurrence of candidiasis in DM patients and related diseases, as well as by reviewing recent and relevant studies on the topic.

2. Particular Features of *Candida* sp. that Increase the Incidence of Candidiasis in Diabetic Patients

2.1. Enzymatic Activity

Several studies have established an association between hydrolytic enzymes activity and an increase in the pathogenic ability of *Candida* sp. [55,56].

It has been demonstrated that, due to higher blood glucose concentration, diabetic *Candida* sp. isolates present significantly higher hemolytic and esterase enzymatic activity, which may contribute to increased enzyme activity among diabetic patients [57–60]. The same authors also hypothesized that these species are more pathogenic under abnormal conditions such as DM [61,62]. Secreted aspartyl proteinases (SAP) capable of degrading numerous substrates that constitute host proteins in the oral cavity have also been studied. These enzymes are thought to help *Candida* sp. to acquire essential nitrogen for growth, to attach to and penetrate oral mucosa, or both [63,64]. They can also cause amplified vascular permeability, leading to inflammatory reactions [65] and clinical symptoms, which may disturb the humoral host defense [66]. Similarly, phospholipase (PL) targets the membrane phospholipids and digests these components, initiating cell lysis and facilitating the penetration of the infecting fungi [67]. This enzyme induces the accumulation of inflammatory cells and plasma proteins, releasing several inflammatory mediators in vivo [67].

Very recently, it was revealed that *C. albicans* hyphae induce both epithelial damage and innate immunity through the secretion of a cytolytic peptide toxin called candidalysin [68,69]. This enzyme is encoded by the hypha-associated *ECE1* gene and is the first peptide toxin to be identified in any human fungal pathogen. Candidalysin induces calcium ion influx and lactate dehydrogenase (LDH) release in oral epithelial cells, which are features of cell damage and membrane destabilization. Importantly, the study also reported that *C. albicans* mutants where the entire *ECE1* gene or the candidalysin-encoding region had been deleted have full invasive potential in vitro but are incapable of inducing tissue damage or cytokine release and are highly weakened in a mouse model of oropharyngeal candidiasis and a zebrafish swim bladder mucosal model [68].

2.2. Biofilm Formation

Biofilms are communities of microorganisms embedded in an extracellular matrix [70,71], which confer substantial resistance to antifungal therapy and increased host immune responses [72,73]. These communities can be formed in both biotic (e.g., mouth mucosae) or abiotic (e.g., catheters) surfaces [74,75]. In fact, candidemia are the most prevalent invasive mycoses worldwide with mortality rates close to 40% [76]. *Candida* sp. are often recognized as the origin of candidemia, urinary tract infections, and hospital pneumonia. In practically all of these cases, the infections are related with the use of a medical device and biofilm formation on its surface [20]. The most frequently colonized medical device is the central venous catheter used for administration of fluids, nutrients, and medicines [77]. The contamination of the catheter or the infusion fluid can arise from the skin of the patient, the hands of health professionals [77], or by migration into the catheter from a pre-existing lesion. Less commonly, if *Candida* sp. that colonize the gastrointestinal tract as a commensal start to develop a pathogenic behavior, they are able to infiltrate the intestinal mucosa and diffuse through the bloodstream. Consequently, circulating yeast may colonize the catheter endogenously. This is more common in cancer patients, as chemotherapy leads to damage to the intestinal mucosa [78]. In the other patients, infected catheters are the most significant source of bloodstream infections, followed by widespread invasive candidiasis. The catheter removal is recommended in patients with disseminated *Candida* sp. infection to enable disinfection of the blood and to increase prognosis [79,80].

Biofilm development of *Candida* sp. (Figure 3) can be explained in four chronological steps: adherence-initial phase in which the yeast in suspension and planktonic cells adhere to the surface (first 1–3 h); intermediate phase-development of biofilm (11–14 h); maturation phase-the polymeric matrix (PEM) completely penetrates all layers of the cells adhered to the surface in a three-dimensional structure (20–48 h); dispersion-the most superficial cells leave the biofilm and colonize areas surrounding the surface (after 24 h) [81]. Hence, a mature biofilm comprises of a dense network of cells in the form of yeasts, hyphae, or pseudohyphae (or not, depending on the *Candida* sp.) involved by PEM and with water channels between the cells. These help in the diffusion of nutrients from the environment through the biomass to the lower layers and also allow the removal of waste [81,82]. Formed using in vivo models, *Candida* sp. biofilms seem to follow the same sequence of in vitro formation [83]. Nonetheless, the maturation step happens more quickly, and the thickness is increased. The final architecture of the biofilm is variable and depends, in part, on the *Candida* sp. involved, the growing conditions, and the substrate on which it is formed [81,84].

High levels of glucose are thought to serve as the carbohydrate energy source necessitated by *Candida* sp. for the biofilm formation and are probably required to produce the polysaccharide matrix [85], which is secreted by sessile cells, providing protection against environmental challenges [86]. Biofilm formation has been shown to be dependent on the *Candida* sp. and its clinical origin. Biofilms are refractory to antifungal drugs and more difficult to treat than infections with planktonic cells [44]. Moreover, it has been verified that *Candida* sp. isolated from patients with DM have a higher pathogenic potential for biofilm-forming [87]. The communities are extremely common on medical devices.

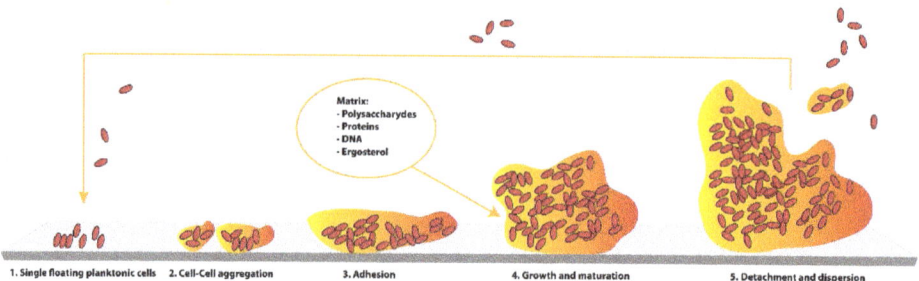

Figure 3. Development of a *Candida* sp. biofilm in a surface.

2.3. Hydrophobicity

In *Candida* sp., the adhesion phenomenon is mediated by agglutinin-like (Als) sequence proteins [88], which are glycosylphosphatidylinositol (GPI)-linked to β-1-6 glucans in the fungal cell wall. Als-dependent cellular adhesion is connected with increases in cell surface hydrophobicity (CSH) [89]. The CSH of *Candida* sp. enhances virulence by promoting adhesion to host tissues [89,90]. *C. albicans* Als3p (hypha-associated) is a major epithelial adhesin that is strongly upregulated during epithelial infection in vitro [90], and the disruption of the *ALS3* gene reduces epithelial adhesion in vitro. Likewise, decreasing the expression of the *ALS2* gene also reduces adhesion [91,92]. On the other side, deletion of the ALS5, ALS6, or ALS7 genes increased adhesion [93], demonstrating that the Als proteins can have opposing roles in fungal attachment to surfaces. Putative homologues of Als proteins have also been identified in NCAC [94]. In *C. glabrata*, for example, epithelial adhesins (Epa) have a comparable structure to the Als proteins [95,96].

Together with adhesion ability, hydrophobicity is a virulent factor that is gene-regulated and usually positively correlated with biofilm metabolic activity [97,98] since hydrophobic interactions seem to be crucial in promoting tissue invasion by the mycelial phase of *Candida* sp. It is presumed that *Candida* sp. can grow under anaerobic conditions, although in these conditions fermentation is the dominant pathway for ATP production [99]. The results of Sardi et al. [100] indicated that 51.97% of diabetic patients' isolates were highly hydrophobic under anaerobic conditions when compared to 21.90% under the aerobic atmosphere [100]. It is recognized that the germ tubes are able to adhere to fibronectin, fibrinogen, and complement via cell surface receptors [101], helping the attachment of filament yeasts to extracellular matrix components (ECM) [102] and producing impairment of phagocytosis, consequently increasing the resistance to blood clearance and the virulence of *Candida* sp. [103].

3. Candidiasis and DM

3.1. Oral Diseases

3.1.1. Oral Candidiasis

The prevalence of oral candidiasis is increasing, as it is one of the most common fungal infections [104]. Oral candidiasis can be diagnosed by the differential patterns of mucosal changes like erythematous, pseudomembranous, and curd-like plaques (biofilms) [105,106]. Higher *Candida* sp. colonization rates were reported in patients with DM type 1 when compared to DM type 2 patients (84% vs. 68%, respectively), while the percentage in nondiabetic subjects was around 27% [18].

The studies also describe how this colonization does not always lead to infection. Nonetheless, it is a prelude to infection when host immunity is compromised and the risk of a disseminated infection is high [107]. Such infections continue to be a major healthcare challenge [108].

The risk factors for oral candidal infection are complex, but it is known that tongue lesions, tobacco smoking, denture wearing, and immunosuppression (e.g., diabetes mellitus) clearly influence oral *Candida* sp. carriage and the upsurge of oral candidiasis [30,109–114]. The causes influencing the higher incidence of oral candidiasis in diabetic patients are presented in Table 1.

Higher expressions in enzymatic activity and the biofilm forming capacity of *Candida* sp. are two of the most important features in oral candidiasis. In a study by Sanitá et al. [115], the virulence of 148 clinical isolates of *C. albicans* from oral candidiasis was characterized by measuring the expression of PL and SAP in healthy subjects (HS), diabetics with oral candidiasis (DOC), and non-diabetics with oral candidiasis (NDOC). For PL, *C. albicans* from NDOC and DOC had the highest enzymatic activity (76.6%); for SAP, *C. albicans* from NDOC exhibited lower enzymatic activity (48.9%). Similar results have been reported in the past [59,87], with percentages greater than 90% for both PL and SAP activity among clinical isolates of *C. albicans* [26,116,117] found. Arlsan and colleagues found 12 different genotypes and compared the virulence factors of several *Candida* sp. isolated from the oral cavities of 142 healthy and diabetic individuals, with and without caries. Although the most isolated species was also *C. albicans*, there were statistical differences in terms of isolated *Candida* frequency between healthy subjects and diabetic patients. DM showed no effect on the activities of virulence factors (biofilm production, proteinase, and phospholipase activity) of *Candida* sp. Yet, different genotypes of *C. albicans* exhibited different virulence activities [118]. Other authors showed that the activity of SAPs suggestively rises in denture wearers with signs of candidiasis compared to denture wearers with a normal palatal mucosa [119]. The inconsistency of results of these reports can be explained by the large variation of intra-and interspecies of *Candida* and deviations in the methodology in most reports [24,26,59,87,116,117,119–123]. A longitudinal study by Sanchés-Vargas et al. [124] quantified biofilms in oral clinical isolates of *Candida* sp. from adults with local and systemic predisposing factors for candidiasis. Between the isolates, authors found *C. albicans*, *C. tropicalis*, *C. glabrata*, *C. krusei*, *C. lusitaniae*, *C. kefyr*, *C. guilliermondii*, and *C. pulcherrima* from the oral mucosa of totally and partially edentulous patients (62.3%) and the oral mucosa of diabetics (37.7%). On average, the oral isolates of *C. glabrata* were considered strong biofilm producers, whereas *C. albicans* (the most common species) and *C. tropicalis* were moderate producers. This might be because *C. glabrata* has been shown to have a higher aggressiveness, producing a great quantity of biofilm matrices yet also increasing chitin concentrations in the cell walls [125–127].

Additional important features are the oral pH and the glycemic control. A study performed by Samaranayake et al. [128] demonstrated that pyruvates and acetates are the major ionic species, generating a quick decrease in pH with *Candida* sp., as found in batch cultures of mixed saliva supplemented with glucose [128].

Other authors indicated that yeasts have a superior ability to adhere to epithelia and denture acrylic surfaces at a low pH of approximately 2–4.14 [31,129]. Balan and colleagues stated that during hyperglycemic episodes, the environmental alteration in the oral cavity increased salivary glucose and acid production, which favored the transition of *Candida* sp. from commensal to pathogen [31]. In another report, while comparing diabetics and non-diabetics, Pallavan et al. [130] verified that 70% of the healthy individuals had lower colonization and 43.3% of the diabetic patients had severe colonization by *Candida* sp., which was also observed in other studies [14,18,21,131]. Prediabetes is a condition where there is an elevation of plasma glucose above the normal range but below that of clinical diabetes [132]. Javed and their colleagues isolated oral *Candida* sp. from 100% of patients with prediabetes and from 65.7% of the controls, observing that the carriage of *C. albicans* was greater among patients with prediabetes (48.7%) than with controls (25.7%) [133]. They also observed that the colonization with *Candida* sp. reduced the salivary flow rate and was independent of glycemic status in patients with prediabetes [132].

In fact, while some studies found a direct significant association between glycosylated hemoglobin and oral *Candida* colonization [134,135], other authors found no relationship between glycosylated hemoglobin and high *Candida*-burden in patients with DM [14,18,136,137]. Furthermore, studies indicate that the concentration of glucose present in the gingival crevicular fluid is related to the blood glucose level [138]. The quality of glycemic control can also partially explain the presence of a significant relationship between subgingival plaque candidal colonization and higher concentrations of glucose [138].

Although most of the scientific community believes that diabetes is a risk factor associated with oral yeast infections, in a recent paper, Costa and colleagues [139] reported that the presence of yeasts in the oral cavity of patients with type 1 DM (60% of total) was not affected by diabetes, metabolic control, duration of the disease, salivary flow rate, or saliva buffer capacity by age, sex, place of residence, number of daily meals, consumption of sweets, or frequency of tooth brushing. *Candida albicans* was the most prevalent yeast species, but a higher number of yeast species was isolated in nondiabetics [139]. The fact that this study was developed exclusively in children may be related to this conclusion.

Table 1. Physiopathology and etiology related to the occurrence of oral candidiasis in diabetics.

	Physiopathology	Reference (s)
Uncontrolled hyperglycemia (high HbA1c) and high glucose levels in saliva	-Uncontrolled hyperglycemia may cause intensification in salivary glucose levels because in diabetics the basement membrane of the parotid salivary gland is more permeable -High glucose levels allow *Candida* sp. to multiply, even in the presence of normal bacterial flora -During hyperglycemic episodes, the chemically reversible glycosylation products with proteins in tissues and the accumulation of glycosylation products on buccal epithelial cells may sequentially increase the number of available receptors for *Candida* sp. -Glucose suppression of the killing capacity of neutrophils, emphasizing colonization (immunosuppression) -Glucose, maltose, and sucrose boost the adhesion of *Candida* to buccal epithelial cells	[15,29,31,52,134,140–147]
Lower salivary pH	-The growth of *Candida* in saliva is accompanied by a rapid decline in pH, which favors their growth and triggers the extracellular phospholipase (PL) and acid proteases, increasing the yeast adhesion to oral mucosal surfaces	[31,128,148]
Tissue response to injury is diminished	-Diabetes mellitus (DM) is known to diminish the host resistance and modify the tissue response to injury. This can result in severe colonization, even in the absence of any clinically evident oral candidiasis and possibly with further dissemination via the blood.	[130,149]
Oral epithelium	-It is most probable that the host oral epithelium of patients with diabetes favors the adhesion of colonization and subsequent infection.	[150,151]
Poor oral hygiene	The lack of control of the oral environment, especially concerning the prevention of dental caries (coronary, root, and periodontal), leads to a higher rate of oral candidiasis, especially in DM older patients	[152–154]
Aging Gender	Diabetic women, orally colonized with *Candida* sp. have higher oral glucose levels than diabetics without oral *Candida* sp.	[134]
Prostheses	Inadequate use of prostheses, together with inadequate hygienization, favours the growth of *Candida* sp.	[155–157]
Drugs	Xerostomia (abnomal lack if saliva): *Candida* sp. stagnation and growth on oral tissues	[30,109–111,136,158,159]

3.1.2. Antifungal Treatment of Oral Candidiasis

Importantly, several reports have stated the importance of the evaluation of the susceptibility of the oral isolates to the antifungal drugs in order to choose proper therapy in diabetic patients to control the fungal diseases. Aitken-Saavedra et al. [160] revealed that 66% of the yeasts isolated in diabetic patients were *C. albicans*, followed by *C. glabrata* (20.7%). In patients with decompensated type 2 DM, higher levels of salivary acidification and a greater diversity and quantity of yeasts of the genus *Candida* were observed. When nystatin was administered in these patients, higher inhibition was observed at a lower pH [160]. The study presented by Lydia Rajakumari and Saravana Kumari [161] showed a lower glycemic control leads to a higher candidal colonization in diabetic patients. The predominant species was *C. albicans*, but among denture wearers, *C. glabrata* was predominant. More importantly, ketoconazole, fluconazole, and itraconazole were effective against the isolated *Candida* sp. [161].

Similarly, Premkumar et al. [162] stated that, although *C. albicans* was the most predominantly isolated species, *C. dubliniensis*, *C. tropicalis*, and *C. parapsilosis* were also observed. The authors showed variable resistance toward amphotericin B, and fluconazole was observed in clinical isolates from diabetics but not from healthy patients. Again, a positive correlation was observed between glycemic control and candidal colonization [162]. In 2011, Bremenkamp et al. [163] found no significant differences in antifungal susceptibility to the tested agents between *Candida* sp. isolates from diabetic and non-diabetic subjects, which was consistent with the study by Manfredi et al. [164]. Furthermore, a high prevalence of *C. dubliniensis* in diabetic patients was found, which may suggest a potential misdiagnosis of its morphologically-related species, *C. albicans*. Other authors found the same two species in DM patients [1,16,57,135]. In yet another study, Sanitá and their colleagues [165] investigated the susceptibility of 198 oral clinical isolates of *Candida* sp. against caspofungin, amphotericin B, itraconazole, and fluconazole. Their findings confirmed the resistant profile of *C. glabrata* isolates against azole antifungals—especially itraconazole—in individuals with diabetes and denture stomatitis. The clinical sources of the isolates were shown to have no effect on the mininum inhibitory concentration (MIC) values obtained for all antifungals tested, which was in accordance with previous reports [26,119]. Additionally, *Candida* sp. isolates with higher rates of resistance to flucytosine, ketoconazole, miconazole, and econazole were confirmed in patients with diabetes when compared to healthy controls [163,166]. The increase in the environment glucose concentration may trigger the expression of several genes responsible for several carbohydrate cell wall and biofilm matrices components, consequently leading to resistant strains. This has been demonstrated before in gene and drug studies [126]. The variability in the susceptibility results may be related to the different antifungal drugs tested in those works.

Using a different approach, Mantri et al. [149] evaluated *Candida* sp. colonization in dentures with a silicone soft liner in diabetic and non-diabetic patients, assessing the antifungal efficacy of chlorhexidine gluconate [149]. The results showed normal oral flora in diabetics and non-diabetics and no difference between groups. They also showed a significant reduction of the colonization after cleaning the dentures with 4% chlorhexidine gluconate. This suggests that this drug has a good antiseptic effect on *Candida* sp. by killing it and preventing new adhesion. In 2015, Indira et al. [167] conducted a study that compared the common opportunistic infections (OIs) between 37 people living with HIV with DM (PLHIV-DM) and 37 people living with HIV without DM (PLHIV). Both of the groups were treated with anti-retroviral therapy (ART) [167]. The most common Ois included oral candidiasis (49% of PLHIV-DM and 35% of PLHIV) and *C. krusei* was the most common *Candida* sp. isolated (50%). No significant difference in the profile of Ois was found between PLHIV with and without DM.

3.1.3. Periodontal Diseases

Periodontal diseases of fungal origin are relatively unusual in healthy individuals but arise more often in immunocompromised people or in cases when normal oral flora has been distressed (e.g., the use of broad-spectrum antibiotics) [168,169]. Diabetes is a stated risk factor for periodontitis, which is the sixth-leading complication of diabetes [170,171]. Alterations in host response, collagen metabolism, vascularity, gingival crevicular fluid, heredity patterns, and immunosuppressive treatment (drugs, dosage, and treatment duration) are known factors that promote periodontitis in diabetes [172,173]. The etiology and pathogenesis of periodontitis is still imprecise, but it is recognized that *Candida* sp. is part of the oral and subgingival microbiota of individuals who suffer from severe periodontal inflammation [174]. The virulence factors of *Candida* sp. simplify the colonization and the proliferation in the periodontal pockets by co-aggregating with bacteria in dental biofilms and adhering to epithelial cells [30], which are essential in the microbial colonization, thereby contributing to the evolution of oral diseases [175,176]. As much as 20% of patients with chronic periodontitis have been shown to have periodontal pockets that are colonized by several species of *Candida* sp., predominantly *C. albicans* [177,178], but *C. dubliniensis* [174], *C. glabrata*, and *C. tropicalis* have been reported too [176,179]. Furthermore, *C. albicans* strains isolated from subgingival sites of diabetic and periodontal patients showed high PL in cases of chronic periodontitis. Environmental oxygen concentration demonstrated influence on the virulence factors [100,180,181]. Sardi et al. [100], in a study using PCR experiments, demonstrated that the quantities of several *Candida* sp. were higher in diabetic patients with a chronic periodontal disease than in patients without diabetes. *C. albicans*, *C. dubliniensis*, *C. tropicalis*, and *C. glabrata* were detected in 57%, 75%, 16%, and 5% of the periodontal pockets, respectively. In non-diabetic patients, *C. albicans* and *C. dubliniensis* were present in 20% and 14%, respectively. Periodontal inflammation has been described to be worse in prediabetics when compared to healthy controls [182–185], assuming that the oxidative stress induced by chronic hyperglycemia with a reduced unstimulated whole salivary flow rate (UWSFR) in these patients may contribute to deteriorating periodontal status [133]. Thus, it has been suggested that glycemic control enhances healing and reduces periodontal inflammation in patients with DM and prediabetes [134,182,185–191]. As a result, some authors believe that it may reduce oral *Candida* sp. carriage in patients with prediabetes [133]. The HbA1c concentration is an important diagnostic tool for monitoring long-term glycemic control [192]. Also, in these cases, higher *Candida* sp. infection levels have also been associated with low diabetic control (HbA1c > 9), occurring less frequently in subjects with well-controlled blood sugar levels (HbA1c < 6).

3.1.4. Denture Prosthetics and Candidiasis

Since the oral cavity is highly populated with several polymicrobial communities, each one occupies very precise niches that diverge in both anatomical location and as well as nutrient availability [193]. A consequence of strong commensal bacteria/yeast colonization is the inhibition of pathogenic microorganism colonization through resistance. The vital function of commensal yeast and bacteria and the harmful effects of commensal depletion through the use of broad spectrum antibiotics [194,195] are well recognized. Recent studies disclosed that commensal microorganisms not only protect the host by niche occupation, but also interact with host tissue, promoting the development of proper tissue structure and function [196,197].

Dentures represent a protective reservoir for oral microorganisms, mostly in biofilm form, favoring yeast proliferation, improving their infective potential, and protecting fungal cells against several medications [198–202]. Elderly edentulous denture wearers, patients with debilitating diseases, and users of acrylic prosthetics have a significant risk of virulent oral yeast infections [124]. Furthermore, elderly patients with diabetes have a 4.4 times higher estimated risk of developing oral candidiasis when compared with individuals without this disease. No statistically significant relation was determined between xerostomia, the use of prosthesis, and oral candidiasis [154], as suggested by some studies [203,204]. Sanitá et al. [199] studied the prevalence of *Candida* sp. in diabetics and non-diabetics with and without denture stomatitis (DS) and found that *C. albicans* was the predominant species isolated in the three groups (81.9%). They also detected *C. tropicalis* (15.71%) and *C. glabrata* (15.24%), as found in previous studies [10,14,15,21,24,57,136,144,173,205–210]. Interestingly, and contrary to other reports, the authors did not detect *C. dubliniensis* among any *Candida* sp. isolates. Even though these results confirm previous findings [10,14,16,21,24,26,136,144,173,207,209,210], this species has been isolated in both diabetic [12,57,206] and non-diabetic [208] patients. This discrepancy among studies may be related to problems with identification techniques, since *C. dubliniensis* and *C. albicans* have similar phenotypic characteristics. The same authors also found that the prevalence of *C. tropicalis* significantly increased, showing the highest degree of inflammation in DS, as observed in previous studies [12,16,24,136,144,173,208–210].

3.1.5. Co-Occurrence of Dental Plaque, Periodontitis, and Gingivitis

The existence of numerous different oral diseases in a single patient is frequent in diabetics. Hammad et al. [29] studied the relationship between the tongue and subgingival plaque *Candida* sp. colonization, as well as its relationship with the quality of glycemic control in type 2 diabetics with periodontitis. The results showed that *Candida* sp. colonized 59% and 48.7% of the patients' tongues and subgingival plaque, respectively. In this cross-sectional study, the authors concluded that poorly controlled type 2 diabetics and female patients with periodontitis showed a higher prevalence of subgingival plaque *Candida* sp. colonization than men, regardless of oral hygiene, tobacco smoking, age, or duration of DM [29]. The authors could not correlate oral candidal colonization and the amount of dental plaque, a patient's gingival status, or oral hygiene, as in other studies [211], but noticed *Candida* sp. present in the dental plaque in the form of biofilm. Remarkably, and compared with the control group, they found that *C. albicans* cells isolated from the subgingival plaque of patients with periodontitis adhered more to epithelial cells [212], suggesting that the oxygen concentration in the periodontal pockets affects the virulence of *C. albicans* [213]. A study that evaluated the effect of *Candida* sp. and general disease- or treatment-related factors on plaque-related gingivitis severity in children and adolescents with Nephrotic syndrome (NS, a clinical condition with a proteinuria level exceeding the body's compensating abilities) and diabetes concluded that poor hygiene control was the main cause of gingivitis. Olczak-Kowalczyk and colleagues [172] showed in their work that *Candida* sp. often occurred in healthy patients, but oral candidiasis was found only in the NS and diabetes groups (9.37% and 11.43%). Their work also showed that gingivitis occurred more frequently in patients with NS/diabetes. Moreover, gingivitis severity was most likely correlated to age, lipid disorders, and an increase in body mass and *Candida* sp. In uncompensated diabetes and in those patients using immunosuppressive treatment, it was assumed that NS would increase the plaque-related gingivitis.

3.1.6. Esophagitis and Oropharyngeal Candidiasis

Candida sp. esophagitis and oropharyngeal are also oral complications found to moderately affect DM patients. Recently, Takahashi et al. [214] determined long-term trends in *Candida* sp. esophagitis (CE) prevalence and associated risk factors for patients with or without HIV infections. A risk analysis revealed that, among other factors, DM is associated with CE. Also, Mojazi and their colleagues [215] identified risk factors for oropharyngeal *Candida* sp. colonization in critically ill patients, with the results confirming DM as a risk factor [215]. Likewise, Owotade and colleagues [216] investigated the role of anti-retroviral (ARV) therapy and other factors related to oral candidiasis. Results demonstrated that 59.4% of the individuals were colonized by yeasts. *C. albicans* was the most common species (71%) and *C. dubliniensis* was the most frequent non-*Candida albicans Candida* species (NCAC). The probabilities of colonization were five times greater in patients with diabetes [216], confirming previous findings [16].

Oral and esophageal candidiasis sometimes leads to mucosal hyperplasia and progresses to carcinoma. There are many reports of the antibacterial effects of probiotics, but consensus about their antifungal effect has not been reached. In order to find alternative therapies, Terayama et al. [217]

investigated whether probiotic (yogurt) containing *Lactobacillus gasseri* OLL2716 (LG21 yogurt) could prevent proliferative and inflammatory changes caused by *C. albicans* in a mucosal candidiasis animal model. Diabetes was induced in eight-week-old WBN/Kob rats by the intravenous administration of alloxan. The results suggested that probiotic (yogurt) containing *L. gasseri* OLL2716 can suppress squamous hyperplastic change and inflammation associated with *C. albicans* infection in the forestomach [217].

3.2. Vulvovaginal Candidiasis

The exact association between DM and vulvovaginal candidiasis (VVC) remains to be clarified, but some investigations propose that the general reduced immune response associated with DM is the main cause of recurrent VVC [218–221]. Additionally, diabetes type, severity, and degree of glucose control are probable risk factors associated with VVC prevalence, and it is acknowledged that the metabolic disorders that predispose to clinical vaginitis can be reduced by performing an appropriate diabetic control [222,223]. *C. albicans* is the most common species isolated, followed by *C. glabrata* in patients both with and without diabetes [219,224,225]. Studies have been reporting an increased frequency of infection by NCAC over time [226,227], especially *C. glabrata*, which is more recurrently associated with VVC in African and Asian countries [228–231]. Table 2 summarizes the metabolic disorders that can predispose one to VVC and those that can be decreased with proper diabetic control.

Several studies explored the association between VVC and DM. Gunther et al. [232] investigated the frequency of total isolation of vaginal *Candida* sp. and its different clinical profiles in women with type 2 DM compared to non-diabetic women in Brazil [232]. Vaginal yeast isolation occurred in 18.8% in the diabetic group and in 11.8% of women in the control group. The diabetic group was shown to be more symptomatic (VVC + recurrent VVC (RVVC) = 66.66%) than colonized women (33.33%), and indicated more colonization, VVC, and RVVC than the controls. Sherry et al. [233] studied the epidemiology of VVC in a cohort in order to find the causative organisms associated with VVC. The authors noticed a shifting prevalence of *Candida* sp. with *C. albicans* as the most common yeast but an increase of NCAC. A heterogeneous biofilm-forming capacity associated with lower antifungal drug sensitivity was also reported.

On the contrary, Ray et al. [234] stated that out of 11 diabetic patients, *C. glabrata* was isolated in 61.3% and *C. albicans* in 28.8% of VVC cases [234]. Other studies have shown similar results in diabetic women [221,235,236]. Results showed a persistent vaginal colonization with *C. glabrata* in estrogenized streptozotocin-induced type 1 diabetic mice, and vaginal polymorphonuclear (PMN) infiltration (constantly low) was found in a murine model study by Nash and colleagues [237]. Contrary to what happens in women and in other in vivo studies, in this case, curiously, biofilm formation was not detected, and co-infection of *C. glabrata* with *C. albicans* did not induce synergistic immunopathogenic effects [237].

Table 2. Physiopathology and etiology related to the occurrence of vulvovaginitis in diabetics.

Condition	Physiopathology	Reference (s)
Uncontrolled hyperglycemia (high HbA1c) and high glucose levels in vaginal mucosae	- The increased serum glucose level is thought to lead to impaired monocyte, granulocyte, and neutrophil adherence, as well as reduced chemotaxis, phagocytosis, and pathogen killing - Diabetics secretions contain glucose, which can be used as a nutrient by yeasts - pH, nutritional substance, temperature, and adherence capacity in the vulvovaginal tissue may induce *Candida* sp. virulence. - The vaginal epithelial cell receptor of fucose supports the adhesion of *Candida* sp. to vaginal epithelial cells - The rise in vaginal glucose and secretions and activities of hydrolytic enzymes [e.g., secreted aspartyl proteinases (SAPs), PL] increases the pathogenicity of *Candida* sp. - Increased levels of glycogen increase colonization and infection by *Candida* sp. by lowering the vaginal pH, facilitating the development of vulvovaginal candidiasis (VVC)	[55,56,59,219,222,224,225,231,238–253]

Table 2. Cont.

Condition	Physiopathology	Reference (s)
Pregnancy	-The increased circulation of estrogen levels and the deposition of glycogen and other substrates in the vagina leads to a 10–50% higher incidence of vaginal colonization by *Candida* sp. -Variability of constitutive defensins (e.g., lactoferrins, peptides) and lysozyme, leading to a poor innate immune response -Hyperglycemia can rise the anaerobic glycolysis in vaginal epithelial cells, increasing lactic acid and acetone production, decreasing the vaginal pH, thus enabling fungal colonization and proliferation	[241,254–260]
Diabetes type	- The incidence of VVC related to the type 1 DM or type 2 DM and is variable among studies	[218,221–223]
Aging	- The older one is, the higher VVC prevalence is	[222,223]

In a different study, Nyirjesy and colleagues evaluated the effects of sodium glucose co-transporter 2 inhibitors (e.g., canagliflozin, dapagliflozin, sitagliptin) used for the treatment of type 2 DM. These drugs improve glycemic control by increasing urinary glucose excretion and are related to increased vaginal colonization with *Candida* sp. and in VVC adverse events in women with type 2 DM [252]. Of the nine subjects with VVC with a positive vaginal culture at the time of the adverse event, six cultures were positive for *C. albicans*, only one was positive for *C. glabrata*, and one was positive for *C. tropicalis*. These findings confirm previous suggestions that *C. glabrata* is less pathogenic than *C. albicans* and more often associated with asymptomatic colonization in VVC [261]. The investigation theorized that urinary glucose excretion and the subsequent deposition of urine on the vulvovaginal tissues with voiding are more significant factors in increasing the risk of VVC in diabetic women than overall glycemic control. In this study, women showed improved glycemic control due to the administration of canagliflozin [262,263] with a higher prevalence of *Candida* sp. colonization and symptomatic infection, which was also detected with dapagliflozin [264]. Also related to SGLT2 inhibitors, the prevalence and risk of VVC before SGLT2 inhibitors was carefully evaluated in real-world practice by Yokoyama and colleagues [265]. They reported that before starting SGLT2 inhibitors, 14.9% of the participants had positive vaginal *Candida* sp. colonization. Younger age and the presence of microangiopathy were significantly associated with the colonization. Moreover, of the 65 participants who were negative for *Candida* sp., 24 participants (36.9%) converted to a positive culture, and 18 participants (15.8%) developed symptomatic vaginitis. The authors concluded that the rates of developing positive colonization and symptomatic vaginitis after starting SGLT2 inhibitors appear to be higher in real-world practice than the rates of 31% and 5–10% in clinical trials, respectively. Risk factors of vaginal *Candida* colonization might be different before and after taking SGLT2 inhibitors [265].

The colonization of the vagina in prepubertal girls with *Candida* sp. is rare, as the low estrogen levels during childhood result in a rich anaerobic vaginal flora which inhibits *Candida* sp. Growth [266,267]. In a recent report, Atabek et al. [219] isolated *Candida* sp. in 39% of children with type 1 DM between 8–16 years in age. The subjects who had *Candida* sp. colonization and candidiasis were considered all acute. *C. albicans* was found in 50% of all cases, followed by *C. glabrata* (36.6%), *C. krusei* (3.3%), and *C. dubliniensis* (3.3%). Patients with VVC had a greater mean HbA1c when compared to those without such infections, and the authors thus suggested that patients with DM should undergo periodic screening for genital candidiasis [219]. Similarly, Sonck et al. [268] studied the anogenital yeast flora of 166 diabetic girls of less than 15 years of age with vulvitis, revealing that 55% were colonized, mostly by *C. albicans*.

Numerous studies have described the higher prevalence of asymptomatic vaginal colonization and symptomatic infection with *Candida* sp. in diabetic women, and some studies suggest pregnancy as an additional risk factor [254–256], although results are inconsistent [28,226].

Several studies have also shown that pregnancy and uncontrolled diabetes increase the infection risk. It is likely that reproductive hormone fluctuations during pregnancy and elevated glucose levels characteristic of diabetes provide the carbon needed for *Candida* overgrowth and infection. However, Sopian IL et al. [269] showed no relationship between diabetes and the occurrence of vaginal yeast infection in pregnant women, showing that there was no significant association between infection and age group, race, or education level [269]. In another report, Zheng et al. [254] studied the diversity of the vaginal fungal flora in healthy non-pregnant women, healthy pregnant women, women with gestational DM, and pregnant women with DM type 1 through an 18S rRNA gene clone library method [254]. Results showed that the most predominant vaginal fungal species belonged to the *Candida* and *Saccharomyces* genera. In a study of 251 women, Nowakowska et al. [270] demonstrated that the probability of vaginal mycosis was 4-fold greater in type 1 DM patients and nearly 2-fold greater in those with gestational DM when compared to healthy pregnant women. The report also highlighted the predominant role of poor glycemic control in the increased prevalence of vaginal candidiasis in pregnant women with type 1 DM [270]. In 2011, Masri et al. [271] determined the prevalence of *Candida* sp. in vaginal swabs of pregnant women from Serdang Hospital, Selangor, Malaysia, and their antifungal susceptibility. Results showed that 17.2% of the specimens were *Candida* sp., with *C. albicans* being the most common species detected (83.5%), followed by *C. glabrata* (16%) and *C. famata* (0.05%). All *C. albicans* and *C. famata* isolates were susceptible to fluconazole, whereas *C. glabrata* isolates had a dose-dependent susceptibility. The authors concluded that the first trimester, the second trimester, and DM were significant risk factors in patients for the vaginal candidiasis ($p < 0.001$). However, other studies noted that DM or impaired glucose tolerance during pregnancy was not connected with vaginal candidiasis [256]. Bassyouni et al. [242] explored the prevalence of VVC in diabetic women versus non-diabetic women and compared the ability of identified *Candida* sp. isolates to secrete PL and SAPs with the characterization of their genetic profile. The study involved 80 females with type 2 DM and 100 non-diabetics within the child-bearing period. Results revealed that VVC was significantly higher among the diabetic group (50%) versus the non-diabetic group (20%), and *C. albicans* was the predominant species in both groups (75% in non-diabetics and 50% in diabetics), followed by *C. glabrata* (20% in non-diabetics and 42.5% in diabetics). They also found that *Candida* sp. isolated from diabetics secreted higher quantities of proteinase than non-diabetics (87.7% and 65%, respectively), especially for *C. albicans* and *C. glabrata*, but non-significant associations between any of the tested proteinase or PL genes and DM were detected. These results were—by some means—in agreement with the ones from other reports [243,244] that also detected *C. parapsilosis* and *C. tropicalis* in a group of diabetic women. Kumari et al. [248] detected poor PL production in the isolated *Candida* sp. (causing vulvovaginitis), of which 81.25% were *C. parapsilosis*, 30.43% *C. albicans*, and 18.75% *C. glabrata*. Moreover, insignificant differences in the expression of *Candida* sp. *PLB1-2* genes and *SAP1–SAP8* genes between diabetic and non-diabetic women were reported by Bassyouni and colleagues [242]. Still, they concluded that the higher prevalence of VVC among diabetics could be directly correlated to increased SAPs production. The discrepancies between the results of different reports may be due to changes in growth conditions and host factors that alter the gene expression qualitatively and quantitatively [59,247], although findings suggest that the expression of hydrolytic enzymes by *Candida* sp. is a multifactorial process in patients with DM and the hyperglycemia level is thus not the only implicated factor.

Lastly, VVC is intimately related to vaginal mucosae biofilms. Mikamo and colleagues studied the involvement of *Candida*'s complement receptor (ICAM-1) in the adhesion of *C. albicans* or *C. glabrata* to the genitourinary epithelial cells in high glucose states. Their results demonstrated that, while the adhesion of *C. albicans* to human vaginal epithelial cells VK2/E6E7 significantly increased in the high glucose, human vulvovaginal epidermal cells A431 did not. ICAM-1 expression was increased in VK2/E6E7 cultured in the high glucose, but the expression level in A431 was not elevated. These data suggested that ICAM-1 is a ligand in the adhesion of *C. albicans* to the vaginal epithelial cells in an environment with high glucose concentration. Moreover, both host immune dysfunction and the adjustment in epithelial cells were considered responsible for VVC in diabetic patients [272].

3.3. Urinary Tract Candidiasis

Around 10% to 15% of in-hospital urinary tract infections (UTIs) are related to *Candida* sp. and the prevalence is still increasing [273]. Some predisposing factors such as DM, urinary retention, urinary stasis, renal transplantation, and hospitalization can increase the risk of candiduria. Specifically, DM has been known to cause severe complicated UTIs as a result of its various changes in the genitourinary system [274]. Since the 1980s, there has been a marked increase in opportunistic fungal infections involving the urinary tract, of which *C. albicans* is the most commonly isolated species, but NCAC sp. is now the majority in many countries worldwide [275,276]. Candiduria (presence of *Candida* sp. in urine) is an increasingly common finding in hospitalized patients [14], and subjects with DM are at a higher risk of developing fungal UTIs. Thus, reducing risk factors such as increasing glycemic control and the removal of urinary catheters can result in the remission of candiduria [273]. Physiopathology and etiology related to the occurrence of UTIs related to *Candida* sp. and DM are presented in Table 3.

According to the results of the Falahati et al. [277] study, there were significant associations between candiduria and the female gender, high fasting blood sugar and urine glucose, uncontrolled diabetes (HbA1c $\geq$ 8), and acidic urine pH ($p < 0.05$). Causative agents were identified as *C. glabrata* (n = 19, 50%), *C. albicans* (n = 12, 31.6%), *C. krusei* (n = 4, 10.5%), *C. tropicalis* (n = 2, 5.3%), and *C. kefyr* (n = 1, 2.6%). The study concluded that when considering the high incidence rate of candiduria in diabetic patients, the control of diabetes, predisposing factors, and causal relationships between diabetes and candiduria should be highlighted [277]. In a 2018 study, Esmailzadeh et al. [276] evaluated candiduria among type 2 diabetic patients. Indeed, the results showed that the rate of candiduria was relatively high in type 2 diabetic patients and they were also suffering from a lack of proper blood glucose control. Although the frequency of NCAC sp. was not significantly higher than *C. albicans*, they obtained more from those with symptomatic candiduria [276]. In a cross-sectional study, Yismaw et al. [273] determined the fungal causative agents of UTIs in asymptomatic and symptomatic diabetic patients and associated risk factors. Significant candiduria was detected in 7.5% and 17.1% of asymptomatic and symptomatic type 2 diabetic patients, respectively. Among the isolated *Candida* sp., 84.2% was observed in the asymptomatic diabetic patients and the remaining 15.8% in symptomatic patients. Rizzi and Trevisan studied the prevalence and significance of UTIs and genital infections (GI) in diabetes and the effects of sodium glucose cotransporter 2 (SGLT-2) inhibitors on these complications. Results presented that diabetic patients are at high risk of UTIs and of GIs. The authors concluded that only GIs were associated with poor glycemic control. Although patients treated with SGLT-2 inhibitors have an increased 3–5 fold risk of GIs, proper medical education may reduce this risk [278].

Diabetes mellitus, indwelling bladder catheter, sex (female), and the use of antibacterial agents have been found as the risk factors identified for both *C. glabrata* and *C. albicans* candiduria [275], as previously reported [27,279]. Emphysematous cystitis, which almost exclusively occurs in diabetic patients, is rare and is seldom the result of a fungal infection [280,281]. This condition is associated with a gas formation that may present itself as cystitis, pyelitis, or pyelonephritis. Uncontrolled DM is a major risk factor for this type of infection, as it provides a favorable microenvironment in which the gas-forming organisms can grow [282,283]. Alansari et al. [284] reported a case in which a patient with uncontrolled DM was diagnosed with emphysematous pyelitis by *C. tropicalis*, while Wang et al. [285] also reported the case of a 53-year-old male patient with fungus ball and emphysematous cystitis caused concurrently by *C. tropicalis*. The predisposing factors were DM and usage of broad-spectrum antibiotics. Garg et al. [286], in a one-year prospective single center study at Dayanand Medical College and Hospital, observed 151 diabetic and non-diabetic female patients diagnosed with UTIs. Uncontrolled diabetes was more commonly associated with severe UTIs like pyelonephritis and emphysematous pyelonephritis.

Table 3. Physiopathology and etiology related to the occurrence of urinary tract infections and systemic candidiasis in diabetics.

Condition	Physiopathology	Reference (s)
Uncontrolled hyperglycemia (high HbA1c) and high glucose levels in urinary tract (UT) mucosae or blood	- Favorable microenvironment for the gas-forming organisms, such as *Candida* sp., to grow	[282,283]
Gender	-An association between candiduria and being female	[27,273,279]
Drugs	-SGLT2 inhibitors (e.g., dapagliflozin, canagliflozin, tofogliflozin) administration leads to a greater susceptibility to urinary tract infection (UTI) -Association with a persistent increase in urine glucose concentration	[287]

Escherichia coli was the most frequently isolated species in both groups, followed by *Klebsiella*, *Pseudomonas*, and *Candida* sp., and the latter was only isolated from the diabetic population. Tumbarello et al. [288] identified DM and urinary catheterization as features that are specifically associated with biofilm-forming *Candida* sp. bloodstream infections. Later, Vaidyanathan et al. [281] related a case of a 58-year-old diabetic paraplegic male with a long-term indwelling urethral catheter that developed a catheter block. Results showed an *E. coli* and *C. albicans* co-infection and HbA1c (glycosylated haemoglobin) was 111 mmol/mol, which is associated with uncontrolled DM. *C. albicans* later disseminated into the bloodstream through the damaged bladder and the urethral mucosa. Moreover, those isolates formed consistently high levels of biofilm formation in vitro and a resistance to voriconazole was also detected [281]. In another report, Suzuki et al. [287] investigated the relationship between UTIs and glucosuria, observing the effect of glucosuria induced by sodium-glucose cotransporter 2 (SGLT2) inhibitors on the progression of UTIs in mice. The results showed that in mice treated with dapagliflozin and canagliflozin (not tofogliflozin), the amount of *C. albicans* colony forming units (CFU) in kidneys increased in accordance with both treatment duration and dosage. The urine glucose concentration (UGC) significantly increased up to 12 (tofogliflozin) to 24 h (dapagliflozin and canagliflozin) after SGLT2 administration, indicating that a greater susceptibility to UTIs is associated with a persistent increase in UGC [287].

3.4. Systemic Candidiasis

It is recognized that DM predisposes one to systemic candidiasis for several factors [289]. Among these factors, the most important are the microvascular disease progression, the low host defense mechanisms, and the diabetic vasculopathy, which exacerbates hypoperfusion and hyperglycemia and may lead to neutrophil and lymphocyte dysfunction with impaired opsonization [11,42,290–322]. Catheter-associated candiduria is a common clinical finding in hospitalized patients, especially in intensive care units [295], and is intimately related to biofilms. Padawer et al. [295] studied demographic and clinical data at an Israeli hospital between 2011 and 2013 on the prevalence of *Candida* sp. in catheterized in-patients and the medical interventions provided to these patients. Their results showed that candiduria was observed in 146 catheterized in-patients out of the 1408 evaluated and was directly associated with DM. *C. albicans* was present in 69.1% of the subjects, followed by *C. parapsilosis* (9.58%), *C. krusei* (7.53%), *C. tropicalis* (6.16%), *C. glabrata* (4.79%), and other species (2.73%). DM was found to be a significant risk factor of infection by *Candida* sp. In another report, Padawer et al. [295] concluded that *Candida* sp. was the second leading pathogen causing catheter-associated urinary tract infections or asymptomatic colonization. Previously, Tambyah et al. [296], Makin and Tambyah [297], and Sievert et al. [298] found similar results.

Muskett et al. [299] performed a systematic review to identify the most prevalent risk factors, looking at published analyses, risk prediction models, and clinical decision rules for invasive fungal disease (IFD) in critically ill adult patients. The authors found studies that had a significant association of DM and IFD on both univariable and multivariable analyses. Paphitou and colleagues [300] established that patients with any combination of DM, new onset hemodialysis, use of total parenteral nutrition, or receipt of broad-spectrum antibiotics had an invasive candidiasis rate of 16.6% compared to a 5.1% rate in patients lacking these characteristics ($p = 0.001$). Also, Michalopuolos et al. [301], in a univariate regression analysis study between 1997 and 2002, confirmed that DM is a significant candidemia-associated factor and an independent candidemia predictor. *C. albicans* (70%), *C. parapsilosis* (10%), *C. glabrata* (6.7%), *C. tropicalis* (6.7%), and *C. krusei* (6.7%) were isolated in patients with candidemia. *C. albicans* was simultaneously isolated from blood (89.5%) and the central venous catheter tip. Among other factors, the authors found that DM was associated with a high 30-day mortality in candidemia. Candidemia due to *C. parapsilosis* was associated with high rates of survival [11], probably due to the fact that adherence and protein secretion do not correlate with strain pathogenicity in this species as opposed to the other *Candida* sp., as had been discussed [323]. Another retrospective study from 2007 to 2015 of candidemia in hospitalized adults was performed by Khatib et al. Most of the isolates (97.5%) were *C. albicans*. *C. glabrata* was more common in diabetics (52.9% vs. 32.0% in non-diabetics; $p = 0.004$) and in abdominal sources. The findings suggested possible species-related differences in colonization dynamics or pathogenicity [324].

Abad et al. [304] carried out a different study to investigate the susceptibilities of clinical fluconazole-resistant and fluconazole-susceptible dose-dependent to caspofungin of 207 *Candida* sp. in Iranian patients. Results showed that only 9.7% of the isolates were non-sensitive to caspofungin and that these isolates were observed in cancer, DM, and AIDS patients [304]. Wu et al. [305] investigated 238 candidemia hospitalized patients between 2009 and 2011 so as to study the incidence rates of candidemia and identify the differences in risk factors of patients with *C. albicans* and NCACs and with *C. guilliermondii* and non-*C. guilliermondii* candidemia. DM was identified as a significant risk factor in patients with candidemia due to *C. albicans* (35.2%) compared to candidemia related to NCACs (13.2%). Although *C. guilliermondii* is an uncommon cause of candidemia, even in immunocompromised hosts [306–311], it was also found to occur in a significant amount of the hospitalized patients. Over the three year period, the percentage of candidemia due to *C. albicans* decreased, while the percentage of candidemia due to *C. parapsilosis* and *C. guilliermondii* increased in more than 80% of all candidemia cases in 2011 [305].

Candida sp. bloodstream infections (CBSI) are the fourth leading cause of nosocomial bloodstream infections in the United States [316,318,325]. CBSIs occur in up to 10% of all bloodstream infections in hospitalized patients [313–315], and the mortality rate is about 40% [316,317]. Normally, this mortality is higher than in bloodstream infections involving bacteria [326,327]. Risk factors for CBSIs include critically ill patients in intensive care units, DM, immunosuppressive states, mechanical ventilation, neutropenia, recent surgical procedures, and prematurity [315,318,319]. In a study by Tumbarello and colleagues [328], it was found that DM is an independent predictor of biofilm-forming *Candida* sp. CBSIs. The use of total parenteral nutrition, hospital mortality, post-CBSI hospital length of stay (LOS), and the costs of antifungal therapy were all significantly greater among patients infected by biofilm-forming isolates when compared to those infected by non-biofilm-forming isolates. It was concluded that biofilm-forming CBSI was significantly related with a high risk of death compared to non-biofilm forming CBSI [328]. Corzo-Leon and colleagues [320] investigated the clinical and epidemiologic characteristics of patients with CBSI in two tertiary care reference medical institutions in Mexico City. Their results showed that CBSIs represented 3.8% of nosocomial bloodstream infections and *C. albicans* was the predominant species (46%), followed by *C. tropicalis* (26%). *C. glabrata* was isolated from 50% of patients with diabetes and elderly patients. Nucci et al. [321] published a paper reporting an incidence of 1.18 episodes of candidemia per 1000 admissions. *C. albicans*, *C. tropicalis*, and *C. parapsilosis* were isolated in 80% of cases and DM was also found in 11% of the total cases.

Gupta et al. [322] reviewed the influence of *C. glabrata* candidemia in intensive care unit (ICU) patients between 2006 and 2010. Results showed that this species was the third most isolated, and DM was a risk factor among 50% of the total cases. Also, urine was the most common source of *C. glabrata* candidemia, while the overall mortality rate was 53.8% [322]. In another report, Wang et al. [42] observed no differences in the distribution of *Candida* sp. between elderly and young patients in China, but the resistance to fluconazole and voriconazole for NCAC in the first group was double the amount of the latter. Host-related risk factors included DM, mechanical ventilation, central vascular and urethral catheter placement, and were more common in elderly patients [42].

3.5. Other Candidiasis

Diabetic patients are highly predisposed to cutaneous fungal infections due to the higher blood sugar levels. These infections are frequently characterized by thick biofilms, and sometimes the use of medical devices to drain these lesions is mandatory. Foot infection (tinea pedis and toenail onychomycosis) is particularly important to diabetic individuals due to the high incidence of diabetic foot in these patients [329,330]. The most significant *Candida* sp. causing onychomycosis are *C. albicans* and *C. parapsilosis* and it is known that DM patients have a high rate of tinea pedis and onychomycosis. Thus, this infection is now considered to be a predictor of diabetic foot syndrome [331]. The predisposing factors for tinea pedis et unguium are presented in Table 4.

Diabetic foot ulcers are a serious cause of diagnostic and therapeutic concern, and Non-*albicans Candida* spp. with potential biofilm forming abilities are emerging as a predominant cause of this problematic condition. Indeed, in a recent study, the prevalence of different *Candida* sp. was identified as *C. tropicalis* (34.6%), *C. albicans* (29.3%), *C. krusei* (16.0%), *C. parapsilosis* (10.6%), and *C. glabrata* (9.33%) [332]. In order to find the frequency of fungal infections among cutaneous lesions of diabetic patients and to investigate azole antifungal agent susceptibility of the isolates, Raiesi et al. [333] studied type 1 and type 2 DM patients with foot ulcers (38.5%) and with skin and nail lesions (61.5%). Results showed that 24.5% had fungal infections and were at a higher frequency in patients with skin and nail lesions (28%) than in foot ulcers (19.1%). *C. albicans* and *Aspergillus flavus* were the most common species isolated, and a high prevalence of fluconazole-resistant *Candida* sp., particularly in diabetic foot ulcers, was determined [333].

Table 4. Physiopathology and etiology related to the occurrence of nail fungal diseases linked to *Candida* sp. in diabetics.

Condition	Physiopathology	Reference (s)
Uncontrolled hyperglycemia (high HbA1c) and high glucose levels in vaginal mucosae	-Circulatory disorders affecting the lower extremities (peripheral circulation), peripheral neuropathy, and retinopathy - Nail thickness is associated with an elevated HbA1c value - Diabetics using hemodialysis exhibit a higher probability of onychomycosis	[329,330,334–338]
Duration of DM	-More time leads to a higher probability of onychomycosis	[336]
Gender Aging	-Being male and being older are directly associated with onychomycosis in diabetics	[331,336]

Diabetics with onychomycosis have a greater risk of having a diabetic foot ulcer [336,337,339,340], as confirmed by numerous studies. In Germany, Eckhard and colleagues [337] found that out of 95 patients with type 1 DM, 84.6% had a fungal infection. The most frequent *Candida* sp. found were *C. albicans*, *C. parapsilosis*, and *C. guilliermondii*, followed by *C. lipolytica*, *C. catenulate*, and *C. famata*. In another study conducted at the Umm Al-Qura University, Makkah, Saudi Arabia from June 2011 to June 2012, the antimicrobial susceptibility of the most common bacterial and fungal infections among infected diabetic patients (foot infections) was determined. All *Candida* sp. showed susceptibility to amphotericin B, econazole, fluconazole, ketoconazole, and nystatin (100% each) [340]. Cases with *Candida* sp. co-infection were also observed in patients with fungal nail infections—both cutaneous and nail infections [337]. Lugo-Somolinos et al. [334] performed a cross-sectional study in Japan and revealed that 51.3% of patients with DM had onychomycosis of the toenails. In this particular case, *C. albicans* was more prevalent in the control group (24% vs. 15% in the DM patients) and nail thickness was significantly associated with an elevated HbA1c value [334]. Gupta et al. [341] reported that there was a 2.77-fold greater risk for diabetic subjects than for healthy individuals to have toenail onychomycosis. In the same year, a previous study in Taiwan reported that 60.5% of onychomycosis was caused by dermatophytes, 31.5% by *Candida* sp., and 8% by non-dermatophyte molds [342]. A total of 20 patients with onychomycosis had concomitant DM. Regarding gender, in diabetic males, the most common pathogens were dermatophytes (58.3%), while in diabetic females, *Candida* sp. was more prevalent (87.5%) [342]. However, on the contrary, Dogra and colleagues found that in Indian diabetics, yeasts were the most common isolate (48.1%), followed by dermatophytes (37%) and non-dermatophyte molds (14.8%) [336]. The authors concluded that diabetics had a 2.5 times greater probability of having onychomycosis when compared to the controls [336]. Chang et al. [331] studied 1245 Taiwanese patients with DM. Among them, 30.76% were reported to suffer from onychomycosis. In this investigation, the diagnosis of onychomycosis was limited to a general histopathologic examination (KOH stain) of the toenails. Therefore, the patients may have been affected by *Candida* sp. and by other fungi. Another study performed by Pierard et al. [335] investigated onychomycosis in 100 DM patients on chronic hemodialysis, showing that 39% of participants had a nail disease. *Candida* sp. was the second most prevalent pathogen (15%), and the authors concluded that diabetics on hemodialysis had about an 88% greater probability of acquiring onychomycosis than non-diabetics [335]. Another report by Wijesuriya and colleagues [338] described the etiological agents causing superficial fungal foot infections (SFFI) in patients with type 2 DM for one year. Their results demonstrated that 295 patients had SFFI and that, among patients with diabetes, more than 10 showed a prevalence of SFFI of 98%. *Aspergillus niger* was the most common pathogen, followed by *C. albicans*. Aging, gender, the duration of diabetes, and less-controlled glycemic levels were significantly associated with SFFIs [338].

A 2018 study explored the differential expression of toll-like receptor 2 (TLR2) and interleukin (IL)-8 secretion by keratinocytes in diabetic patients when challenged with *C. albicans*. Wang et al. [343] determined that the expression levels of both TLR2 and IL-8 increased and then decreased in the control and the diabetic groups, but in different dynamics. The observations revealed that TLR2 and IL-8 act on the keratinocytes interacting with *C. albicans*, and high glucose status can distress the function of HaCaT cells by reducing the secretion of IL-8 and TLR2. The study clearly supports the immunosuppression state that diabetic patients live in [343].

Adherence to the vascular endothelium, neutrophil chemotaxis, phagocytosis and opsonization, intracellular bactericidal activity, and cell-mediated immunity are all decreased in DM patients with hyperglycemia [344,345]. Regarding this matter, Souza et al. [346] treated diabetic rats with aminoguanidine (AMG, an inhibitor of protein glycation) and evaluated neutrophil reactive oxygen species (ROS) generation and *C. albicans* killing ability in order to evaluate the effects of hyperglycemia and the glycation of proteins on the NOX2 (phagocyte NADPH oxidase) activity of neutrophils and its implications for cellular physiology. The authors indicated that AMG increased the NOX2 response and microbicidal activity by neutrophils of the diabetic status. AMG seems to be a promising therapeutic answer for these patients [346].

In another interesting recent in vivo report, the interference of diabetic conditions in diabetic mice and the relation to the progress of *C. albicans* infection and anti-inflammatory response was evaluated. Compared to non-diabetic mice, diabetic mice indicated a significantly lower density of F4/80 and M2 macrophages, higher fungal burden, and deficiency in cytokine responses. *C. albicans* also increased tissue injury, highlighting significant deviations in diabetic animal responses to *C. albicans* infection that may be critical to the pathophysiological processes supporting cutaneous candidiasis in diabetic patients [347].

Several other pathologies related to *Candida* sp. have also been linked to a DM predisposition. Researchers often recognize the importance of DM in the development of the pathology due to immunosuppression issues [348]. The reports are summarized in Table 5.

Table 5. Physiopathology and etiology related to the occurrence of other diseases linked to *Candida* sp. in diabetics.

Condition	Physiopathology	*Candida* sp. Found in the Study	Reference (s)
Arterial infection	-Direct invasion or haematogenous spread of *Candida* sp. to the vessels wall (less common): a. infection of a pre-existing aneurysm (most possible from atherosclerotic) with fungi after an episode of candidemia b. contained fungal infection of the arterial wall (linked mostly to intravenous drug abuse).	*C. albicans* *C. tropicalis* *C. parapsilosis* Other *Candida* sp. (*not specified*)	[348–357]
Endophthalmitis	- Uncontrolled DM concomitant with other co-morbidities	*C. albicans*	[358]
Cholecystitis	- Uncontrolled DM concomitant with other co-morbidities	*C. famata*	[359]
Skin abscesses	- Uncontrolled DM concomitant with other co-morbidities	*C. albicans*	[360,361]
Brain abscesses	-Immunocompromised states and poorly-controlled diabetes (the role of DM as an immunosuppressive condition in this particular case is uncertain)	*C. albicans* *C. parapsilosis* *C. tropicalis* *C. guilliermondi* Other *Candida* sp. (*not specified*)	[362–364]
Fungal infections after liver transplantation	- Chronically high blood sugar may be a predisposing factor (among other factors)	*C. albicans*	[365]
Peritonitis		*C. haemulonii* *C. glabrata* Other *Candida* sp. (*not specified*)	[366–368]
Penile prosthesis Infections	- Uncontrolled DM concomitant with other co-morbidities	Other *Candida* sp. (*not specified*)	[369–372]
Balanitis		*C. albicans*	[373]
Fournier's gangrene		*Candida* sp. (*not specified*)	[374]
Chronic obstructive pulmonary disease		*C. ciferrii*	[375]

4. Diabetes Mellitus In Vivo Models

Diabetes mellitus is a serious epidemic disease, and the research for new therapies is becoming critical. Thus, the correct choice of the animal models is of vital importance for the validity of the reported studies.

In DM type 1, the choices range from chemical ablation of the pancreatic β-cells to animals with spontaneously developing autoimmune diabetes. In DM type 2, the animal models can be both obese and non-obese animals with varying degrees of insulin resistance and beta cell failure [376]. The animal models (e.g., species, strain, gender, genetic) of DM type 1 and type 2 have diverse purposes, and the choice of a model depends on the purpose of the study (e.g., applied for pharmacological or genetics studies and understanding disease mechanisms) [376–381]. Table 6 summarizes the main animal models used in diabetes mellitus in vivo studies.

Table 6. Main animal models used in diabetes mellitus studies [376].

Diabetes Mellitus	Model/Induction	Studies	Features
Type 1	*Chemical induction*		
	High dose streptozotocin	New formulations of insulin	Hyperglicaemia model
	Alloxan	Transplantation	Induced insulitis
	Multiple low dose streptozotocin	Treatment to prevent β-cell death	
	Spontaneous autoimmune		
	NOD mice	Understanding genetic mechanisms	Autoimmune β-cell destruction
	BB rats		
	LEW.1AR1/-iddm rats	Treatment to prevent β-cell death or to manipulate autoimmune processes	
	Genetically Induced		
	AKITA rats*	New formulations of insulin Transplantation Treatment to prevent ER stress	β-cell destruction due to ER + Insulin dependent
	Virally induction		
	Coxsackie B virus		
	Encephalomyocarditis virus	Study of potencial role of viruses in DM type 1	Viral β-cell destruction
	Kilham rat virus		
	Lymphocytic choriomeningitis virus (LCMV) under insulin promoter		
Type 2	*Monogenic—obese models*		
		Obese-induced hyperglycemia	
	$Lep^{ob/ob}$ mice	Treatment to improve insulin resistance	
	$Lepr^{db/db}$ mice	Treatment to improve β-cell resistance	
	KDF rats		
	Polygenic—obese models		
	KK mice	Treatment to insulin resistance	
	OLEFT rat	Treatment to improve β-cell function	
	NZO mice	Some models show diabetic complications	
	TallyHO/Jng mice		
	NoncNZO10/l LtJ mice		
	Induced obesity		
	High fat feeding (mice or rats)	Treatment to insulin resistance	
	Nile grass rat	Treatment to prevent diet-induced obesity	
	Desert gerbil	Treatment to improve β-cell function	

* can be also used as a DM type 2 model.

5. Conclusions

Diabetes mellitus is a severe metabolic chronic disease that is most prevalent in developed countries. The general immunocompromised state with an often-poor glucose control often leads to secondary diseases in DM individuals. The biofilm fungal infections in diabetic patients are recognized to be more complicated to treat than they are in healthy patients, especially if related to medical devices. Among the candidiasis, oral diseases are the most frequent infections that occur in DM patients, as well as VVC and, more seriously, systemic candidiasis. The reports of these cases and the results of the elected therapeutic are extremely important if we are to continue to treat these patients in the most effective manner.

Author Contributions: C.F.R. and M.E.R. made the literature review and analyzed the data; C.F.R., M.E.R., and M.H. wrote the paper.

Funding: This study was supported by the Portuguese Foundation for Science and Technology (FCT) under the scope of: the strategic funding of UID/BIO/04469/2013 unit, COMPETE 2020 (POCI-01-0145-FEDER-006684) and BioTecNorte operation (NORTE-01-0145-FEDER-000004) funded by the European Regional Development Fund under the scope of Norte2020-Programa Operacional Regional do Norte, financially supported by project UID/EQU/00511/2019 - Laboratory for Process Engineering, Environment, Biotechnology and Energy – LEPABE funded by national funds through FCT/MCTES (PIDDAC), and by Célia F. Rodrigues' [SFRH/BD/93078/2013] PhD grant and M. Elisa Rodrigues [SFRH/BPD/95401/2013] post-doc grant.

Acknowledgments: The authors would like to thank Liliana Araújo, from the Imperial College, London, for reviewing the English.

Conflicts of Interest: The authors declare no conflict of interest. The founding sponsors had no role in the design of the study, in the collection, analyses, or interpretation of data, in the writing of the manuscript, or in the decision to publish the results.

References

1. Willis, A.M.; Coulter, W.A.; Fulton, C.R.; Hayes, J.R.; Bell, P.M.; Lamey, P.J. Oral candidal carriage and infection in insulin-treated diabetic patients. *Diabet. Med. J. Br. Diabet. Assoc.* **1999**, *16*, 675–679. [CrossRef]
2. Karaa, A.; Goldstein, A. The spectrum of clinical presentation, diagnosis, and management of mitochondrial forms of diabetes. *Pediatr. Diabetes* **2015**, *16*, 1–9. [CrossRef] [PubMed]
3. Calvet, H.M.; Yoshikawa, T.T. Infections in diabetes. *Infect. Dis. Clin. N. Am.* **2001**, *15*, 407–421. [CrossRef]
4. Type 2 Diabetes: Prevention in People at High Risk | NICE Public Health Guideline 38—NICE. Available online: https://www.nice.org.uk/guidance/ph38/resources/type-2-diabetes-prevention-in-people-at-high-risk-pdf-1996304192197 (accessed on 11 September 2018).
5. Blake, R.; Trounce, I.A. Mitochondrial dysfunction and complications associated with diabetes. *Biochim. Biophys. Acta Gen. Subj.* **2014**, *1840*, 1404–1412. [CrossRef] [PubMed]
6. Tang, X.; Luo, Y.-X.; Chen, H.-Z.; Liu, D.-P. Mitochondria, endothelial cell function, and vascular diseases. *Front. Physiol.* **2014**, *5*, 175. [CrossRef] [PubMed]
7. Martin, S.D.; McGee, S.L. The role of mitochondria in the aetiology of insulin resistance and type 2 diabetes. *Biochim. Biophys. Acta Gen. Subj.* **2014**, *1840*, 1303–1312. [CrossRef]
8. King, H.; Aubert, R.E.; Herman, W.H. Global burden of diabetes, 1995-2025: Prevalence, numerical estimates, and projections. *Diabetes Care* **1998**, *21*, 1414–1431. [CrossRef]
9. Agarwal, S.; Raman, R.; Paul, P.G.; Rani, P.K.; Uthra, S.; Gayathree, R.; McCarty, C.; Kumaramanickavel, G.; Sharma, T. Sankara Nethralaya—Diabetic Retinopathy Epidemiology and Molecular Genetic Study (SN—DREAMS 1): Study Design and Research Methodology. *Ophthalmic Epidemiol.* **2005**, *12*, 143–153. [CrossRef]
10. De Resende, M.A.; de Sousa, L.V.N.F.; de Oliveira, R.C.B.W.; Koga-Ito, C.Y.; Lyon, J.P. Prevalence and Antifungal Susceptibility of Yeasts Obtained from the Oral Cavity of Elderly Individuals. *Mycopathologia* **2006**, *162*, 39–44. [CrossRef]
11. Guimarães, T.; Nucci, M.; Mendonça, J.S.; Martinez, R.; Brito, L.R.; Silva, N.; Moretti, M.L.; Salomão, R.; Colombo, A.L. Epidemiology and predictors of a poor outcome in elderly patients with candidemia. *Int. J. Infect. Dis.* **2012**, *16*, 442–447. [CrossRef]
12. Khosravi, A.R.; Yarahmadi, S.; Baiat, M.; Shokri, H.; Pourkabireh, M. Factors affecting the prevalence of yeasts in the oral cavity of patients with diabetes mellitus. *J. Mycol. Médicale J. Med. Mycol.* **2008**, *18*, 83–88. [CrossRef]
13. Tang, H.J.; Liu, W.L.; Lin, H.L.; Lai, C.C. Epidemiology and prognostic factors of candidemia in elderly patients. *Geriatr. Gerontol. Int.* **2015**, *15*, 688–693. [CrossRef]
14. Belazi, M.; Velegraki, A.; Fleva, A.; Gidarakou, I.; Papanaum, L.; Baka, D.; Daniilidou, N.; Karamitsos, D. Candidal overgrowth in diabetic patients: Potential predisposing factors. *Mycoses* **2005**, *48*, 192–196. [CrossRef] [PubMed]

15. Darwazeh, A.M.G.; Lamey, P.-J.; Samaranayake, L.P.; Macfarlane, T.W.; Fisher, B.M.; Macrury, S.M.; Maccuish, A.C. The relationship between colonisation, secretor status and in-vitro adhesion of Candida albicans to buccal epithelial cells from diabetics. *J. Med. Microbiol.* **1990**, *33*, 43–49. [CrossRef] [PubMed]
16. Gonçalves, R.H.P.; Miranda, E.T.; Zaia, J.E.; Giannini, M.J.S.M. Species diversity of yeast in oral colonization of insulin-treated diabetes mellitus patients. *Mycopathologia* **2006**, *162*, 83–89. [CrossRef] [PubMed]
17. Gudlaugsson, O.; Gillespie, S.; Lee, K.; Vande Berg, J.; Hu, J.; Messer, S.; Herwaldt, L.; Pfaller, M.; Diekema, D. Attributable mortality of nosocomial candidemia, revisited. *Clin. Infect. Dis.* **2003**, *37*, 1172–1177. [CrossRef] [PubMed]
18. Kumar, B.V.; Padshetty, N.S.; Bai, K.Y.; Rao, M.S. Prevalence of Candida in the oral cavity of diabetic subjects. *J. Assoc. Physicians India* **2005**, *53*, 599–602. [PubMed]
19. Davenport, J.C. The oral distribution of candida in denture stomatitis. *Br. Dent. J.* **1970**, *129*, 151–156. [CrossRef]
20. Flier, J.S.; Underhill, L.H.; Brownlee, M.; Cerami, A.; Vlassara, H. Advanced Glycosylation End Products in Tissue and the Biochemical Basis of Diabetic Complications. *N. Engl. J. Med.* **1988**, *318*, 1315–1321. [CrossRef]
21. Kadir, T.; Pisiriciler, R.; Akyüz, S.; Yarat, A.; Emekli, N.; Ipbüker, A. Mycological and cytological examination of oral candidal carriage in diabetic patients and non-diabetic control subjects: Thorough analysis of local aetiologic and systemic factors. *J. Oral Rehabil.* **2002**, *29*, 452–457. [CrossRef]
22. Wilson, R.M.; Reeves, W.G. Neutrophil phagocytosis and killing in insulin-dependent diabetes. *Clin. Exp. Immunol.* **1986**, *63*, 478–484. [PubMed]
23. Duggan, S.; Essig, F.; Hünniger, K.; Mokhtari, Z.; Bauer, L.; Lehnert, T.; Brandes, S.; Häder, A.; Jacobsen, I.D.; Martin, R.; et al. Neutrophil activation by Candida glabrata but not Candida albicans promotes fungal uptake by monocytes. *Cell. Microbiol.* **2015**, *17*, 1259–1276. [CrossRef] [PubMed]
24. Motta-Silva, A.C.; Aleva, N.A.; Chavasco, J.K.; Armond, M.C.; França, J.P.; Pereira, L.J. Erythematous Oral Candidiasis in Patients with Controlled Type II Diabetes Mellitus and Complete Dentures. *Mycopathologia* **2010**, *169*, 215–223. [CrossRef] [PubMed]
25. Calderone, R.A.; Fonzi, W.A. Virulence factors of Candida albicans. *Trends Microbiol.* **2001**, *9*, 327–335. [CrossRef]
26. Pinto, E.; Ribeiro, I.C.; Ferreira, N.J.; Fortes, C.E.; Fonseca, P.A.; Figueiral, M.H. Correlation between enzyme production, germ tube formation and susceptibility to fluconazole in Candida species isolated from patients with denture-related stomatitis and control individuals. *J. Oral Pathol. Med.* **2008**, *37*, 587–592. [CrossRef]
27. Dorko, E.; Baranová, Z.; Jenča, A.; Kizek, P.; Pilipčinec, E.; Tkáčiková, L. Diabetes mellitus and candidiases. *Folia Microbiol.* **2005**, *50*, 255–261. [CrossRef]
28. Nowakowska, D.; Kurnatowska, A.; Stray-Pedersen, B.; Wilczyński, J. Species distribution and influence of glycemic control on fungal infections in pregnant women with diabetes. *J. Infect.* **2004**, *48*, 339–346. [CrossRef]
29. Hammad, M.M.; Darwazeh, A.M.G.; Idrees, M.M. The effect of glycemic control on Candida colonization of the tongue and the subgingival plaque in patients with type II diabetes and periodontitis. *Oral Surg. Oral Med. Oral Pathol. Oral Radiol.* **2013**, *116*, 321–326. [CrossRef]
30. Al Mubarak, S.; Robert, A.A.; Baskaradoss, J.K.; Al-Zoman, K.; Al Sohail, A.; Alsuwyed, A.; Ciancio, S. The prevalence of oral Candida infections in periodontitis patients with type 2 diabetes mellitus. *J. Infect. Public Health* **2013**, *6*, 296–301.
31. Balan, P.; Castelino, R.L.; Fazil Areekat, B.K. Candida Carriage Rate and Growth Characteristics of Saliva in Diabetes Mellitus Patients: A Case-Control Study. *J. Dent. Res. Dent. Clin. Dent. Prospect.* **2015**, *9*, 274–279. [CrossRef]
32. Gürsoy, S.; Koçkar, T.; Atik, S.U.; Önal, Z.; Önal, H.; Adal, E. Autoimmunity and intestinal colonization by Candida albicans in patients with type 1 diabetes at the time of the diagnosis. *Korean J. Pediatr.* **2018**, *61*, 217–220. [CrossRef] [PubMed]
33. Bommanavar, S.; Gugwad, S.; Malik, N. Phenotypic switch: The enigmatic white-gray-opaque transition system of Candida albicans. *J. Oral Maxillofac. Pathol.* **2017**, *21*, 82. [CrossRef] [PubMed]
34. Vaarala, O.; Atkinson, M.A.; Neu, J. The "Perfect Storm" for Type 1 Diabetes: The Complex Interplay Between Intestinal Microbiota, Gut Permeability, and Mucosal Immunity. *Diabetes* **2008**, *57*, 2555–2562. [CrossRef] [PubMed]

35. Sapone, A.; de Magistris, L.; Pietzak, M.; Clemente, M.G.; Tripathi, A.; Cucca, F.; Lampis, R.; Kryszak, D.; Cartenì, M.; Generoso, M.; et al. Zonulin upregulation is associated with increased gut permeability in subjects with type 1 diabetes and their relatives. *Diabetes* **2006**, *55*, 1443–1449. [CrossRef] [PubMed]
36. Gosiewski, T.; Salamon, D.; Szopa, M.; Sroka, A.; Malecki, M.T.; Bulanda, M. Quantitative evaluation of fungi of the genus Candida in the feces of adult patients with type 1 and 2 diabetes—A pilot study. *Gut Pathog.* **2014**, *6*, 43. [CrossRef]
37. Soyucen, E.; Gulcan, A.; Aktuglu-Zeybek, A.C.; Onal, H.; Kiykim, E.; Aydin, A. Differences in the gut microbiota of healthy children and those with type 1 diabetes. *Pediatr. Int.* **2014**, *56*, 336–343. [CrossRef] [PubMed]
38. Kowalewska, B.; Zorena, K.; Szmigiero-Kawko, M.; Wąż, P.; Myśliwiec, M. High Interleukin-12 Levels May Prevent an Increase in the Amount of Fungi in the Gastrointestinal Tract during the First Years of Diabetes Mellitus Type 1. *Dis. Mark.* **2016**, *2016*, 1–10. [CrossRef]
39. Abelson, J.A.; Moore, T.; Bruckner, D.; Deville, J.; Nielsen, K. Frequency of Fungemia in Hospitalized Pediatric Inpatients Over 11 Years at a Tertiary Care Institution. *Pediatrics* **2005**, *116*, 61–67. [CrossRef]
40. Costa, S.F.; Marinho, I.; Araújo, E.A.; Manrique, A.E.; Medeiros, E.A.; Levin, A.S. Nosocomial fungaemia: A 2-year prospective study. *J. Hosp. Infect.* **2000**, *45*, 69–72. [CrossRef]
41. Lopes Colombo, A.; Nucci, M.; Salomão, R.; Branchini, M.L.M.; Richtmann, R.; Derossi, A.; Wey, S.B. High rate of non-albicans candidemia in Brazilian tertiary care hospitals. *Diagn. Microbiol. Infect. Dis.* **1999**, *34*, 281–286. [CrossRef]
42. Wang, H.; Liu, N.; Yin, M.; Han, H.; Yue, J.; Zhang, F.; Shan, T.; Guo, H.; Wu, D. The epidemiology, antifungal use and risk factors of death in elderly patients with candidemia: A multicentre retrospective study. *BMC Infect. Dis.* **2014**, *14*, 609. [CrossRef] [PubMed]
43. Rodrigues, C.F.; Rodrigues, M.; Silva, S.; Henriques, M. Candida glabrata Biofilms: How Far Have We Come? *J. Fungi* **2017**, *3*, 11. [CrossRef]
44. Silva, S.; Rodrigues, C.F.; Araújo, D.; Rodrigues, M.; Henriques, M. Candida Species Biofilms' Antifungal Resistance. *J. Fungi* **2017**, *3*, 8. [CrossRef] [PubMed]
45. Pappas, P.G.; Kauffman, C.A.; Andes, D.R.; Clancy, C.J.; Marr, K.A.; Ostrosky-Zeichner, L.; Reboli, A.C.; Schuster, M.G.; Vazquez, J.A.; Walsh, T.J.; et al. Clinical Practice Guideline for the Management of Candidiasis: 2016 Update by the Infectious Diseases Society of America. *Clin. Infect. Dis.* **2015**, *62*, e1–e50. [CrossRef] [PubMed]
46. Hedayati, M.T.; Tavakoli, M.; Zakavi, F.; Shokohi, T.; Mofarrah, R.; Ansari, S.; Armaki, M.T. In vitro antifungal susceptibility of Candida speciesisolated from diabetic patients. *Rev. Soc. Bras. Med. Trop.* **2018**, *51*, 542–545. [CrossRef] [PubMed]
47. Puig-Asensio, M.; Padilla, B.; Garnacho-Montero, J.; Zaragoza, O.; Aguado, J.M.; Zaragoza, R.; Montejo, M.; Muñoz, P.; Ruiz-Camps, I.; Cuenca-Estrella, M.; et al. Epidemiology and predictive factors for early and late mortality in Candida bloodstream infections: A population-based surveillance in Spain. *Clin. Infect. Dis.* **2014**, *20*, O245–O254. [CrossRef] [PubMed]
48. Meunier-Carpentier, F.; Kiehn, T.E.; Armstrong, D. Fungemia in the immunocompromised host. Changing patterns, antigenemia, high mortality. *Am. J. Med.* **1981**, *71*, 363–370. [CrossRef]
49. Dimopoulos, G.; Karabinis, A.; Samonis, G.; Falagas, M.E. Candidemia in immunocompromised and immunocompetent critically ill patients: A prospective comparative study. *Eur. J. Clin. Microbiol. Infect. Dis.* **2007**, *26*, 377–384. [CrossRef]
50. Man, A.; Ciurea, C.N.; Pasaroiu, D.; Savin, A.-I.; Toma, F.; Sular, F.; Santacroce, L.; Mare, A. New perspectives on the nutritional factors influencing growth rate of Candida albicans in diabetics. An in vitro study. *Mem. Inst. Oswaldo Cruz* **2017**, *112*, 587–592. [CrossRef]
51. Barnett, J.A. The Utilization of Disaccharides and Some Other Sugars RY Yeasts. *Adv. Carbohydr. Chem. Biochem.* **1981**, *39*, 347–404.
52. Rodrigues, C.F.; Henriques, M. Oral mucositis caused by Candida glabrata biofilms: Failure of the concomitant use of fluconazole and ascorbic acid. *Ther. Adv. Infect. Dis.* **2017**, *1*, 1–8. [CrossRef] [PubMed]
53. Mandal, S.M.; Mahata, D.; Migliolo, L.; Parekh, A.; Addy, P.S.; Mandal, M.; Basak, A. Glucose directly promotes antifungal resistance in the fungal pathogen, Candida spp. *J. Biol. Chem.* **2014**, *289*, 25468–25473. [CrossRef] [PubMed]

54. Rodaki, A.; Bohovych, I.M.; Enjalbert, B.; Young, T.; Odds, F.C.; Gow, N.A.R.; Brown, A.J.P. Glucose Promotes Stress Resistance in the Fungal Pathogen Candida albicans. *Mol. Biol. Cell* **2009**, *20*, 4845–4855. [CrossRef] [PubMed]
55. Bramono, K.; Yamazaki, M.; Tsuboi, R.; Ogawa, H. Comparison of proteinase, lipase and alpha-glucosidase activities from the clinical isolates of Candida species. *Jpn. J. Infect. Dis.* **2006**, *59*, 73–76.
56. Ingham, C.J.; Boonstra, S.; Levels, S.; de Lange, M.; Meis, J.F.; Schneeberger, P.M. Rapid Susceptibility Testing and Microcolony Analysis of Candida spp. Cultured and Imaged on Porous Aluminum Oxide. *PLoS ONE* **2012**, *7*, e33818. [CrossRef]
57. Manfredi, M.; McCullough, M.J.; Al-Karaawi, Z.M.; Hurel, S.J.; Porter, S.R. The isolation, identification and molecular analysis of Candida spp. isolated from the oral cavities of patients with diabetes mellitus. *Oral Microbiol. Immunol.* **2002**, *17*, 181–185. [CrossRef]
58. Soysa, N.S.; Samaranayake, L.P.; Ellepola, A.N.B. Diabetes mellitus as a contributory factor in oral candidosis. *Diabet. Med.* **2006**, *23*, 455–459. [CrossRef] [PubMed]
59. Tsang, C.S.P.; Chu, F.C.S.; Leung, W.K.; Jin, L.J.; Samaranayake, L.P.; Siu, S.C. Phospholipase, proteinase and haemolytic activities of Candida albicans isolated from oral cavities of patients with type 2 diabetes mellitus. *J. Med. Microbiol.* **2007**, *56*, 1393–1398. [CrossRef] [PubMed]
60. Manns, J.M.; Mosser, D.M.; Buckley, H.R. Production of a hemolytic factor by Candida albicans. *Infect. Immun.* **1994**, *62*, 5154–5156.
61. Fatahinia, M.; Poormohamadi, F.; Mahmoudabadi, A.Z. Comparative study of esterase and hemolytic activities in clinically important Candida species, isolated from oral cavity of diabetic and non-diabetic individuals. *Jundishapur J. Microbiol.* **2015**, *8*, 3–6. [CrossRef]
62. Shimizu, M.T.; Almeida, N.Q.; Fantinato, V.; Unterkircher, C.S. Studies on hyaluronidase, chondroitin sulphatase, proteinase and phospholipase secreted by Candida species. *Mycoses* **1996**, *39*, 161–167. [CrossRef] [PubMed]
63. Naglik, J.R.; Challacombe, S.J.; Hube, B. Candida albicans secreted aspartyl proteinases in virulence and pathogenesis. *Microbiol. Mol. Biol. Rev.* **2003**, *67*, 400–428. [CrossRef] [PubMed]
64. Naglik, J.; Albrecht, A.; Bader, O.; Hube, B. Candida albicans proteinases and host/pathogen interactions. *Cell. Microbiol.* **2004**, *6*, 915–926. [CrossRef] [PubMed]
65. Kaminishi, H.; Tanaka, M.; Cho, T.; Maeda, H.; Hagihara, Y. Activation of the plasma kallikrein-kinin system by Candida albicans proteinase. *Infect. Immun.* **1990**, *58*, 2139–2143. [PubMed]
66. Kaminishi, H.; Miyaguchi, H.; Tamaki, T.; Suenaga, N.; Hisamatsu, M.; Mihashi, I.; Matsumoto, H.; Maeda, H.; Hagihara, Y. Degradation of humoral host defense by Candida albicans proteinase. *Infect. Immun.* **1995**, *63*, 984–988.
67. Ghannoum, M.A. Potential role of phospholipases in virulence and fungal pathogenesis. *Clin. Microbiol. Rev.* **2000**, *13*, 122–143. [CrossRef] [PubMed]
68. Moyes, D.L.; Wilson, D.; Richardson, J.P.; Mogavero, S.; Tang, S.X.; Wernecke, J.; Höfs, S.; Gratacap, R.L.; Robbins, J.; Runglall, M.; et al. Candidalysin is a fungal peptide toxin critical for mucosal infection. *Nature* **2016**, *532*, 64. [CrossRef]
69. Naglik, J.R.; König, A.; Hube, B.; Gaffen, S.L. Candida albicans–epithelial interactions and induction of mucosal innate immunity. *Curr. Opin. Microbiol.* **2017**, *40*, 104–112. [CrossRef]
70. Costerton, J.W.; Lewandowski, Z.; Caldwell, D.E.; Korber, D.R.; Lappin-Scott, H.M. Microbial Biofilms. *Annu. Rev. Microbiol.* **1995**, *49*, 711–745. [CrossRef]
71. Donlan, R.; Costerton, J. Biofilms: Survival mechanisms of clinically relevant microorganisms. *Clin. Microbiol. Rev.* **2002**, *15*, 167–193. [CrossRef]
72. Fonseca, E.; Silva, S.; Rodrigues, C.F.; Alves, C.; Azeredo, J.; Henriques, M. Effects of fluconazole on Candida glabrata biofilms and its relationship with ABC transporter gene expression. *Biofouling* **2014**, *30*, 447–457. [CrossRef] [PubMed]
73. Rodrigues, C.F.; Silva, S.; Henriques, M. Candida glabrata: A review of its features and resistance. *Eur. J. Clin. Microbiol. Infect. Dis.* **2014**, *33*, 673–688. [CrossRef] [PubMed]
74. Chandra, J.; Mukherjee, P.K. Candida Biofilms: Development, Architecture, and Resistance. *Microbiol. Spectr.* **2015**, *3*, 157–176. [CrossRef] [PubMed]

75. Kojic, E.M.E.M.; Darouiche, R.O.R.O. Candida infections of medical devices. *Clin. Microbiol. Rev.* **2004**, *17*, 255–267. [CrossRef] [PubMed]
76. Falagas, M.E.; Roussos, N.; Vardakas, K.Z. Relative frequency of albicans and the various non-albicans Candida spp among candidemia isolates from inpatients in various parts of the world: A systematic review. *Int. J. Infect. Dis.* **2010**, *14*, e954–e966. [CrossRef] [PubMed]
77. Seneviratne, C.J.; Jin, L.; Samaranayake, L.P. Biofilm lifestyle of Candida: A mini review. *Oral Dis.* **2008**, *14*, 582–590. [CrossRef] [PubMed]
78. Douglas, L.J. Candida biofilms and their role in infection. *Trends Microbiol.* **2003**, *11*, 30–36. [CrossRef]
79. Mermel, L.A.; Allon, M.; Bouza, E.; Craven, D.E.; Flynn, P.; O'Grady, N.P.; Raad, I.I.; Rijnders, B.J.A.; Sherertz, R.J.; Warren, D.K. Clinical practice guidelines for the diagnosis and management of intravascular catheter-related infection: 2009 Update by the Infectious Diseases Society of America. *Clin. Infect. Dis.* **2009**, *49*, 1–45. [CrossRef]
80. Nucci, M.; Anaissie, E.; Betts, R.F.; Dupont, B.F.; Wu, C.; Buell, D.N.; Kovanda, L.; Lortholary, O. Early Removal of Central Venous Catheter in Patients with Candidemia Does Not Improve Outcome: Analysis of 842 Patients from 2 Randomized Clinical Trials. *Clin. Infect. Dis.* **2010**, *51*, 295–303. [CrossRef] [PubMed]
81. Chandra, J.; Kuhn, D.; Mukherjee, P.; Hoyer, L.; McCormick, T.; Ghannoum, M. Biofilm formation by the fungal pathogen Candida albicans: Development, architecture, and drug resistance. *J. Bacteriol.* **2001**, *183*, 5385–5394. [CrossRef] [PubMed]
82. Ramage, G.; Saville, S.P.; Thomas, D.P.; López-Ribot, J.L. Candida biofilms: An update. *Eukaryot. Cell* **2005**, *4*, 633–638. [CrossRef] [PubMed]
83. Andes, D.; Nett, J.; Oschel, P.; Albrecht, R.; Marchillo, K.; Pitula, A. Development and characterization of an in vivo central venous catheter Candida albicans biofilm model. *Infect. Immun.* **2004**, *72*, 6023–6031. [CrossRef] [PubMed]
84. Mukherjee, P.K.; Chandra, J. Candida biofilm resistance. *Drug Resist. Updat.* **2004**, *7*, 301–309. [CrossRef] [PubMed]
85. Nett, J.; Lepak, A.; Marchillo, K.; Andes, D. Time course global gene expression analysis of an in vivo Candida biofilm. *J. Infect. Dis.* **2009**, *200*, 307–313. [CrossRef] [PubMed]
86. Pierce, C.; Vila, T.; Romo, J.; Montelongo-Jauregui, D.; Wall, G.; Ramasubramanian, A.; Lopez-Ribot, J. The Candida albicans Biofilm Matrix: Composition, Structure and Function. *J. Fungi* **2017**, *3*, 14. [CrossRef] [PubMed]
87. Rajendran, R.; Robertson, D.P.; Hodge, P.J.; Lappin, D.F.; Ramage, G. Hydrolytic Enzyme Production is Associated with Candida Albicans Biofilm Formation from Patients with Type 1 Diabetes. *Mycopathologia* **2010**, *170*, 229–235. [CrossRef]
88. Hoyer, L.L.; Cota, E. Candida albicans agglutinin-like sequence (Als) family vignettes: A review of als protein structure and function. *Front. Microbiol.* **2016**, *7*, 280. [CrossRef]
89. Rauceo, J.M.; Gaur, N.K.; Lee, K.-G.; Edwards, J.E.; Klotz, S.A.; Lipke, P.N. Global Cell Surface Conformational Shift Mediated by a Candida albicans Adhesin. *Infect. Immun.* **2004**, *72*, 4948–4955. [CrossRef]
90. Zakikhany, K.; Naglik, J.R.; Schmidt-Westhausen, A.; Holland, G.; Schaller, M.; Hube, B. In vivo transcript profiling of Candida albicans identifies a gene essential for interepithelial dissemination. *Cell. Microbiol.* **2007**, *9*, 2938–2954. [CrossRef]
91. Zhao, X.; Oh, S.-H.; Cheng, G.; Green, C.B.; Nuessen, J.A.; Yeater, K.; Leng, R.P.; Brown, A.J.P.; Hoyer, L.L. ALS3 and ALS8 represent a single locus that encodes a Candida albicans adhesin; functional comparisons between Als3p and Als1p. *Microbiology* **2004**, *150*, 2415–2428. [CrossRef]
92. Zhao, X.; Oh, S.-H.; Yeater, K.M.; Hoyer, L.L. Analysis of the Candida albicans Als2p and Als4p adhesins suggests the potential for compensatory function within the Als family. *Microbiology* **2005**, *151*, 1619–1630. [CrossRef] [PubMed]
93. Zhao, X.; Oh, S.-H.; Hoyer, L.L. Deletion of *ALS5*, *ALS6* or *ALS7* increases adhesion of *Candida albicans* to human vascular endothelial and buccal epithelial cells. *Med. Mycol.* **2007**, *45*, 429–434. [CrossRef] [PubMed]
94. Richardson, J.; Ho, J.; Naglik, J. Candida–Epithelial Interactions. *J. Fungi* **2018**, *4*, 22. [CrossRef] [PubMed]
95. De Las Peñas, A.; Pan, S.-J.; Castaño, I.; Alder, J.; Cregg, R.; Cormack, B.P. Virulence-related surface glycoproteins in the yeast pathogen Candida glabrata are encoded in subtelomeric clusters and subject to RAP1- and SIR-dependent transcriptional silencing. *Genes Dev.* **2003**, *17*, 2245–2258. [CrossRef] [PubMed]

96. Castano, I.; Pan, S.; Zupancic, M.; Hennequin, C.; Dujon, B.; Cormack, B. Telomere length control and transcriptional regulation of subtelomeric adhesins in Candida glabrata. *Mol. Microbiol.* **2005**, *55*, 1246–1258. [CrossRef]
97. Silva-Dias, A.; Miranda, I.M.; Branco, J.; Monteiro-Soares, M.; Pina-Vaz, C.; Rodrigues, A.G. Adhesion, biofilm formation, cell surface hydrophobicity, and antifungal planktonic susceptibility: Relationship among Candida spp. *Front. Microbiol.* **2015**, *6*, 205. [CrossRef] [PubMed]
98. De Groot, P.W.J.; Kraneveld, E.A.; Yin, Q.Y.; Dekker, H.L.; Gross, U.; Crielaard, W.; de Koster, C.G.; Bader, O.; Klis, F.M.; Weig, M. The cell wall of the human pathogen Candida glabrata: Differential incorporation of novel adhesin-like wall proteins. *Eukaryot. Cell* **2008**, *7*, 1951–1964. [CrossRef] [PubMed]
99. Ogasawara, A.; Odahara, K.; Toume, M.; Watanabe, T.; Mikami, T.; Matsumoto, T. Change in the respiration system of Candida albicans in the lag and log growth phase. *Biol. Pharm. Bull.* **2006**, *29*, 448–450. [CrossRef]
100. Sardi, J.C.O.; Duque, C.; Höfling, J.F.; Gonçalves, R.B. Genetic and phenotypic evaluation of Candida albicans strains isolated from subgingival biofilm of diabetic patients with chronic periodontitis. *Med. Mycol.* **2012**, *50*, 467–475. [CrossRef]
101. Calderone, R.A.; Braun, P.C. Adherence and receptor relationships of Candida albicans. *Microbiol. Rev.* **1991**, *55*, 1–20.
102. Silva, T.M.; Glee, P.M.; Hazen, K.C. Influence of cell surface hydrophobicity on attachment of Candida albicans to extracellular matrix proteins. *J. Med. Vet. Mycol.* **1995**, *33*, 117–122. [CrossRef] [PubMed]
103. Rodrigues, A.G.; Mårdh, P.A.; Pina-Vaz, C.; Martinez-de-Oliveira, J.; Fonseca, A.F. Germ tube formation changes surface hydrophobicity of Candida cells. *Infect. Dis. Obstet. Gynecol.* **1999**, *7*, 222–226. [CrossRef] [PubMed]
104. Akpan, A.; Morgan, R. Oral candidiasis. *Postgrad. Med. J.* **2002**, *78*, 455–459. [CrossRef] [PubMed]
105. Neville, B.W.; Damm, D.D.; Allen, C.M.; Chi, A.C. Oral and maxillofacial pathology. In *In Fungal and Protozoal Diseases*; Elsevier: London, UK, 2011; pp. 213–221.
106. Regezi, J.A.; Sciubba, J.J.; Jordan, R.C.K. Oral pathology clinical pathologic correlations. In *White Lesions*; Elsevier: St. Louis, MO, USA, 2008; pp. 98–102.
107. Lott, T.J.; Holloway, B.P.; Logan, D.A.; Fundyga, R.; Arnold, J. Towards understanding the evolution of the human commensal yeast Candida albicans. *Microbiology* **1999**, *145*, 1137–1143. [CrossRef] [PubMed]
108. Van der Meer, J.W.M.; van de Veerdonk, F.L.; Joosten, L.A.B.; Kullberg, B.-J.; Netea, M.G. Severe Candida spp. infections: New insights into natural immunity. *Int. J. Antimicrob. Agents* **2010**, *36*, S58–S62. [CrossRef] [PubMed]
109. Javed, F.; Klingspor, L.; Sundin, U.; Altamash, M.; Klinge, B.; Engström, P.-E. Periodontal conditions, oral Candida albicans and salivary proteins in type 2 diabetic subjects with emphasis on gender. *BMC Oral Health* **2009**, *9*, 12. [CrossRef]
110. Lamey, P.J.; Darwaza, A.; Fisher, B.M.; Samaranayake, L.P.; Macfarlane, T.W.; Frier, B.M. Secretor status, candidal carriage and candidal infection in patients with diabetes mellitus. *J. Oral Pathol.* **1988**, *17*, 354–357. [CrossRef]
111. Mulu, A.; Kassu, A.; Anagaw, B.; Moges, B.; Gelaw, A.; Alemayehu, M.; Belyhun, Y.; Biadglegne, F.; Hurissa, Z.; Moges, F.; et al. Frequent detection of 'azole' resistant Candida species among late presenting AIDS patients in northwest Ethiopia. *BMC Infect. Dis.* **2013**, *13*, 82. [CrossRef]
112. Goregen, M.; Miloglu, O.; Buyukkurt, M.C.; Caglayan, F.; Aktas, A.E. Median rhomboid glossitis: A clinical and microbiological study. *Eur. J. Dent.* **2011**, *5*, 367–372.
113. Arendorf, T.M.; Walker, D.M. Tobacco smoking and denture wearing as local aetiological factors in median rhomboid glossitis. *Int. J. Oral Surg.* **1984**, *13*, 411–415. [CrossRef]
114. Flaitz, C.M.; Nichols, C.M.; Hicks, M.J. An overview of the oral manifestations of AIDS-related Kaposi's sarcoma. *Compend. Contin. Educ. Dent.* **1995**, *16*, 136–138. [PubMed]
115. Sanitá, P.V.; Zago, C.E.; Pavarina, A.C.; Jorge, J.H.; Machado, A.L.; Vergani, C.E. Enzymatic activity profile of a Brazilian culture collection of Candida albicans isolated from diabetics and non-diabetics with oral candidiasis. *Mycoses* **2014**, *57*, 351–357. [PubMed]
116. Samaranayake, L.P.; Raeside, J.M.; MacFarlane, T.W. Factors affecting the phospholipase activity of Candida species in vitro. *Sabouraudia* **1984**, *22*, 201–207. [CrossRef]

117. Lyon, J.P.; de Resende, M.A. Correlation between adhesion, enzyme production, and susceptibility to fluconazole in Candida albicans obtained from denture wearers. *Oral Surg. Oral Med. Oral Pathol. Oral Radiol. Endodontol.* **2006**, *102*, 632–638. [CrossRef]
118. Arslan, S.; Koç, A.N.; Şekerci, A.E.; Tanriverdi, F.; Sav, H.; Aydemir, G.; Diri, H. Genotypes and virulence factors of Candida species isolated from oralcavities of patients with type 2 diabetes mellitus. *Turkish J. Med. Sci.* **2016**, *46*, 18–27. [CrossRef] [PubMed]
119. Koga-Ito, C.Y.; Lyon, J.P.; Vidotto, V.; de Resende, M.A. Virulence Factors and Antifungal Susceptibility of Candida albicans Isolates from Oral Candidosis Patients and Control Individuals. *Mycopathologia* **2006**, *161*, 219–223. [CrossRef] [PubMed]
120. D'Eça Júnior, A.; Silva, A.F.; Rosa, F.C.; Monteiro, S.G.; de Maria Silva Figueiredo, P.; de Andrade Monteiro, C. In vitro differential activity of phospholipases and acid proteinases of clinical isolates of Candida. *Rev. Soc. Bras. Med. Trop.* **2011**, *44*, 334–338. [CrossRef] [PubMed]
121. Manfredi, M.; McCullough, M.J.; Al-Karaawi, Z.M.; Vescovi, P.; Porter, S.R. In vitro evaluation of virulence attributes of Candida spp. isolated from patients affected by diabetes mellitus. *Oral Microbiol. Immunol.* **2006**, *21*, 183–189. [CrossRef]
122. De Menezes Thiele, M.C.; de Paula E Carvalho, A.; Gursky, L.C.; Rosa, R.T.; Samaranayake, L.P.; Rosa, E.A.R. The role of candidal histolytic enzymes on denture-induced stomatitis in patients living in retirement homes. *Gerodontology* **2008**, *25*, 229–236. [CrossRef]
123. Negri, M.; Martins, M.; Henriques, M.; Svidzinski, T.I.E.; Azeredo, J.; Oliveira, R. Examination of Potential Virulence Factors of Candida tropicalis Clinical Isolates From Hospitalized Patients. *Mycopathologia* **2010**, *169*, 175–182. [CrossRef]
124. Sánchez-Vargas, L.O.; Estrada-Barraza, D.; Pozos-Guillen, A.J.; Rivas-Caceres, R. Biofilm formation by oral clinical isolates of Candida species. *Arch. Oral Biol.* **2013**, *58*, 1318–1326. [CrossRef] [PubMed]
125. Rodrigues, C.F.; Rodrigues, M.; Henriques, M. Susceptibility of Candida glabrata biofilms to echinocandins: Alterations in the matrix composition. *Biofouling* **2018**, *34*, 569–578. [CrossRef] [PubMed]
126. Rodrigues, C.F.; Henriques, M. Portrait of Matrix Gene Expression in Candida glabrata Biofilms with Stress Induced by Different Drugs. *Genes* **2018**, *9*, 205. [CrossRef] [PubMed]
127. Walker, L.A.; Gow, N.A.R.; Munro, C.A. Elevated chitin content reduces the susceptibility of Candida species to caspofungin. *Antimicrob. Agents Chemother.* **2013**, *57*, 146–154. [CrossRef] [PubMed]
128. Samaranayake, L.P.; Hughes, A.; Weetman, D.A.; MacFarlane, T.W. Growth and acid production of Candida species in human saliva supplemented with glucose. *J. Oral Pathol.* **1986**, *15*, 251–254. [CrossRef] [PubMed]
129. Samaranayake, L.P.; MacFarlane, T.W. An in-vitro study of the adherence of Candida albicans to acrylic surfaces. *Arch. Oral Biol.* **1980**, *25*, 603–609. [CrossRef]
130. Pallavan, B.; Ramesh, V.; Dhanasekaran, B.P.; Oza, N.; Indu, S.; Govindarajan, V. Comparison and correlation of candidal colonization in diabetic patients and normal individuals. *J. Diabetes Metab. Disord.* **2014**, *13*, 66. [CrossRef]
131. Zomorodian, K.; Kavoosi, F.; Pishdad, G.R.; Mehriar, P.; Ebrahimi, H.; Bandegani, A.; Pakshir, K. Prevalence of oral Candida colonization in patients with diabetes mellitus. *J. Mycol. Med.* **2016**, *26*, 103–110. [CrossRef]
132. Buysschaert, M.; Medina, J.L.; Bergman, M.; Shah, A.; Lonier, J. Prediabetes and associated disorders. *Endocrine* **2015**, *48*, 371–393. [CrossRef]
133. Javed, F.; Ahmed, H.B.; Mehmood, A.; Saeed, A.; Al-Hezaimi, K.; Samaranayake, L.P. Association between glycemic status and oral Candida carriage in patients with prediabetes. *Oral Surg. Oral Med. Oral Pathol. Oral Radiol.* **2014**, *117*, 53–58. [CrossRef]
134. Darwazeh, A.M.; MacFarlane, T.W.; McCuish, A.; Lamey, P.J. Mixed salivary glucose levels and candidal carriage in patients with diabetes mellitus. *J. Oral Pathol. Med.* **1991**, *20*, 280–283. [CrossRef] [PubMed]
135. Yar Ahmadi, S.; Khosravi, A.; Larijani, B.; Baiat, M.; Mahmoudi, M.; Baradar Jalili, R. Assessment of the fungal flora and the prevalence of fungal infections in the mouth of diabetics. *Iran. J. Endocrinol. Metab.* **2002**, *4*, 105–109.
136. Fisher, B.M.; Lamey, P.J.; Samaranayake, L.P.; MacFarlane, T.W.; Frier, B.M. Carriage of Candida species in the oral cavity in diabetic patients: Relationship to glycaemic control. *J. Oral Pathol.* **1987**, *16*, 282–284. [CrossRef] [PubMed]
137. Sahin, I.; Oksuz, S.; Sencan, I.; Gulcan, A.; Karabay, O.; Gulcan, E.; Yildiz, O. Prevalance and risk factors for yeast colonization in adult diabetic patients. *Ethiop. Med. J.* **2005**, *43*, 103–109. [PubMed]

138. Kjellman, O. Secretion rate and buffering action of whole mixed saliva in subjects with insulin-treated diabetes mellitus. *Odontol. Revy* **1970**, *21*, 159–168.
139. Costa, A.L.; Silva, B.M.A.; Soares, R.; Mota, D.; Alves, V.; Mirante, A.; Ramos, J.C.; Maló de Abreu, J.; Santos-Rosa, M.; Caramelo, F.; et al. Type 1 diabetes in children is not a predisposing factor for oral yeast colonization. *Med. Mycol.* **2016**, *55*, 358–367. [CrossRef]
140. Reinhart, H.; Muller, G.; Sobel, J.D. Specificity and mechanism of in vitro adherence of Candida albicans. *Ann. Clin. Lab. Sci.* **1985**, *15*, 406–413.
141. Samaranayake, L.P.; Macfarlane, T.W. The Effect of Dietary Carbohydrates on the In-vitro Adhesion of Candida Albicans to Epithelial Cells. *J. Med. Microbiol.* **1982**, *15*, 511–517. [CrossRef]
142. Naik, R.; Ahmed Mujib, B.R.; Raaju, U.R.; Telagi, N. Assesing oral candidal carriage with mixed salivary glucose levels as non-invasive diagnostic tool in type-2 Diabetics of Davangere, Karnataka, India. *J. Clin. Diagn. Res.* **2014**, *8*, 69–72.
143. Sashikumar, R.; Kannan, R. Salivary glucose levels and oral candidal carriage in type II diabetics. *Oral Surg. Oral Med. Oral Pathol. Oral Radiol. Endodontol.* **2010**, *109*, 706–711. [CrossRef]
144. Geerlings, S.E.; Hoepelman, A.I. Immune dysfunction in patients with diabetes mellitus (DM). *FEMS Immunol. Med. Microbiol.* **1999**, *26*, 259–265. [CrossRef] [PubMed]
145. Ferguson, D. The physiology and biology of saliva. In *Color Atlas and Text of Salivary Gland: Disease, Disorders and Surgery*; deBurgh Norman, J., McGurk, M., Eds.; Mosby-Wolfe: London, UK, 1995; pp. 40–48.
146. Panchbhai, A.S.; Degwekar, S.S.; Bhowte, R.R. Estimation of salivary glucose, salivary amylase, salivary total protein and salivary flow rate in diabetics in India. *J. Oral Sci.* **2010**, *52*, 359–368. [CrossRef] [PubMed]
147. Dorocka-Bobkowska, B.; Budtz-Jörgensen, E.; Włoch, S. Non-insulin-dependent diabetes mellitus as a risk factor for denture stomatitis. *J. Oral Pathol. Med.* **1996**, *25*, 411–415. [CrossRef] [PubMed]
148. Samaranayake, L.P.; MacFarlane, T.W. Factors affecting the in-vitro adherence of the fungal oral pathogen Candida albicans to epithelial cells of human origin. *Arch. Oral Biol.* **1982**, *27*, 869–873. [CrossRef]
149. Mantri, S.P.S.S.P.; Parkhedkar, R.D.; Mantri, S.P.S.S.P. Candida colonisation and the efficacy of chlorhexidine gluconate on soft silicone-lined dentures of diabetic and non-diabetic patients. *Gerodontology* **2013**, *30*, 288–295. [CrossRef] [PubMed]
150. Knight, L.; Fletcher, J. Growth of Candida albicans in saliva: Stimulation by glucose associated with antibiotics, corticosteroids, and diabetes mellitus. *J. Infect. Dis.* **1971**, *123*, 371–377. [CrossRef] [PubMed]
151. Malic, S.; Hill, K.E.; Ralphs, J.R.; Hayes, A.; Thomas, D.W.; Potts, A.J.; Williams, D.W. Characterization of Candida albicans infection of an in vitro oral epithelial model using confocal laser scanning microscopy. *Oral Microbiol. Immunol.* **2007**, *22*, 188–194. [CrossRef]
152. Wang, J.; Ohshima, T.; Yasunari, U.; Namikoshi, S.; Yoshihara, A.; Miyazaki, H.; Maeda, N. The carriage of Candida species on the dorsal surface of the tongue: The correlation with the dental, periodontal and prosthetic status in elderly subjects. *Gerodontology* **2006**, *23*, 157–163. [CrossRef]
153. Maria Beatriz Ribeiro Cardoso; Eliana Campêlo Lago. Oral Changes in Elderly from an Association Center. *Rev. Para. Med. V* **2010**, *24*, 35–41.
154. Bianchi, C.M.; Bianchi, H.A.; Tadano, T.; Depaula, C.R.; Hoffmann-Santos, H.D.; Leite, D.P.; Hahn, R.C. Factors related to oral candidiasis in elderly users and non-users of removable dental prostheses. *Rev. Inst. Med. Trop. Sao Paulo* **2016**, *58*, 6–10. [CrossRef]
155. Prado Leite, D.; Rabello Piva, M.; Ricardo Saquete Martins-Filho, P. Identification of Candida species in patients with denture stomatitis and evaluation of susceptibility to miconazole and photodynamic therapy. *Rev. Odontol. UNESP* **2015**, *44*, 12–17.
156. Da Silva Santos, J.; Batista, S.A.; Silva, A., Jr.; Ferreira, M.F.; Agostini, M.; Torres, S.R. Oral candidiasis in patients admitted to ICU. *Rev. Bras. Odontol.* **2014**, *71*, 176–179.
157. Scalercio, M.; Valente, T.; Israel, M.S.; Ramos, M.E. Denture stomatitis associated with candidiasis: Diagnosis and treatment. *RGO* **2007**, *44*, 395–398.
158. Khovidhunkit, S.P.; Suwantuntula, T.; Thaweboon, S.; Mitrirattanakul, S.; Chomkhakhai, U.; Khovidhunkit, W. Xerostomia, hyposalivation, and oral microbiota in type 2 diabetic patients: A preliminary study. *J. Med. Assoc. Thail.* **2009**, *92*, 1220–1228.
159. Sudbery, P.; Gow, N.; Berman, J. The distinct morphogenic states of Candida albicans. *Trends Microbiol.* **2004**, *12*, 317–324. [CrossRef] [PubMed]

160. Aitken-Saavedra, J.; Lund, R.G.; González, J.; Huenchunao, R.; Perez-Vallespir, I.; Morales-Bozo, I.; Urzúa, B.; Tarquinio, S.C.; Maturana-Ramírez, A.; Martos, J.; et al. Diversity, frequency and antifungal resistance of *Candida* species in patients with type 2 diabetes mellitus. *Acta Odontol. Scand.* **2018**, *76*, 580–586. [CrossRef]
161. Lydia Rajakumari, M.; Saravana Kumari, P. Prevalence of Candida species in the buccal cavity of diabetic and non-diabetic individuals in and around Pondicherry. *J. Mycol. Med.* **2016**, *26*, 359–367. [CrossRef]
162. Premkumar, J.; Ramani, P.; Chandrasekar, T.; Natesan, A.; Premkumar, P. Detection of species diversity in oral candida colonization and anti-fungal susceptibility among non-oral habit adult diabetic patients. *J. Nat. Sci. Biol. Med.* **2014**, *5*, 148. [CrossRef]
163. Bremenkamp, R.M.; Caris, A.R.; Jorge, A.O.C.; Back-Brito, G.N.; Mota, A.J.; Balducci, I.; Brighenti, F.L.; Koga-Ito, C.Y. Prevalence and antifungal resistance profile of Candida spp. oral isolates from patients with type 1 and 2 diabetes mellitus. *Arch. Oral Biol.* **2011**, *56*, 549–555. [CrossRef]
164. Manfredi, M.; McCullough, M.J.; Polonelli, L.; Conti, S.; Al-Karaawi, Z.M.; Vescovi, P.; Porter, S.R. In vitro antifungal susceptibility to six antifungal agents of 229 Candida isolates from patients with diabetes mellitus. *Oral Microbiol. Immunol.* **2006**, *21*, 177–182. [CrossRef]
165. Sanitá, P.V.; De Oliveira Mima, E.G.; Pavarina, A.C.; Jorge, J.H.; Machado, A.L.; Vergani, C.E. Susceptibility profile of a Brazilian yeast stock collection of Candida species isolated from subjects with Candida-associated denture stomatitis with or without diabetes. *Oral Surg. Oral Med. Oral Pathol. Oral Radiol.* **2013**, *116*, 562–569. [CrossRef] [PubMed]
166. Al-Attas, S.; Amro, S. Candidal colonization, strain diversity, and antifungal susceptibility among adult diabetic patients. *Ann. Saudi Med.* **2010**, *30*, 101. [CrossRef] [PubMed]
167. Indira, P.; Kumar, P.M.; Shalini, S.; Vaman, K. Opportunistic infections among People Living with HIV (PLHIV) with Diabetes Mellitus (DM) attending a tertiary care hospital in coastal city of South India. *PLoS ONE* **2015**, *10*, 4–11. [CrossRef]
168. Scully, C.; Monteil, R.; Sposto, M.R. Infectious and tropical diseases affecting the human mouth. *Periodontology 2000* **1998**, *18*, 47–70. [CrossRef] [PubMed]
169. Stanford, T.W.; Rivera-Hidalgo, F. Oral mucosal lesions caused by infective microorganisms. II. Fungi and parasites. *Periodontology 2000* **1999**, *21*, 125–144. [CrossRef] [PubMed]
170. Löe, H. Periodontal disease. The sixth complication of diabetes mellitus. *Diabetes Care* **1993**, *16*, 329–334. [CrossRef] [PubMed]
171. Cullinan, M.; Ford, P.; Seymour, G. Periodontal disease and systemic health: Current status. *Aust. Dent. J.* **2009**, *54*, S62–S69. [CrossRef] [PubMed]
172. Olczak-Kowalczyk, D.; Pyrżak, B.; Dąbkowska, M.; Pańczyk-Tomaszewska, M.; Miszkurka, G.; Rogozińska, I.; Swoboda-Kopeć, E.; Gozdowski, D.; Kalińska, A.; Piróg, A.; et al. Candida spp. and gingivitis in children with nephrotic syndrome or type 1 diabetes. *BMC Oral Health* **2015**, *15*, 57. [CrossRef]
173. Lotfi-Kamran, M.H.; Jafari, A.A.; Falah-Tafti, A.; Tavakoli, E.; Falahzadeh, M.H. Candida Colonization on the Denture of Diabetic and Non-diabetic Patients. *Dent. Res. J.* **2009**, *6*, 23–27.
174. Urzúa, B.; Hermosilla, G.; Gamonal, J.; Morales-Bozo, I.; Canals, M.; Barahona, S.; Cóccola, C.; Cifuentes, V. Yeast diversity in the oral microbiota of subjects with periodontitis: *Candida albicans* and *Candida dubliniensis* colonize the periodontal pockets. *Med. Mycol.* **2008**, *46*, 783–793. [CrossRef]
175. Sardi, J.; Duque, C.; Mariano, F.; Peixoto, I.; Hofling, J.; Gonçalves, R.B. Candida spp. in periodontal disease: A brief review. *J. Oral Sci.* **2010**, *52*, 177–185. [CrossRef] [PubMed]
176. Järvensivu, A.; Hietanen, J.; Rautemaa, R.; Sorsa, T.; Richardson, M. Candida yeasts in chronic periodontitis tissues and subgingival microbial biofilms in vivo. *Oral Dis.* **2004**, *10*, 106–112. [CrossRef] [PubMed]
177. Slots, J.; Rams, T.E.; Listgarten, M.A. Yeasts, enteric rods and pseudomonads in the subgingival flora of severe adult periodontitis. *Oral Microbiol. Immunol.* **1988**, *3*, 47–52. [CrossRef] [PubMed]
178. Reynaud, A.H.; Nygaard-Østby, B.; Bøygard, G.K.; Eribe, E.R.; Olsen, I.; Gjermo, P. Yeasts in periodontal pockets. *J. Clin. Periodontol.* **2001**, *28*, 860–864. [CrossRef] [PubMed]
179. Ergun, S.; Cekici, A.; Topcuoglu, N.; Migliari, D.-A.; Külekçi, G.; Tanyeri, H.; Isik, G. Oral status and Candida colonization in patients with Sjögren's Syndrome. *Med. Oral Patol. Oral Cir. Bucal* **2010**, *15*, e310–e315. [CrossRef] [PubMed]

180. Sardi, J.C.O.; Duque, C.; Camargo, G.A.C.G.; Hofling, J.F.; Gonçalves, R.B. Periodontal conditions and prevalence of putative periodontopathogens and Candida spp. in insulin-dependent type 2 diabetic and non-diabetic patients with chronic periodontitis—A pilot study. *Arch. Oral Biol.* **2011**, *56*, 1098–1105. [CrossRef] [PubMed]
181. Barros, L.M.; Boriollo, M.F.G.; Alves, A.C.B.A.; Klein, M.I.; Gonçalves, R.B.; Höfling, J.F. Genetic diversity and exoenzyme activities of Candida albicans and Candida dubliniensis isolated from the oral cavity of Brazilian periodontal patients. *Arch. Oral Biol.* **2008**, *53*, 1172–1178. [CrossRef] [PubMed]
182. Javed, F.; Thafeed AlGhamdi, A.S.; Mikami, T.; Mehmood, A.; Ahmed, H.B.; Samaranayake, L.P.; Tenenbaum, H.C. Effect of Glycemic Control on Self-Perceived Oral Health, Periodontal Parameters, and Alveolar Bone Loss Among Patients With Prediabetes. *J. Periodontol.* **2014**, *85*, 234–241. [CrossRef] [PubMed]
183. Javed, F.; Samaranayake, L.P.; Al-Askar, M.; Al-Hezaimi, K. Periodontal Disease in Habitual Cigarette Smokers and Nonsmokers With and Without Prediabetes. *Am. J. Med. Sci.* **2013**, *345*, 94–98. [CrossRef] [PubMed]
184. Javed, F.; Tenenbaum, H.C.; Nogueira-Filho, G.; Nooh, N.; O'Bello Correa, F.; Warnakulasuriya, S.; Dasanayake, A.P.; Al-Hezaimi, K. Periodontal Inflammatory Conditions Among Gutka Chewers and Non-chewers With and Without Prediabetes. *J. Periodontol.* **2013**, *84*, 1158–1164. [CrossRef] [PubMed]
185. Javed, F.; Al-Askar, M.; Al-Rasheed, A.; Al-Hezaimi, K.; Babay, N.; Galindo-Moreno, P. Comparison of Self-Perceived Oral Health, Periodontal Inflammatory Conditions and Socioeconomic Status in Individuals With and Without Prediabetes. *Am. J. Med. Sci.* **2012**, *344*, 100–104. [CrossRef] [PubMed]
186. Javed, F.; Näsström, K.; Benchimol, D.; Altamash, M.; Klinge, B.; Engström, P.-E. Comparison of Periodontal and Socioeconomic Status Between Subjects With Type 2 Diabetes Mellitus and Non-Diabetic Controls. *J. Periodontol.* **2007**, *78*, 2112–2119. [CrossRef]
187. Javed, F.; Romanos, G.E. Impact of Diabetes Mellitus and Glycemic Control on the Osseointegration of Dental Implants: A Systematic Literature Review. *J. Periodontol.* **2009**, *80*, 1719–1730. [CrossRef] [PubMed]
188. Bader, M.S.; Hinthorn, D.; Lai, S.M.; Ellerbeck, E.F. Hyperglycaemia and mortality of diabetic patients with candidaemia. *Diabet. Med.* **2005**, *22*, 1252–1257. [CrossRef]
189. Oztürkcan, S.; Oztürkcan, S.; Topçu, S.; Akinci, S.; Bakici, M.Z.; Yalçin, N. Incidence of oral candidiasis in diabetic patients. *Mikrobiyol. Bülteni* **1993**, *27*, 352–356.
190. Rodero, L.; Davel, G.; Soria, M.; Vivot, W.; Córdoba, S.; Canteros, C.E.; Saporiti, A.; EMIFN. [Multicenter study of fungemia due to yeasts in Argentina]. *Rev. Argent. Microbiol.* **2005**, *37*, 189–195. [PubMed]
191. Saes Busato, I.M.; Bittencourt, M.S.; Machado, M.Â.N.; Grégio, A.M.T.; Azevedo-Alanis, L.R. Association between metabolic control and oral health in adolescents with type 1 diabetes mellitus. *Oral Surg. Oral Med. Oral Pathol. Oral Radiol. Endodontol.* **2010**, *109*, e51–e56. [CrossRef]
192. Weykamp, C. HbA1c: A review of analytical and clinical aspects. *Ann. Lab. Med.* **2013**, *33*, 393–400. [CrossRef]
193. Marsh, P.D. Microbial Ecology of Dental Plaque and its Significance in Health and Disease. *Adv. Dent. Res.* **1994**, *8*, 263–271. [CrossRef]
194. Brook, I. Bacterial Interference. *Crit. Rev. Microbiol.* **1999**, *25*, 155–172. [CrossRef]
195. He, X.; McLean, J.S.; Guo, L.; Lux, R.; Shi, W. The social structure of microbial community involved in colonization resistance. *ISME J.* **2014**, *8*, 564–574. [CrossRef]
196. Roberts, F.A.; Darveau, R.P. Microbial protection and virulence in periodontal tissue as a function of polymicrobial communities: Symbiosis and dysbiosis. *Periodontology 2000* **2015**, *69*, 18–27. [CrossRef]
197. Ley, R.E.; Hamady, M.; Lozupone, C.; Turnbaugh, P.J.; Ramey, R.R.; Bircher, J.S.; Schlegel, M.L.; Tucker, T.A.; Schrenzel, M.D.; Knight, R.; et al. Evolution of Mammals and Their Gut Microbes. *Science* **2008**, *320*, 1647–1651. [CrossRef] [PubMed]
198. Mima, E.G.G.; Vergani, C.E.E.; Machado, A.L.L.; Massucato, E.M.S.M.S.; Colombo, A.L.L.; Bagnato, V.S.S.; Pavarina, A.C.C. Comparison of Photodynamic Therapy versus conventional antifungal therapy for the treatment of denture stomatitis: A randomized clinical trial. *Clin. Microbiol. Infect.* **2012**, *18*, E380–E388. [CrossRef] [PubMed]
199. Sanit, P.V.; Pavarina, A.C.; Giampaolo, E.T.; Silva, M.M.; De Oliveira Mima, E.G.; Ribeiro, D.G.; Vergani, C.E. Candida spp. prevalence in well controlled type 2 diabetic patients with denture stomatitis. *Oral Surg. Oral Med. Oral Pathol. Oral Radiol. Endodontol.* **2011**, *111*, 726–733. [CrossRef] [PubMed]

200. Sanita, P.V.; Machado, A.L.; Pavarina, A.C.; Massucato, E.M.S.; Colombo, A.L.; Vergani, C.E. Microwave denture disinfection versus nystatin in treating patients with well-controlled type 2 diabetes and denture stomatitis: A randomized clinical trial. *Int. J. Prosthodont.* **2012**, *25*, 232–244.
201. Silva, M.M.; Mima, E.G.; Colombo, A.L.; Sanitá, P.V.; Jorge, J.H.; Massucato, E.M.S.; Vergani, C.E. Comparison of denture microwave disinfection and conventional antifungal therapy in the treatment of denture stomatitis: A randomized clinical study. *Oral Surg. Oral Med. Oral Pathol. Oral Radiol.* **2012**, *114*, 469–479. [CrossRef]
202. Melo, A.S.; Bizerra, F.C.; Freymüller, E.; Arthington-Skaggs, B.A.; Colombo, A.L. Biofilm production and evaluation of antifungal susceptibility amongst clinical *Candida* spp. isolates, including strains of the *Candida parapsilosis* complex. *Med. Mycol.* **2011**, *49*, 253–262. [CrossRef]
203. Iacopino, A.M.; Wathen, W.F. Oral candidal infection and denture stomatitis: A comprehensive review. *J. Am. Dent. Assoc.* **1992**, *123*, 46–51. [CrossRef]
204. Artico, G.; Freitas, R.; Santos Filho, A.; Benard, G.; Romiti, R.; Migliari, D. Prevalence of *Candida* spp., xerostomia, and hyposalivation in oral lichen planus—A controlled study. *Oral Dis.* **2014**, *20*, e36–e41. [CrossRef]
205. Willis, A.M.; Coulter, W.A.; Sullivan, D.J.; Coleman, D.C.; Hayes, J.R.; Bell, P.M.; Lamey, P.J. Isolation of C. dubliniensis from insulin-using diabetes mellitus patients. *J. Oral Pathol. Med.* **2000**, *29*, 86–90. [CrossRef] [PubMed]
206. Coco, B.J.; Bagg, J.; Cross, L.J.; Jose, A.; Cross, J.; Ramage, G. Mixed Candida albicans and Candida glabrata populations associated with the pathogenesis of denture stomatitis. *Oral Microbiol. Immunol.* **2008**, *23*, 377–383. [CrossRef] [PubMed]
207. Marcos-Arias, C.; Vicente, J.L.; Sahand, I.H.; Eguia, A.; De-Juan, A.; Madariaga, L.; Aguirre, J.M.; Eraso, E.; Quindós, G. Isolation of Candida dubliniensis in denture stomatitis. *Arch. Oral Biol.* **2009**, *54*, 127–131. [CrossRef] [PubMed]
208. Vanden Abbeele, A.; de Meel, H.; Ahariz, M.; Perraudin, J.-P.; Beyer, I.; Courtois, P. Denture contamination by yeasts in the elderly. *Gerodontology* **2008**, *25*, 222–228. [CrossRef] [PubMed]
209. Webb, B.C.; Thomas, C.J.; Whittle, T. A 2-year study of Candida-associated denture stomatitis treatment in aged care subjects. *Gerodontology* **2005**, *22*, 168–176. [CrossRef] [PubMed]
210. Fongsmut, T.; Deerochanawong, C.; Prachyabrued, W. Intraoral candida in Thai diabetes patients. *J. Med. Assoc. Thail.* **1998**, *81*, 449–453.
211. Darwazeh, A.-G.; Hammad, M.; Al-Jamaei, A. The relationship between oral hygiene and oral colonization with *Candida* species in healthy adult subjects. *Int. J. Dent. Hyg.* **2010**, *8*, 128–133. [CrossRef] [PubMed]
212. Machado, A.G.; Komiyama, E.Y.; Dos Santos, S.S.F.; Jorge, A.O.C.; Brighenti, F.L.; Koga-Ito, C.Y. In vitro adherence of Candida albicans isolated from patients with chronic periodontitis. *J. Appl. Oral Sci.* **2011**, *19*, 384–387. [CrossRef]
213. Rosa, E.A.R.; Rached, R.N.; Ignacio, S.A.; Rosa, R.T.; Jose da Silva, W.; Yau, J.Y.Y.; Samaranayake, L.P. Phenotypic evaluation of the effect of anaerobiosis on some virulence attributes of Candida albicans. *J. Med. Microbiol.* **2008**, *57*, 1277–1281. [CrossRef]
214. Takahashi, Y.; Nagata, N.; Shimbo, T.; Nishijima, T.; Watanabe, K.; Aoki, T.; Sekine, K.; Okubo, H.; Watanabe, K.; Sakurai, T.; et al. Long-term trends in esophageal candidiasis prevalence and associated risk factors with or without HIV infection: Lessons from an endoscopic study of 80,219 patients. *PLoS ONE* **2015**, *10*, 1–13. [CrossRef]
215. Mojazi Amiri, H.; Frandah, W.; Colmer-Hamood, J.; Raj, R.; Nugent, K. Risk factors of Candida colonization in the oropharynx of patients admitted to an intensive care unit. *J. Mycol. Med.* **2012**, *22*, 301–307. [CrossRef] [PubMed]
216. Owotade, F.J.; Patel, M.; Ralephenya, T.R.M.D.R.; Vergotine, G. Oral candida colonization in HIV-positive women: Associated factors and changes following antiretroviral therapy. *J. Med. Microbiol.* **2013**, *62*, 126–132. [CrossRef] [PubMed]
217. Terayama, Y.; Matsuura, T.; Uchida, M.; Narama, I.; Ozaki, K. Probiotic (yogurt) containing Lactobacillus gasseri OLL2716 is effective for preventing Candida albicans-induced mucosal inflammation and proliferation in the forestomach of diabetic rats. *Histol. Histopathol.* **2016**, *31*, 689–697. [PubMed]

218. Malazy, O.T.; Shariat, M.; Heshmat, R.; Majlesi, F.; Alimohammadian, M.; Tabari, N.K.; Larijani, B. Vulvovaginal candidiasis and its related factors in diabetic women. *Taiwan J. Obstet. Gynecol.* **2007**, *46*, 399–404. [CrossRef]
219. Atabek, M.E.; Akyürek, N.; Eklioglu, B.S. Frequency of Vaginal Candida Colonization and Relationship between Metabolic Parameters in Children with Type 1 Diabetes Mellitus. *J. Pediatr. Adolesc. Gynecol.* **2013**, *26*, 257–260. [CrossRef] [PubMed]
220. Bohannon, N.J. V Treatment of Vulvovaginal Candidiasis in Patients With Diabetes. *Diabetes Care* **1998**, *21*, 451. [CrossRef] [PubMed]
221. De Leon, E.M.; Jacober, S.J.; Sobel, J.D.; Foxman, B. Prevalence and risk factors for vaginal Candida colonization in women with type 1 and type 2 diabetes. *BMC Infect. Dis.* **2002**, *2*, 1. [CrossRef]
222. Reed, B.D. Risk factors for Candida vulvovaginitis. *Obstet. Gynecol. Surv.* **1992**, *47*, 551–560. [CrossRef]
223. Hoeltge, G. *Clinical Laboratory Technical Procedure Manuals*, 3rd ed.; NCCLS: Wayne, PA, USA, 1996; ISBN 9781562383152.
224. Saporiti, A.M.; Gómez, D.; Levalle, S.; Galeano, M.; Davel, G.; Vivot, W.; Rodero, L. [Vaginal candidiasis: Etiology and sensitivity profile to antifungal agents in clinical use]. *Rev. Argent. Microbiol.* **2001**, *33*, 217–222.
225. Sobel, J.D.; Chaim, W. Treatment of Torulopsis glabrata vaginitis: Retrospective review of boric acid therapy. *Clin. Infect. Dis.* **1997**, *24*, 649–652. [CrossRef]
226. Goswami, R.; Dadhwal, V.; Tejaswi, S.; Datta, K.; Paul, A.; Haricharan, R.N.; Banerjee, U.; Kochupillai, N.P. Species-specific prevalence of vaginal candidiasis among patients with diabetes mellitus and its relation to their glycaemic status. *J. Infect.* **2000**, *41*, 162–166. [CrossRef] [PubMed]
227. Nagesha, C.N.; Ananthakrishna, N.C. Clinical and laboratory study of monilial vaginitis. *Am. J. Obstet. Gynecol.* **1970**, *107*, 1267–1268. [CrossRef]
228. Grigoriou, O.; Baka, S.; Makrakis, E.; Hassiakos, D.; Kapparos, G.; Kouskouni, E. Prevalence of clinical vaginal candidiasis in a university hospital and possible risk factors. *Eur. J. Obstet. Gynecol. Reprod. Biol.* **2006**, *126*, 121–125. [CrossRef] [PubMed]
229. Achkar, J.M.; Fries, B.C. Candida infections of the genitourinary tract. *Clin. Microbiol. Rev.* **2010**, *23*, 253–273. [CrossRef] [PubMed]
230. Deorukhkar, S.C.; Saini, S.; Mathew, S. Non-albicans Candida Infection: An Emerging Threat. *Interdiscip. Perspect. Infect. Dis.* **2014**, *2014*, 615958. [CrossRef] [PubMed]
231. Lattif, A.A.; Mukhopadhyay, G.; Banerjee, U.; Goswami, R.; Prasad, R. Molecular typing and in vitro fluconazole susceptibility of Candida species isolated from diabetic and nondiabetic women with vulvovaginal candidiasis in India. *J. Microbiol. Immunol. Infect.* **2011**, *44*, 166–171. [CrossRef]
232. Gunther, L.S.A.; Martins, H.P.R.; Gimenes, F.; De Abreu, A.L.P.; Consolaro, M.E.L.; Svidzinski, T.I.E. Prevalence of Candida albicans and non-albicans isolates from vaginal secretions: Comparative evaluation of colonization, vaginal candidiasis and recurrent vaginal candidiasis in diabetic and non-diabetic women. *Sao Paulo Med. J.* **2014**, *132*, 116–120. [CrossRef]
233. Sherry, L.; Kean, R.; McKloud, E.; O'Donnell, L.E.; Metcalfe, R.; Jones, B.L.; Ramage, G. Biofilms Formed by Isolates from Recurrent Vulvovaginal Candidiasis Patients Are Heterogeneous and Insensitive to Fluconazole. *Antimicrob. Agents Chemother.* **2017**, *61*, e01065-17. [CrossRef]
234. Ray, D.; Goswami, R.; Banerjee, U.; Dadhwal, V.; Goswami, D.; Mandal, P.; Sreenivas, V.; Kochupillai, N. Prevalence of Candida glabrata and Its Response to Boric Acid Vaginal Suppositories in Comparison With Oral Fluconazole in Patients With Diabetes and Vulvovaginal Candidiasis. *Diabetes Care* **2007**, *30*, 312–317. [CrossRef]
235. Peer, A.K.; Hoosen, A.A.; Seedat, M.A.; van den Ende, J.; Omar, M.A. Vaginal yeast infections in diabetic women. *S. Afr. Med. J.* **1993**, *83*, 727–729.
236. Nyirjesy, P.; Sobel, J.D. Genital Mycotic Infections in Patients With Diabetes. *Postgrad. Med.* **2013**, *125*, 33–46. [CrossRef] [PubMed]
237. Nash, E.E.; Peters, B.M.; Lilly, E.A.; Noverr, M.C.; Fidel, P.L. A Murine Model of Candida glabrata Vaginitis Shows No Evidence of an Inflammatory Immunopathogenic Response. *PLoS ONE* **2016**, *11*, e0147969. [CrossRef] [PubMed]
238. Corrêa, P.R.; David, P.R.; Peres, N.P.; da Cunha, K.C.; de Almeida, M.T.G. [Phenotypic characterization of yeasts isolated from the vaginal mucosa of adult women]. *Rev. Bras. Ginecol. Obstet.* **2009**, *31*, 177–181.

239. Carrara, M.A.; Bazotte, R.B.; Donatti, L.; Svidzinski, T.I.E.; Consolaro, M.E.L.; Patussi, E.V.; Batista, M.R. Effect of experimental diabetes on the development and maintenance of vulvovaginal candidiasis in female rats. *Am. J. Obstet. Gynecol.* **2009**, *200*, 659.e1–659.e4. [CrossRef] [PubMed]
240. Bassyouni, R.H.; Wegdan, A.A.; Abdelmoneim, A.; Said, W.; Aboelnaga, F. Phospholipase and aspartyl proteinase activities of candida species causing vulvovaginal candidiasis in patients with type 2 diabetes mellitus. *J. Microbiol. Biotechnol.* **2015**, *25*, 1734–1741. [CrossRef] [PubMed]
241. Faraji, R.; Rahimi, A.; Rezvanmadani, F.; Hashemi, M. Prevalence of vaginal candidiasis infection in diabetic women. *Afr. J. Microbiol. Res.* **2012**, *6*, 2773–2778.
242. Yildirim, Z.; Kilic, N.; Kalkanci, A. Fluorometric determination of acid proteinase activity in Candida albicans strains from diabetic patients with vulvovaginal candidiasis. *Mycoses* **2011**, *54*, e463–e467. [CrossRef]
243. Chaffin, W.L. Candida albicans cell wall proteins. *Microbiol. Mol. Biol. Rev.* **2008**, *72*, 495–544. [CrossRef]
244. Yang, Y.-L. Virulence factors of Candida species. *J. Microbiol. Immunol. Infect.* **2003**, *36*, 223–228.
245. Samaranayake, Y.H.; Dassanayake, R.S.; Cheung, B.P.K.; Jayatilake, J.A.M.S.; Yeung, K.W.S.; Yau, J.Y.Y.; Samaranayake, L.P. Differential phospholipase gene expression by *Candida albicans* in artificial media and cultured human oral epithelium. *APMIS* **2006**, *114*, 857–866. [CrossRef]
246. Tilak, R.; Kumari, V.; Banerjee, T.; Kumar, P.; Pandey, S. Emergence of non-albicans Candida among candidal vulvovaginitis cases and study of their potential virulence factors, from a tertiary care center, North India. *Indian J. Pathol. Microbiol.* **2013**, *56*, 144. [CrossRef] [PubMed]
247. Kuştimur, S.; El-Nahi, H.; Altan, N. Virulence of Proteinase-Positive and Proteinase-Negative Candida Albicans to Mouse and Killing of the Yeast by Normal Human Leukocytes. In *Candida and Candidamycosis*; Springer US: Boston, MA, USA, 1991; pp. 159–166.
248. Kendirci, M.; Koç, A.N.; Kurtoglu, S.; Keskin, M.; Kuyucu, T. Vulvovaginal candidiasis in children and adolescents with type 1 diabetes mellitus. *J. Pediatr. Endocrinol. Metab.* **2004**, *17*, 1545–1549. [CrossRef] [PubMed]
249. Kelekci, S.; Kelekci, H.; Cetin, M.; Inan, I.; Tokucoglu, S. Glucose tolerance in pregnant women with vaginal candidiasis. *Ann. Saudi Med.* **2004**, *24*, 350–353. [CrossRef] [PubMed]
250. Nyirjesy, P.; Zhao, Y.; Ways, K.; Usiskin, K. Evaluation of vulvovaginal symptoms and Candida colonization in women with type 2 diabetes mellitus treated with canagliflozin, a sodium glucose co-transporter 2 inhibitor. *Curr. Med. Res. Opin.* **2012**, *28*, 1173–1178. [CrossRef] [PubMed]
251. Raith, L.; Csató, M.; Dobozy, A. Decreased Candida albicans killing activity of granulocytes from patients with diabetes mellitus. *Mykosen* **1983**, *26*, 557–564. [CrossRef]
252. Paramythiotou, E.; Frantzeskaki, F.; Flevari, A.; Armaganidis, A.; Dimopoulos, G. Invasive Fungal Infections in the ICU: How to Approach, How to Treat. *Molecules* **2014**, *19*, 1085–1119. [CrossRef]
253. Sobel, J.D.; Myers, P.G.; Kaye, D.; Levison, M.E. Adherence of Candida albicans to human vaginal and buccal epithelial cells. *J. Infect. Dis.* **1981**, *143*, 76–82. [CrossRef]
254. Zheng, N.N.; Guo, X.C.; Lv, W.; Chen, X.X.; Feng, G.F. Characterization of the vaginal fungal flora in pregnant diabetic women by 18S rRNA sequencing. *Eur. J. Clin. Microbiol. Infect. Dis.* **2013**, *32*, 1031–1040. [CrossRef]
255. Nowakowska, D.; Kurnatowska, A.; Stray-Pedersen, B.; Wilczyński, J. Activity of hydrolytic enzymes in fungi isolated from diabetic pregnant women: Is there any relationship between fungal alkaline and acid phosphatase activity and glycemic control? *APMIS* **2004**, *112*, 374–383. [CrossRef] [PubMed]
256. Guzel, A.B.; Ilkit, M.; Burgut, R.; Urunsak, İ.F.; Ozgunen, F.T. An Evaluation of Risk Factors in Pregnant Women with Candida Vaginitis and the Diagnostic Value of Simultaneous Vaginal and Rectal Sampling. *Mycopathologia* **2011**, *172*, 25–36. [CrossRef] [PubMed]
257. Hay, P.; Czeizel, A.E. Asymptomatic trichomonas and candida colonization and pregnancy outcome. *Best Pract. Res. Clin. Obstet. Gynaecol.* **2007**, *21*, 403–409. [CrossRef] [PubMed]
258. Spinillo, A.; Capuzzo, E.; Acciano, S.; De Santolo, A.; Zara, F. Effect of antibiotic use on the prevalence of symptomatic vulvovaginal candidiasis. *Am. J. Obstet. Gynecol.* **1999**, *180*, 14–17. [CrossRef]
259. Cotch, M.F.; Hillier, S.L.; Gibbs, R.S.; Eschenbach, D.A. Epidemiology and outcomes associated with moderate to heavy Candida colonization during pregnancy. Vaginal Infections and Prematurity Study Group. *Am. J. Obstet. Gynecol.* **1998**, *178*, 374–380. [CrossRef]
260. French, W.; Gad, A. The frequency of Candida infections in pregnancy and their treatment with clotrimazole. *Curr. Med. Res. Opin.* **1977**, *4*, 640–644. [CrossRef] [PubMed]

261. Huang, A.J.; Moore, E.E.; Boyko, E.J.; Scholes, D.; Lin, F.; Vittinghoff, E.; Fihn, S.D. Vaginal symptoms in postmenopausal women. *Menopause* **2010**, *17*, 121–126. [CrossRef]
262. Rosenstock, J.; Polidori, D.; Zhao, Y.; Al, E. Canagliflozin, an inhibitor of sodium glucose co-transporter 2, improves glycemic control, lowers body weight, and improves beta-cell function in subjects with type 2 diabetes on background metformin. In Proceedings of the 46th Annual Meeting of the European Association for the Study of Diabetes, Stockholm, Sweden, 20–24 September 2010.
263. Rosenstock, J.; Aggarwal, N.; Polidori, D.; Zhao, Y.; Arbit, D.; Usiskin, K.; Capuano, G.; Canovatchel, W. Canagliflozin DIA 2001 Study Group Dose-Ranging Effects of Canagliflozin, a Sodium-Glucose Cotransporter 2 Inhibitor, as Add-On to Metformin in Subjects With Type 2 Diabetes. *Diabetes Care* **2012**, *35*, 1232–1238. [CrossRef] [PubMed]
264. Bailey, C.J.; Gross, J.L.; Pieters, A.; Bastien, A.; List, J.F. Effect of dapagliflozin in patients with type 2 diabetes who have inadequate glycaemic control with metformin: A randomised, double-blind, placebo-controlled trial. *Lancet* **2010**, *375*, 2223–2233. [CrossRef]
265. Yokoyama, H.; Nagao, A.; Watanabe, S.; Honjo, J. Incidence and risk of vaginal candidiasis associated with sodium-glucose cotransporter 2 inhibitors in real-world practice for women with type 2 diabetes. *J. Diabetes Investig.* **2018**. [CrossRef]
266. Banerjee, K.; Curtis, E.; San Lazaro, C.; Graham, J.C. Low prevalence of genital candidiasis in children. *Eur. J. Clin. Microbiol. Infect. Dis.* **2004**, *23*, 696–698. [CrossRef]
267. Schaaf, V.M.; Perez-Stable, E.J.; Borchardt, K. The limited value of symptoms and signs in the diagnosis of vaginal infections. *Arch. Intern. Med.* **1990**, *150*, 1929–1933. [CrossRef]
268. Sonck, C.E.; Somersalo, O. The yeast flora of the anogenital region in diabetic girls. *Arch. Dermatol.* **1963**, *88*, 846–852. [CrossRef] [PubMed]
269. Sopian, I.L.; Shahabudin, S.; Ahmed, M.A.; Lung, L.T.T.; Sandai, D. Yeast Infection and Diabetes Mellitus among Pregnant Mother in Malaysia. *Malays. J. Med. Sci.* **2016**, *23*, 27–34. [PubMed]
270. Nowakowska, D.; Kurnatowska, A.; Stray-Pedersen, B.; Wilczynski, J. Prevalence of fungi in the vagina, rectum and oral cavity in pregnant diabetic women: Relation to gestational age and symptoms. *Acta Obstet. Gynecol. Scand.* **2004**, *83*, 251–256. [CrossRef] [PubMed]
271. Masri, S.N.; Noor, S.M.; Mat Nor, L.A.; Osman, M.; Rahman, M.M. Candida isolates from pregnant women and their antifungal susceptibility in a Malaysian tertiary-care hospital. *Pakistan J. Med. Sci.* **2015**, *31*, 658–661.
272. Mikamo, H.; Yamagishi, Y.; Sugiyama, H.; Sadakata, H.; Miyazaki, S.; Sano, T.; Tomita, T. High glucose-mediated overexpression of ICAM-1 in human vaginal epithelial cells increases adhesion of *Candida albicans*. *J. Obstet. Gynaecol.* **2018**, *38*, 226–230. [CrossRef]
273. Yismaw, G.; Asrat, D.; Woldeamanuel, Y.; Unakal, C. Prevalence of candiduria in diabetic patients attending Gondar University Hospital, Gondar, Ethiopia. *Iran. J. Kidney Dis.* **2013**, *7*, 102–107. [PubMed]
274. Mnif, M.F.; Kamoun, M.; Kacem, F.H.; Bouaziz, Z.; Charfi, N.; Mnif, F.; Ben Naceur, B.; Rekik, N.; Abid, M. Complicated urinary tract infections associated with diabetes mellitus: Pathogenesis, diagnosis and management. *Indian J. Endocrinol. Metab.* **2013**, *17*, 442–445.
275. Sobel, J.D. Vaginitis. *N. Engl. J. Med.* **1997**, *337*, 1896–1903. [CrossRef]
276. Esmailzadeh, A.; Zarrinfar, H.; Fata, A.; Sen, T. High prevalence of candiduria due to non- albicans Candida species among diabetic patients: A matter of concern? *J. Clin. Lab. Anal.* **2018**, *32*, e22343. [CrossRef]
277. Falahati, M.; Farahyar, S.; Akhlaghi, L.; Mahmoudi, S.; Sabzian, K.; Yarahmadi, M.; Aslani, R. Characterization and identification of candiduria due to Candida species in diabetic patients. *Curr. Med. Mycol.* **2016**, *2*, 10–14. [CrossRef]
278. Rizzi, M.; Trevisan, R. Genitourinary infections in diabetic patients in the new era of diabetes therapy with sodium-glucose cotransporter-2 inhibitors. *Nutr. Metab. Cardiovasc. Dis.* **2016**, *26*, 963–970. [CrossRef]
279. Jarvis, W.R. Epidemiology of nosocomial fungal infections, with emphasis on Candida species. *Clin. Infect. Dis.* **1995**, *20*, 1526–1530. [CrossRef]
280. Bartkowski, D.P.; Lanesky, J.R. Emphysematous prostatitis and cystitis secondary to Candida albicans. *J. Urol.* **1988**, *139*, 1063–1065. [CrossRef]
281. Vaidyanathan, S.; Soni, B.; Hughes, P.; Ramage, G.; Sherry, L.; Singh, G.; Mansour, P. Candida albicans Fungaemia following Traumatic Urethral Catheterisation in a Paraplegic Patient with Diabetes Mellitus and Candiduria Treated by Caspofungin. *Case Rep. Infect. Dis.* **2013**, *2013*, 693480. [PubMed]

282. Huang, J.J.; Tseng, C.C. Emphysematous pyelonephritis: Clinicoradiological classification, management, prognosis, and pathogenesis. *Arch. Intern. Med.* **2000**, *160*, 797–805. [CrossRef] [PubMed]
283. Grupper, M.; Kravtsov, A.; Potasman, I. Emphysematous Cystitis. *Medicine* **2007**, *86*, 47–53. [CrossRef]
284. Alansari, A.; Borras, M.D.; Boma, N. "I have chicken fat in my urine!" A case of Candida tropicalis induced emphysematous pyelitis. *Med. Mycol. Case Rep.* **2015**, *10*, 27–28. [CrossRef]
285. Wang, L.; Ji, X.; Sun, G.; Qin, Y.; Gong, M.; Zhang, J.; Li, N.; Na, Y. Fungus ball and emphysematous cystitis secondary to Candida tropicalis: A case report. *Can. Urol. Assoc. J.* **2015**, *9*, E683–E686. [CrossRef]
286. Garg, V. Comparison of Clinical Presentation and Risk Factors in Diabetic and Non- Diabetic Females with Urinary Tract Infection Assessed as Per the European Association of Urology Classification. *J. Clin. Diagnostic Res.* **2015**, *9*, PC12–PC14. [CrossRef] [PubMed]
287. Suzuki, M.; Hiramatsu, M.; Fukazawa, M.; Matsumoto, M.; Honda, K.; Suzuki, Y.; Kawabe, Y. Effect of SGLT2 inhibitors in a murine model of urinary tract infection with Candida albicans. *Diabetes Obes. Metab.* **2014**, *16*, 622–627. [CrossRef] [PubMed]
288. Tumbarello, M.; Posteraro, B.; Trecarichi, E.; Al, E. Biofilm production by Candida species and inadequate antifungal therapy as predictors of mortality for patients with candidemia. *J. Clin. Microbiol.* **2007**, *45*, 1843–1850. [CrossRef]
289. Michalopoulos, A.; Kriaras, J.; Geroulanos, S. Systemic candidiasis in cardiac surgery patients. *Eur. J. Cardiothorac. Surg.* **1997**, *11*, 728–731. [CrossRef]
290. Sievert, D.M.; Ricks, P.; Edwards, J.R.; Schneider, A.; Patel, J.; Srinivasan, A.; Kallen, A.; Limbago, B.; Fridkin, S.; National Healthcare Safety Network (NHSN) Team and Participating NHSN Facilities. Antimicrobial-Resistant Pathogens Associated with HealthcareAssociated Infections: Summary of Data Reported to the National Healthcare Safety Network at the Centers for Disease Control and Prevention, 2009–2010. *Infect. Control Hosp. Epidemiol.* **2013**, *34*, 1–14. [PubMed]
291. Muskett, H.; Shahin, J.; Eyres, G.; Harvey, S.; Rowan, K.; Harrison, D. Risk factors for invasive fungal disease in critically ill adult patients: A systematic review. *Crit. Care* **2011**, *15*, R287. [CrossRef] [PubMed]
292. Paphitou, N.I.; Ostrosky-Zeichner, L.; Rex, J.H. Rules for identifying patients at increased risk for candidal infections in the surgical intensive care unit: Approach to developing practical criteria for systematic use in antifungal prophylaxis trials. *Med. Mycol.* **2005**, *43*, 235–243. [CrossRef] [PubMed]
293. Michalopoulos, A.S.; Geroulanos, S.; Mentzelopoulos, S.D. Determinants of Candidemia and Candidemia-Related Death in Cardiothoracic ICU Patients. *Clin. Investig. Crit. Care* **2003**, *124*, 2244–2255. [CrossRef]
294. Wu, J.-Q.; Zhu, L.-P.; Ou, X.-T.; Xu, B.; Hu, X.-P.; Wang, X.; Weng, X.-H. Epidemiology and risk factors for non- Candida albicans candidemia in non-neutropenic patients at a Chinese teaching hospital. *Med. Mycol.* **2010**, *49*, 1–4. [CrossRef]
295. Pfaller, M.; Jones, R.; Doern, G.; Fluit, A.; Verhoef, J.; Sader, H.; Messer, S.; Houston, A.; Coffman, S.; Hollis, R. International surveillance of blood stream infections due to Candida species in the European SENTRY Program: Species distribution and antifungal susceptibility including the investigational triazole and echinocandin agents. SENTRY Participant Group (Euro). *Diagn. Microbiol. Infect. Dis.* **1999**, *35*, 19–25. [CrossRef]
296. Shekari Ebrahim Abad, H.; Zaini, F.; Kordbacheh, P.; Mahmoudi, M.; Safara, M.; Mortezaee, V. In Vitro Activity of Caspofungin Against Fluconazole-Resistant Candida Species Isolated From Clinical Samples in Iran. *Jundishapur J. Microbiol.* **2015**, *8*, 4–7. [CrossRef]
297. Wu, Z.; Liu, Y.; Feng, X.; Liu, Y.; Wang, S.; Zhu, X.; Chen, Q.; Pan, S. Candidemia: Incidence rates, type of species, and risk factors at a tertiary care academic hospital in China. *Int. J. Infect. Dis.* **2014**, *22*, 4–8. [CrossRef]
298. Barchiesi, F.; Spreghini, E.; Tomassetti, S.; Della Vittoria, A.; Arzeni, D.; Manso, E.; Scalise, G. Effects of caspofungin against Candida guilliermondii and Candida parapsilosis. *Antimicrob. Agents Chemother.* **2006**, *50*, 2719–2727. [CrossRef]
299. Zepelin, M.B.-V.; Kunz, L.; Ruchel, R.; Reichard, U.; Weig, M.; Gross, U. Epidemiology and antifungal susceptibilities of Candida spp. to six antifungal agents: Results from a surveillance study on fungaemia in Germany from July 2004 to August 2005. *J. Antimicrob. Chemother.* **2007**, *60*, 424–428. [CrossRef] [PubMed]

300. Golden, S.H.; Peart-Vigilance, C.; Kao, W.H.; Brancati, F.L. Perioperative glycemic control and the risk of infectious complications in a cohort of adults with diabetes. *Diabetes Care* **1999**, *22*, 1408–1414. [CrossRef] [PubMed]
301. Desnos-Ollivier, M.; Ragon, M.; Robert, V.; Raoux, D.; Gantier, J.-C.; Dromer, F. Debaryomyces hansenii (Candida famata), a Rare Human Fungal Pathogen Often Misidentified as Pichia guilliermondii (Candida guilliermondii). *J. Clin. Microbiol.* **2008**, *46*, 3237–3242. [CrossRef] [PubMed]
302. Savini, V.; Catavitello, C.; Di Marzio, I.; Masciarelli, G.; Astolfi, D.; Balbinot, A.; Bianco, A.; Pompilio, A.; Di Bonaventura, G.; D'Amario, C.; et al. Pan-azole-Resistant Candida guilliermondii from a Leukemia Patient's Silent Funguria. *Mycopathologia* **2010**, *169*, 457–459. [CrossRef] [PubMed]
303. Savini, V.; Catavitello, C.; Onofrillo, D.; Masciarelli, G.; Astolfi, D.; Balbinot, A.; Febbo, F.; D'Amario, C.; D'Antonio, D. What do we know about Candida guilliermondii? A voyage throughout past and current literature about this emerging yeast. *Mycoses* **2011**, *54*, 434–441. [CrossRef]
304. Hamilton, H.C.; Foxcroft, D. Central venous access sites for the prevention of venous thrombosis, stenosis and infection in patients requiring long-term intravenous therapy. In *Cochrane Database of Systematic Reviews*; Hamilton, H.C., Ed.; John Wiley & Sons, Ltd.: Chichester, UK, 2007; p. CD004084.
305. Ma, X.; Sun, W.; Liu, T. [Clinical characteristics of Candida septicemia seen in a neonatal intensive care unit: Analysis of 9 cases]. *Zhonghua er ke za zhi = Chin. J. Pediatr.* **2006**, *44*, 694–697.
306. Patel, G.P.; Simon, D.; Scheetz, M.; Crank, C.W.; Lodise, T.; Patel, N. The Effect of Time to Antifungal Therapy on Mortality in Candidemia Associated Septic Shock. *Am. J. Ther.* **2009**, *16*, 508–511. [CrossRef] [PubMed]
307. Colombo, A.L.; Nucci, M.; Park, B.J.; Nouér, S.A.; Arthington-Skaggs, B.; da Matta, D.A.; Warnock, D.; Morgan, J.; Brazilian Network Candidemia Study, for the B.N.C. Epidemiology of candidemia in Brazil: A nationwide sentinel surveillance of candidemia in eleven medical centers. *J. Clin. Microbiol.* **2006**, *44*, 2816–2823. [CrossRef] [PubMed]
308. Horn, D.L.; Neofytos, D.; Anaissie, E.J.; Fishman, J.A.; Steinbach, W.J.; Olyaei, A.J.; Marr, K.A.; Pfaller, M.A.; Chang, C.; Webster, K.M. Epidemiology and Outcomes of Candidemia in 2019 Patients: Data from the Prospective Antifungal Therapy Alliance Registry. *Clin. Infect. Dis.* **2009**, *48*, 1695–1703. [CrossRef] [PubMed]
309. Pfaller, M.A.; Diekema, D.J. Epidemiology of invasive candidiasis: A persistent public health problem. *Clin. Microbiol. Rev.* **2007**, *20*, 133–163. [CrossRef] [PubMed]
310. Nucci, M.; Queiroz-Telles, F.; Tobón, A.M.; Restrepo, A.; Colombo, A.L. Epidemiology of Opportunistic Fungal Infections in Latin America. *Clin. Infect. Dis.* **2010**, *51*, 561–570. [CrossRef] [PubMed]
311. Ryan, T.; Mc Carthy, J.F.; Rady, M.Y.; Serkey, J.; Gordon, S.; Starr, N.J.; Cosgrove, D.M. Early bloodstream infection after cardiopulmonary bypass: Frequency rate, risk factors, and implications. *Crit. Care Med.* **1997**, *25*, 2009–2014. [CrossRef] [PubMed]
312. Leroy, O.; Gangneux, J.-P.; Montravers, P.; Mira, J.-P.; Gouin, F.; Sollet, J.-P.; Carlet, J.; Reynes, J.; Rosenheim, M.; Regnier, B.; et al. Epidemiology, management, and risk factors for death of invasive Candida infections in critical care: A multicenter, prospective, observational study in France (2005–2006). *Crit. Care Med.* **2009**, *37*, 1612–1618. [CrossRef] [PubMed]
313. Shorr, A.F.; Lazarus, D.R.; Sherner, J.H.; Jackson, W.L.; Morrel, M.; Fraser, V.J.; Kollef, M.H. Do clinical features allow for accurate prediction of fungal pathogenesis in bloodstream infections? Potential implications of the increasing prevalence of non-albicans candidemia. *Crit. Care Med.* **2007**, *35*, 1077–1083. [CrossRef] [PubMed]
314. Corzo-leon, D.E.; Alvarado-matute, T.; Colombo, A.L.; Cornejo-juarez, P.; Cortes, J.; Echevarria, J.I.; Macias, A.E.; Nucci, M.; Ostrosky-Zeichner, L.; Ponce-de-Leon, A.; et al. Surveillance of Candida spp Bloodstream Infections: Epidemiological Trends and Risk Factors of Death in Two Mexican Tertiary Care Hospitals. *PLoS ONE* **2014**, *9*, 1–6. [CrossRef] [PubMed]
315. Nucci, M.; Queiroz-Telles, F.; Alvarado-Matute, T.; Tiraboschi, I.N.; Cortes, J.; Zurita, J.; Guzman-Blanco, M.; Santolaya, M.E.; Thompson, L.; Sifuentes-Osornio, J.; et al. Epidemiology of Candidemia in Latin America: A Laboratory-Based Survey. *PLoS ONE* **2013**, *8*, e59373. [CrossRef] [PubMed]
316. Gupta, A.; Gupta, A.; Varma, A. Candida glabrata candidemia: An emerging threat in critically ill patients. *Indian J. Crit. Care Med.* **2015**, *19*, 151–154. [CrossRef] [PubMed]
317. Pozzilli, P.; Leslie, R.D. Infections and diabetes: Mechanisms and prospects for prevention. *Diabet. Med.* **1994**, *11*, 935–941. [CrossRef] [PubMed]

318. MacCuish, A.C.; Urbaniak, S.J.; Campbell, C.J.; Duncan, L.J.; Irvine, W.J. Phytohemagglutinin transformation and circulating lymphocyte subpopulations in insulin-dependent diabetic patients. *Diabetes* **1974**, *23*, 708–712. [CrossRef] [PubMed]
319. Hostetter, M.K. Handicaps to host defense. Effects of hyperglycemia on C3 and Candida albicans. *Diabetes* **1990**, *39*, 271–275. [CrossRef] [PubMed]
320. Padawer, D.; Pastukh, N.; Nitzan, O.; Labay, K.; Aharon, I.; Brodsky, D.; Glyatman, T.; Peretz, A. Catheter-associated candiduria: Risk factors, medical interventions, and antifungal susceptibility. *Am. J. Infect. Control* **2015**, *43*, e19–e22. [CrossRef] [PubMed]
321. Tambyah, P.A.; Halvorson, K.T.; Maki, D.G. A Prospective Study of Pathogenesis of Catheter-Associated Urinary Tract Infections. *Mayo Clin. Proc.* **1999**, *74*, 131–136. [CrossRef] [PubMed]
322. Maki, D.G.; Tambyah, P.A. Engineering out the risk for infection with urinary catheters. *Emerg. Infect. Dis.* **2001**, *7*, 342–347. [CrossRef] [PubMed]
323. Kuhn, D.M.; Mikherjee, P.K.; Clark, T.A.; Pujol, C.; Chandra, J.; Hajjeh, R.A.; Warnock, D.W.; Soil, D.R.; Ghannoum, M.A. Candida parapsilosis characterization in an outbreak setting. *Emerg. Infect. Dis.* **2004**, *10*, 1074–1081. [CrossRef] [PubMed]
324. Khatib, R.; Johnson, L.B.; Fakih, M.G.; Riederer, K.; Briski, L. Current trends in candidemia and species distribution among adults: *Candida glabrata* surpasses *C. albicans* in diabetic patients and abdominal sources. *Mycoses* **2016**, *59*, 781–786. [CrossRef] [PubMed]
325. Lipsett, P.A. Surgical critical care: Fungal infections in surgical patients. *Crit. Care Med.* **2006**, *34*, S215–S224. [CrossRef]
326. Hattori, H.; Maeda, M.; Nagatomo, Y.; Takuma, T.; Niki, Y.; Naito, Y.; Sasaki, T.; Ishino, K. Epidemiology and risk factors for mortality in bloodstream infections: A single-center retrospective study in Japan. *Am. J. Infect. Control* **2018**, *46*, e75–e79. [CrossRef]
327. Zhao, S.J.; Fu, Y.Q.; Zhu, M.X.; Zhou, H.; Xu, M.; Yan, R.L.; Shui, Y.X.; Zhou, J.Y. [Patients of Escherichia coli bloodstream infection: Analysis of antibiotic resistance and predictors of mortality]. *Zhonghua Yi Xue Za Zhi* **2017**, *97*, 2496–2500.
328. Tumbarello, M.; Fiori, B.; Trecarichi, E.M.; Posteraro, P.; Losito, A.R.; de Luca, A.; Sanguinetti, M.; Fadda, G.; Cauda, R.; Posteraro, B. Risk factors and outcomes of candidemia caused by biofilm-forming isolates in a tertiary care hospital. *PLoS ONE* **2012**, *7*, 1–9. [CrossRef]
329. Bristow, I.R.; Spruce, M.C. Fungal foot infection, cellulitis and diabetes: A review. *Diabet. Med.* **2009**, *26*, 548–551. [CrossRef] [PubMed]
330. Tchernev, G.; Penev, P.K.; Nenoff, P.; Zisova, L.G.; Cardoso, J.C.; Taneva, T.; Ginter-Hanselmayer, G.; Ananiev, J.; Gulubova, M.; Hristova, R.; et al. Onychomycosis: Modern diagnostic and treatment approaches. *Wiener Medizinische Wochenschrift* **2013**, *163*, 1–12. [CrossRef] [PubMed]
331. Chang, S.-J.; Hsu, S.-C.; Tien, K.-J.; Hsiao, J.-Y.; Lin, S.-R.; Chen, H.-C.; Hsieh, M.-C. Metabolic syndrome associated with toenail onychomycosis in Taiwanese with diabetes mellitus. *Int. J. Dermatol.* **2008**, *47*, 467–472. [CrossRef] [PubMed]
332. Kumar, D.; Banerjee, T.; Chakravarty, J.; Singh, S.; Dwivedi, A.; Tilak, R. Identification, antifungal resistance profile, in vitro biofilm formation and ultrastructural characteristics of Candida species isolated from diabetic foot patients in Northern India. *Indian J. Med. Microbiol.* **2016**, *34*, 308.
333. Raiesi, O.; Siavash, M.; Mohammadi, F.; Chabavizadeh, J.; Mahaki, B.; Maherolnaghsh, M.; Dehghan, P. Frequency of Cutaneous Fungal Infections and Azole Resistance of the Isolates in Patients with Diabetes Mellitus. *Adv. Biomed. Res.* **2017**, *6*, 71. [PubMed]
334. Lugo-Somolinos, A.; Sánchez, J.L. Prevalence of dermatophytosis in patients with diabetes. *J. Am. Acad. Dermatol.* **1992**, *26*, 408–410. [CrossRef]
335. Pierard, G.E.; Pierard-Franchimont, C. The nail under fungal siege in patients with type II diabetes mellitus. *Mycoses* **2005**, *48*, 339–342. [CrossRef]
336. Dogra, S.; Kumar, B.; Bhansali, A.; Chakrabarty, A. Epidemiology of onychomycosis in patients with diabetes mellitus in India. *Int. J. Dermatol.* **2002**, *41*, 647–651. [CrossRef]
337. Eckhard, M.; Lengler, A.; Liersch, J.; Bretzel, R.G.; Mayser, P. Fungal foot infections in patients with diabetes mellitus-results of two independent investigations. *Mycoses* **2007**, *50*, 14–19. [CrossRef]

338. Wijesuriya, T.M.; Weerasekera, M.M.; Kottahachchi, J.; Ranasinghe, K.N.P.; Dissanayake, M.S.S.; Prathapan, S.; Gunasekara, T.D.C.P.; Nagahawatte, A.; Guruge, L.D.; Bulugahapitiya, U.; et al. Proportion of lower limb fungal foot infections in patients with type 2 diabetes at a tertiary care hospital in Sri Lanka. *Indian J. Endocrinol. Metab.* **2014**, *18*, 63–69.
339. Boyko, E.J.; Ahroni, J.H.; Cohen, V.; Nelson, K.M.; Heagerty, P.J. Prediction of Diabetic Foot Ulcer Occurrence Using Commonly Available Clinical Information: The Seattle Diabetic Foot Study. *Diabetes Care* **2006**, *29*, 1202–1207. [CrossRef] [PubMed]
340. Johargy, A.K. Antimicrobial susceptibility of bacterial and fungal infections among infected diabetic patients. *J. Pak. Med. Assoc.* **2016**, *66*, 1291–1295. [PubMed]
341. Gupta, A.K.; Konnikov, N.; Macdonald, P.; Rich, P.; Rodger, N.W.; Edmonds, M.W.; Mcmanus, R.; Summerbell, R.C. Prevalence and epidemiology of toenail onychomycosis in diabetic subjects: A multicentre survey. *Br. J. Dermatol.* **1998**, *139*, 665–671. [CrossRef]
342. Chi, C.-C.; Wang, S.-H.; Chou, M.-C. The causative pathogens of onychomycosis in southern Taiwan. *Mycoses* **2005**, *48*, 413–420. [CrossRef] [PubMed]
343. Wang, D.; Jiang, Y.; Li, Z.; Xue, L.; Li, X.; Liu, Y.; Li, C.; Wang, H. The Effect of Candida albicans on the Expression Levels of Toll-like Receptor 2 and Interleukin-8 in HaCaT Cells Under High- and Low-glucose Conditions. *Indian J. Dermatol.* **2018**, *63*, 201–207. [PubMed]
344. Delamaire, M.; Maugendre, D.; Moreno, M.; Le Goff, M.-C.; Allannic, H.; Genetet, B. Impaired Leucocyte Functions in Diabetic Patients. *Diabet. Med.* **1997**, *14*, 29–34. [CrossRef]
345. Llorente, L.; De La Fuente, H.; Richaud-Patin, Y.; Alvarado-De La Barrera, C.; Diaz-Borjón, A.; López-Ponce, A.; Lerman-Garber, I.; Jakez-Ocampo, J. Innate immune response mechanisms in non-insulin dependent diabetes mellitus patients assessed by flow cytoenzymology. *Immunol. Lett.* **2000**, *74*, 239–244. [CrossRef]
346. De Souza Ferreira, C.; Pennacchi, P.C.; Araújo, T.H.; Taniwaki, N.N.; De Araújo Paula, F.B.; Da Silveira Duarte, S.M.; Rodrigues, M.R. Aminoguanidine treatment increased NOX2 response in diabetic rats: Improved phagocytosis and killing of Candida albicans by neutrophils. *Eur. J. Pharmacol.* **2016**, *772*, 83–91. [CrossRef]
347. Pupim, A.C.E.; Campois, T.G.; Araújo, E.J.A.; Svidizinski, T.I.E.; Felipe, I. Infection and tissue repair of experimental cutaneous candidiasis in diabetic mice. *J. Med. Microbiol.* **2017**, *66*, 808–815. [CrossRef]
348. Rubin, B.G.; German, M.L.; Louis, S. Candida infection with aneurysm formation in the juxtarenal aorta. *J. Vasc. Surg.* **1994**, *20*, 311–314. [CrossRef]
349. King, A.J.F. The use of animal models in diabetes research. *Br. J. Pharmacol.* **2012**, *166*, 877–894. [CrossRef] [PubMed]
350. Brosius, F.C.; Alpers, C.E.; Bottinger, E.P.; Breyer, M.D.; Coffman, T.M.; Gurley, S.B.; Harris, R.C.; Kakoki, M.; Kretzler, M.; Leiter, E.H.; et al. Mouse Models of Diabetic Nephropathy. *J. Am. Soc. Nephrol.* **2009**, *20*, 2503–2512. [CrossRef] [PubMed]
351. Sullivan, K.A.; Hayes, J.M.; Wiggin, T.D.; Backus, C.; Su Oh, S.; Lentz, S.I.; Brosius, F.; Feldman, E.L. Mouse models of diabetic neuropathy. *Neurobiol. Dis.* **2007**, *28*, 276–285. [CrossRef] [PubMed]
352. Sullivan, K.A.; Lentz, S.I.; Roberts, J.L., Jr.; Feldman, E.L. Criteria for Creating and Assessing Mouse Models of Diabetic Neuropathy. *Curr. Drug Targets* **2008**, *9*, 3. [PubMed]
353. Franconi, F.; Seghieri, G.; Canu, S.; Straface, E.; Campesi, I.; Malorni, W. Are the available experimental models of type 2 diabetes appropriate for a gender perspective? *Pharmacol. Res.* **2008**, *57*, 6–18. [CrossRef]
354. Inada, A.; Arai, H.; Nagai, K.; Miyazaki, J.; Yamada, Y.; Seino, Y.; Fukatsu, A. Gender Difference in ICER Iγ Transgenic Diabetic Mouse. *Biosci. Biotechnol. Biochem.* **2007**, *71*, 1920–1926. [CrossRef]
355. Hassan, A.; Poon, W.; Baker, M.; Linton, C.; Mühlschlegel, F.A. Confirmed Candida albicans endogenous fungal endophthalmitis in a patient with chronic candidiasis. *Med. Mycol. Case Rep.* **2012**, *1*, 42–44. [CrossRef] [PubMed]
356. Woodrum, D.T.; Welke, K.F.; Fillinger, M.F. Candida infection associated with a solitary mycotic common iliac artery aneurysm. *J. Vasc. Surg.* **2001**, *34*, 166–168. [CrossRef]
357. Dowling, R.D.; Baladi, N.; Zenati, M.; Dummer, J.S.; Kormos, R.L.; Armitage, J.M.; Yousem, S.A.; Hardesty, R.L.; Griffith, B.P. Disruption of the aortic anastomosis after heart-lung transplantation. *Ann. Thorac. Surg.* **1990**, *49*, 118–122. [CrossRef]

358. Laouad, I.; Buchler, M.; Noel, C.; Sadek, T.; Maazouz, H.; Westeel, P.F.; Lebranchu, Y. Renal Artery Aneurysm Secondary to Candida albicans in Four Kidney Allograft Recipients. *Transplant. Proc.* **2005**, *37*, 2834–2836. [CrossRef]
359. Mai, H.; Champion, L.; Ouali, N.; Hertig, A.; Peraldi, M.-N.; Glotz, D.; Rondeau, E.; Costa, M.-A.; Snanoudj, R.; Benoit, G.; et al. Candida albicans Arteritis Transmitted by Conservative Liquid After Renal Transplantation: A Report of Four Cases and Review of the Literature. *Transplantation* **2006**, *82*, 1163–1167. [CrossRef] [PubMed]
360. Valentine, R.J.; Chung, J. Primary Vascular Infection. *Curr. Probl. Surg.* **2012**, *49*, 128–182. [CrossRef] [PubMed]
361. Chapuis-Taillard, C.; Manuel, O.; Bille, J.; Calandra, T.; Rotman, S.; Tarr, P.E. Candida Arteritis in Patients Who Have Not Received Organ Transplants: Case Report and Review of the Literature. *Clin. Infect. Dis.* **2008**, *46*, e106–e111. [CrossRef] [PubMed]
362. Brown, S.L.; Busuttil, R.W.; Baker, J.D.; Machleder, H.I.; Moore, W.S.; Barker, W.F. Bacteriologic and surgical determinants of survival in patients with mycotic aneurysms. *J. Vasc. Surg.* **1984**, *1*, 541–547. [CrossRef]
363. Potti, A.; Danielson, B.; Sen, K. "True" mycotic aneurysm of a renal artery allograft. *Am. J. Kidney Dis.* **1998**, *31*, E3. [CrossRef] [PubMed]
364. Oderich, G.S.; Panneton, J.M.; Bower, T.C.; Cherry, K.J., Jr.; Rowland, C.M.; Noel, A.A.; Hallett, J.W., Jr.; Gloviczk, P. Infected aortic aneurysms: Aggressive presentation, complicated early outcome, but durable results. *J. Vasc. Surg.* **2001**, *34*, 900–908. [CrossRef]
365. Sergio, P.; De Araujo, R.; Medeiros, Z.; Melo, F.L. De Case Report Candida famata- induced fulminating cholecystitis. *Rev Soc Bras Med Trop.* **2013**, *46*, 795–796.
366. Kakeya, H.; Izumikawa, K.; Yamada, K.; Narita, Y.; Nishino, T.; Obata, Y.; Takazono, T.; Kurihara, S.; Kosai, K.; Morinaga, Y.; et al. Concurrent subcutaneous candidal abscesses and pulmonary cryptococcosis in a patient with diabetes mellitus and a history of corticosteroid therapy. *Intern Med.* **2014**, *53*, 1385–1390. [CrossRef]
367. Florescu, D.F.; Brostrom, S.E.; Dumitru, I.; Kalil, A.C. Candida albicans Skin Abscess in a Heart Transplant Recipient. *Infect. Dis. Clin. Pract.* **2010**, *18*, 243–246. [CrossRef]
368. Neves, N.; Santos, L.; Reis, C.; Sarmento, A. Candida albicans brain abscesses in an injection drug user patient: A case report. *BMC Res. Notes* **2014**, *7*, 837. [CrossRef]
369. Honda, H.; Warren, D.K. Central Nervous System Infections: Meningitis and Brain Abscess. *Infect. Dis. Clin. N. Am.* **2009**, *23*, 609–623. [CrossRef] [PubMed]
370. Fennelly, A.M.; Slenker, A.K.; Murphy, L.C.; Moussouttas, M.; DeSimone, J.A. Candida cerebral abscesses: A case report and review of the literature. *Med. Mycol.* **2013**, *51*, 779–784. [CrossRef] [PubMed]
371. Yang, C.-H.; He, X.-S.; Chen, J.; Ouyang, B.; Zhu, X.-F.; Chen, M.-Y.; Xie, W.-F.; Chen, L.; Zheng, D.-H.; Zhong, Y.; et al. Fungal infection in patients after liver transplantation in years 2003 to 2012. *Ann. Transplant.* **2012**, *17*, 59–63. [PubMed]
372. Abraham, G.; Kumar, V.; Nayak, K.S.; Ravichandran, R.; Srinivasan, G.; Krishnamurthy, M.; Prasath, A.K.; Kumar, S.; Thiagarajan, T.; Mathew, M.; et al. Predictors of long-term survival on peritoneal dialysis in south india: A multicenter study. *Perit. Dial. Int.* **2010**, *30*, 29–34. [CrossRef]
373. Yuvaraj, A.; Rohit, A.; Koshy, P.J.; Nagarajan, P.; Nair, S.; Abraham, G. Rare occurrence of fatal Candida haemulonii peritonitis in a diabetic CAPD patient. *Ren. Fail.* **2014**, *36*, 1466–1467. [CrossRef] [PubMed]
374. Zappella, N.; Desmard, M.; Chochillon, C.; Ribeiro-Parenti, L.; Houze, S.; Marmuse, J.P.; Montravers, P. Positive peritoneal fluid fungal cultures in postoperative peritonitis after bariatric surgery. *Clin. Microbiol. Infect.* **2015**, *21*, 853.e1–853.e3. [CrossRef] [PubMed]
375. Mulcahy, J.J. Long-term experience with salvage of infected penile implants. *J. Urol.* **2000**, *163*, 481–482. [CrossRef]
376. Peppas, D.S.; Moul, J.W.; McLeod, D.G. Candida albicans corpora abscess following penile prosthesis placement. *J. Urol.* **1988**, *140*, 1541–1542. [CrossRef]
377. Mulcahy, J.J.; Carson, C.C. Long-Term Infection Rates in Diabetic Patients Implanted With Antibiotic-Impregnated Versus Nonimpregnated Inflatable Penile Prostheses: 7-Year Outcomes. *Eur. Urol.* **2011**, *60*, 167–172. [CrossRef]
378. Cotta, B.H.; Butcher, M.; Welliver, C.; Mcvary, K.; Köhler, T. Two Fungal Infections of Inflatable Penile Prostheses in Diabetics. *Sex. Med.* **2015**, *3*, 339–342. [CrossRef]

379. Maatouk, I.; Hajjar, M.; Moutran, R. Candida albicans and Streptococcus pyogenes balanitis: Diabetes or STI? *Int. J. Std Aids* **2015**, *26*, 755–756. [CrossRef] [PubMed]
380. Wróblewska, M.; Kuzaka, B.; Borkowski, T.; Kuzaka, P.; Kawecki, D.; Radziszewski, P. Fournier's Gangrene—Current Concepts. *Polish J. Microbiol.* **2014**, *63*, 267–273.
381. Saha, K.; Sit, N.K.; Maji, A.; Jash, D. Recovery of fluconazole sensitive Candida ciferrii in a diabetic chronic obstructive pulmonary disease patient presenting with pneumonia. *Lung India* **2013**, *30*, 338–340. [CrossRef] [PubMed]

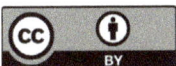

© 2019 by the authors. Licensee MDPI, Basel, Switzerland. This article is an open access article distributed under the terms and conditions of the Creative Commons Attribution (CC BY) license (http://creativecommons.org/licenses/by/4.0/).

MDPI
St. Alban-Anlage 66
4052 Basel
Switzerland
Tel. +41 61 683 77 34
Fax +41 61 302 89 18
www.mdpi.com

Journal of Clinical Medicine Editorial Office
E-mail: jcm@mdpi.com
www.mdpi.com/journal/jcm

www.ingramcontent.com/pod-product-compliance
Lightning Source LLC
LaVergne TN
LVHW070726100526
838202LV00013B/1181